PRAISE FOR

Reflections of a Military Psychiatrist

"Dr. Marietta unlocks the black box of military mental health and reveals its secrets as no one else has ever done. This is an insider's look from the perspective of a military and mental health professional. Incredibly insightful, and based on firsthand experience, it's a must-read for anyone seeking to know the real deal when it comes to military and veterans' mental health. Dr. Marietta has done a phenomenal service to our nation, our military, and the medical profession."

—Major General Gregg F. Martin, PhD, US Army (retired), author of *BIPOLAR GENERAL: My Forever War with Mental Illness*

"Dr. Marietta's book offers a compelling exploration of the complexities surrounding military mental health care. Beneath the surface, providers navigate a maze of challenges, including conflicting roles, dual relationships, inconsistent guidance, undue influence, and hospital politics. This work masterfully summarizes these issues, shedding light on the diverse approaches to mental health, the role of command, and the expectations shaping care delivery.

"While no single book can capture every service member's experience, Dr. Marietta provides a balanced perspective, blending program descriptions, embedded care models, and the realities of military culture. As a physician, I see patients grappling with their military past and the lingering effects of their treatment. Many have urged me to 'write a book about it.' Now I can point them to this one. Dr. Marietta captures the struggles of both providers and patients, offering insight into why certain decisions were made. For some, this book will bring closure; for others, it may highlight ongoing frustrations with a system that sometimes leaves them behind.

"This book is a vital insider's look at the unseen challenges of military mental health care, offering clarity and understanding to those willing to see both sides."

—Greg Henderson, MD, CDR, US Navy (retired)

"Reading this book confirmed many of my own experiences with the Department of Defense and its manpower resiliency shortfalls. It is a serious depiction of the military's challenges to addressing mental health, including the complexities of developing and implementing programs that have lasting impacts for all service members. Having founded the Defense Suicide Prevention Office, I experienced firsthand the bureaucratic dysfunction that stalled progress. The Pentagon and the services often fail to align, leading to lost data, redundancies in some areas, and gaps in others, while promising programs and initiatives are canceled. The Pentagon felt like a mix of a combat zone and a hostile work environment, and, like Dr. Marietta, the story of another program and policy champion who is gaslit, marginalized, and shunned while service members suffer from lost resources and ineffective policies that do not help them endure."

—Dr. Jacqueline Garrick, founder of Whistleblowers of America, Workplace Promise Institute

"In this bold and necessary exposé, *Reflections of a Military Psychiatrist* shines a light on the often-overlooked cracks in our military mental health system. Dr. Marietta writes with the kind of unflinching honesty and lived experience that only comes from someone who has been embedded in the work, boots on the ground directly serving our military members.

"I had the opportunity to work alongside Dr. Marietta at one of the DoD facilities mentioned in this book. His portrayal of the systemic barriers, cultural stigma, and human cost we witnessed is not only accurate but urgent. This book challenges us to do better, both as providers and as a system. It's an essential read for policymakers, clinicians, and anyone who claims to support our military community."

>—Jesalyn Moore, LCSW, LSATP, CAADC, EMS health and wellness manager, Virginia Beach, former DoD clinician and military spouse

"*Reflections of a Military Psychiatrist* is a much-needed road map in the complex world of military mental health. Dr. Marietta, with his extensive experience across multiple branches, provides an invaluable insider's perspective. While honestly acknowledging the challenges within the system, his book ultimately serves as a practical guide for navigating those challenges, promoting positive change, and offering hope for both service members and providers. It's packed with actionable insights and real-world examples, making it an essential resource for anyone seeking to understand and improve the well-being of our military community."

>—CDR Sarah Garrett, LCSW, BCD, CSAC, CSOTP, US Coast Guard/USPHS

"A powerful and unflinching exposé of the military's mental health system—this book pulls no punches. It shines a glaring light on the systemic failures, while still honoring the dedicated professionals doing their best in an under-resourced, overburdened system. The cross-branch comparisons are eye-opening, the stories of those left behind are heartbreaking, and the overlooked solutions are deeply frustrating. More than just critique, this is a clarion call to action—a reminder that we must do better for those who serve. We owe them more than gratitude—we owe them real support."

—Theresa Carpenter, host of the *Stories of Service* podcast

"*Reflections of a Military Psychiatrist* is a must-read for all mental health providers who work with military members, past or present. I also hope all members of the Armed Services Committee read this book to ensure mental health services are funded and provided to all those who serve for the USA."

—Jacqueline O'Connell-Bagnati, LCSW, Air Force veteran

"Dr. Robert Marietta pulls back the veil on military mental health care with his compelling account of his time as a Navy psychiatrist. The differences in quality of care and philosophies of care among the military services that he recounts are both fascinating and appalling. My old service, the US Air Force, seems to be the gold standard. This is a great read for anyone with a connection to the military and to mental health care and for everyone else who cares to learn more about mental health.

—Brian J. Morra, award-winning author of *The Able Archers* and *The Righteous Arrows*

"As someone who has never served in the military, this book opened the door to a world I hadn't yet encountered: the field of military mental health. With over forty-eight years of experience in public health across both national and international arenas, I recognized many striking parallels between military mental health services and the systems I've long worked within. This book provided a powerful, eye-opening journey into a field that remains largely underexamined. Aside from the widely reported suicide clusters over the past decade, there's been limited public discourse or literature addressing the challenges within military mental health. *Reflections of a Military Psychiatrist* is not just a compelling read—it's an essential starting point for reimagining and revitalizing how we approach mental health in the armed forces in the twenty-first century."

> —Dr. Daniel S. Gerber, MPH, EdD, faculty member in the Community Health Program of the School of Public Health and Health Sciences at the University of Massachusetts/Amherst, (formerly the associate dean for Academic Affairs, 2010 to 2020, of the School of Public Health and Health Sciences at the University of Massachusetts/Amherst)

"As a ten-and-a-half-year Air Force veteran and mental health professional with over fourteen years of experience, including roles as a trauma therapist and senior social worker at Virginia Veterans Affairs, I deeply resonate with Dr. Marietta's insights in *Reflections of a Military Psychiatrist*. His extensive experience across the Marines, Navy, Air Force, Coast Guard, and Veterans Affairs uniquely positions him to advocate for a shift from mission-oriented to recovery-oriented mental health care. Dr. Marietta's action-focused solutions highlight the need for effective, robust mental health services to support our active-duty members, moving beyond superficial care to foster true recovery."

> —Christian Allen Kreuzberger, LCSW, independent certified licensed provider

"Having lived through the failures of the military mental health system myself during my time at the US Air Force Academy, I felt a deep connection to every page of *Reflections of a Military Psychiatrist*. Dr. Marietta's honesty and compassion shine through in a way that's both refreshing and urgently needed. He doesn't sugarcoat the issues—he lays them bare with stories and insights that hit close to home for anyone who's seen how broken things can get when service members reach out for help and find the system working against them.

"What really sets this book apart is how Dr. Marietta moves past just exposing problems and focuses on real, practical solutions. He talks about why working together—commanders, doctors, and service members—matters so much and how early support can actually save lives before things spiral. His suggestions for change aren't pipe dreams; they're based on what he's lived and learned over decades in uniform.

"If you've ever wondered why so many in the military struggle in silence or why things don't seem to change, this book will open your eyes. I can't recommend it enough—and I hope it inspires others to demand the changes we so desperately need."

—CPT Adam DeRito, MS, US Army Civil Affairs, USAFA class of 2010

"As a woman veteran who has carried the unforgettable weight of military transition, medical separation, and the long, often painful process of medical boarding and discharge—along with the complex journey of healing within the challenging VA system—*Reflections of a Military Psychiatrist* resonated with me on a deeply personal level. Dr. Robert Marietta, a Navy veteran and military psychiatrist, brings a rare depth of knowledge and insight across all branches of service, offering a perspective that is both informed and compassionate. While some parts of this book were personally triggering for me—bringing up painful memories tied to my own experiences with discharge and navigating the VA—I believe that speaks to how deeply he captures the emotional and psychological toll this system can take. He does a remarkable job grasping the broader picture of what we go through as individuals, especially the profound loss of identity that often comes with leaving the uniform behind. He masterfully weaves together history, clinical expertise, and real-life experiences with clarity and heart. This book is more than a reflection; it's a vital and timely resource that I believe every service member, family, and policymaker should read."

> —Jami Raishbrook, USAF veteran and advocate for women veterans

Reflections of a Military Psychiatrist
by Robert G. Marietta, MD, MPH

© Copyright 2025 Robert G. Marietta, MD, MPH

ISBN 979-8-88824-794-5

All rights reserved. No part of this publication may be reproduced, stored in a retrieval system, or transmitted in any form or by any means—electronic, mechanical, photocopy, recording, or any other—except for brief quotations in printed reviews, without the prior written permission of the author.

Published by

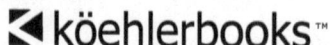

3705 Shore Drive
Virginia Beach, VA 23455
800–435–4811
www.koehlerbooks.com

Reflections of a Military Psychiatrist

Robert G. Marietta, MD, MPH

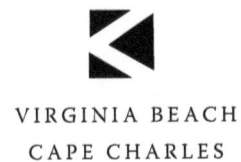

VIRGINIA BEACH
CAPE CHARLES

All views are mine alone and do not represent the DoD, Navy, or any other organization.

Table of Contents

Foreword 1

Introduction 7

Chapter 1: Leyte 11

Chapter 2: Flagship 21

Chapter 3: Slave Ship 27

Chapter 4: Air Force 34

Chapter 5: Coast Guard 40

Chapter 6: Navy a Second Time Through 46

Chapter 7: *USS George Washington* and
    MARMC Suicide Clusters 56

Chapter 8: Navy Mental Health Case Examples 80

Chapter 9: Fight to Deliver Mental Health Services 100

Chapter 10: The Doctor, Patient, and Military Relationship
    Triangle 129

Chapter 11: Information Technology Issues 155

Chapter 12: Obstacles the Military Faces Addressing Mental
    Health Issues 167

Chapter 13: Challenges in Assisting Service Members ... 192

Chapter 14: How the Military Environment Impacts Personnel ... 204

Chapter 15: Mental Health and Support Resources ... 222

Chapter 16: Common Issues Service Members Face ... 236

Chapter 17: Essential Coping Skills to Thrive in the Military ... 268

Chapter 18: Clinical Pearls, Tips, and Techniques ... 280

Chapter 19: Burnout and Compassion Fatigue ... 296

Chapter 20: Public Health Service ... 316

Chapter 21: That Time I Became a Whistleblower ... 321

Chapter 22: Veterans Affairs ... 329

Chapter 23: Future Reforms ... 337

Chapter 24: Closing Thoughts ... 372

References ... 377

FOREWORD

IF YOU HAD ASKED me five years ago if the landscape of people advocating for military mental health would resemble what it does today, I probably would not have believed you. As someone who experienced most of the negative sides of what Dr. Marietta talks about in this book, I have such a deep appreciation for hearing "the other side" of mental health in the military. I have met my fair share of social workers, military psychiatrists, and psychologists. What sets Dr. Marietta apart from most is his passion to share the raw truth about the system, but not from a place of malice or anger, rather from a solution-based narrative that offers tangible options to an organization that has needed an overhaul for years.

I went to A School in Pensacola, Florida, to become an aviation electronics technician (AT). Shortly after I arrived, I was warned about a group of Marines who had a game of sorts to see how many new female sailors they could sleep with. I had friends who were sexually and physically assaulted, there were suicides, and excessive amounts of drinking took place on that base in the short eight months that I was there. My experience at A School set the tone for the rest of my Navy experience. Boot camp made me feel like the Navy might be a safe place where men and women respect each other. A School taught me to keep to myself in my own little bubble because anything outside of that bubble was dangerous and could impact my career.

When I arrived at my first duty station, I was sexually assaulted. When I brought it up at work the next day, I was immediately shut down and told it was my fault. My work center was a cesspool of inappropriate touching, inappropriate jokes, and being the minority (one of a handful of females), and as an E2, I didn't feel I had a voice.

I went to C School to study the Consolidated Automated Support System aviation maintenance system and started to recognize my own mental health challenges. I confided in an instructor and was encouraged to go to Medical to seek help for my intense anxiety. Command Medical had a bad reputation for helping sailors with mental health issues, and that made it all the more difficult to muster up the courage to seek help. The first thing I was told by the corpsman I saw was "You cannot be in the Navy with anxiety." I was prescribed an antihistamine (hydroxyzine) and was referred to a psychologist in the primary care clinic. It was recommended to me to keep my mental health issues at the lowest level possible, as to not reflect "poorly" on my medical record and impact my career. After meeting with the psychologist a few times and expressing that I needed different medication because my anxiety was preventing therapy from being effective, she discouraged me. She told me, "You can either be on medication for the rest of your life or do therapy. You have to pick one. You cannot do both." After that visit, I never saw that psychologist again.

That experience almost discouraged me from ever seeking mental treatment again, but one of my friends convinced me to try going straight to Mental Health on base. I spoke to the front desk clerk at the clinic. She said she was looking out for me by scheduling me with the ununiformed psychiatrist because the Navy psychiatrist "isn't going to want to help you." Thankfully, the nonuniformed psychiatrist did help me with a medication adjustment, but I was disappointed when the therapist I was set up with was not a good fit. I didn't feel seen or heard. I focused on getting to the root of what was wrong, but she focused on coping mechanisms. It was draining to have to tell my story over and over to different people, and I took a break from therapy. A couple years later, when I attempted to pick it back up, I was told I needed to see the *same* therapist—who I already knew was not a good fit—a dreaded thirty-plus days later. I tried to go to Fleet and Family Services, but they were booked. Military OneSource referred me back to Mental Health on base. I asked for help with the network deferral process. I was told an off-base provider would take weeks longer than waiting for someone on base; however, that wasn't the case. I was able to find a mental health provider who could see me even sooner than the base. I was met with extreme resistance. The psychiatrist was rude and threw his hands in the air. I did end up obtaining an off-base referral for therapy from a nonmilitary provider, and she was great. I felt I could be more open with her. I felt she was looking out for my best interests, and I did not have to be scared of negative career implications. After what I experienced from the Navy mental health system, I concluded there was no way I could open up and discuss sensitive issues with a military provider, especially military sexual assault. I went to a base all-call, where mental health was being discussed. I told the TRICARE representative my story about the network deferral issues, and she tried to provide a justification that "we like to take care of our own." I don't agree with that. My needs weren't met. I had to find and fight for my own therapist, even though the clinic did not have availability.

Throughout the time I saw my psychiatrist at mental health, I was diagnosed with adjustment disorder. I knew there was something more. Every time I saw him, I would fish for answers beyond that blanket diagnosis. It wasn't until I separated from the Navy that I got my posttraumatic stress disorder (PTSD) diagnosis from Veterans Affairs and started on a path toward recovery. In the Navy mental health system, I felt unseen, unheard, and invalidated by my Navy psychiatrist. Every time I saw him, he had difficulty remembering simple details about my life. He made me feel like another check in the box.

Navy culture was harsh. Initially, I loved the Navy, was excited, and wanted to succeed, but my chain of command and working conditions took the wind out of my sails. Sailors worked long hours, had erratic sleep schedules, lived off vending machine food, and were told "your family did not come in your seabag." My chain of command made things as hard as possible. They made it difficult for me to get my qualifications, and it felt like they sabotaged me. We were given pointless tasks to complete. It was like it was all part of some elaborate hazing ritual. Sailors worked really hard, drank to oblivion, and smoked excessively to cope. Mental health issues were widespread but not addressed or talked about. Sailors joked about suicide because the topic was uncomfortable. The harsh working conditions, chain of command issues, and poor mental health care compounded to make life harder. It's no wonder why suicide has been such a large issue among servicemembers.

I lost three friends in the Navy to suicide. The first died in 2019, and the other two died in 2020. The third suicide hit me the hardest. I can distinctly remember the day when I received a phone call to come in to work early. I worked "midcheck," the third shift overnight, and was slightly annoyed that I had to show up earlier than usual. My work center chief and leading petty officer gathered the entire shop in our tiny space and informed us all that AT1 had taken his life over the weekend. What my chain of command did not know is that I had spoken with AT1 right before the weekend kicked off, and he was not his usual self. I carried an immense amount of guilt surrounding his death and could not step foot in that work center due to intense panic attacks. I tried to work with my chain of command to come up with a better option, but they refused. I approached the mental health clinic for help, but the only person willing to stick his neck out for me was the flight doc in my squadron. I am grateful for him to this day. He wrote me a *sick-in-quarters* chit for two whole weeks until my limited duty paperwork finished processing. That man likely saved my life.

I was so moved by military mental health issues in 2019, spanning from an instance on a detachment where I almost took my own life, I created a petition to the master chief petty officer of the Navy (https://chng.it/PRzstCwDPG) pleading to improve mental health conditions in the Navy. In 2021, when I reached the end of service, I started a military mental health podcast, *Your Story Doesn't End Here*. I thought that if the civilian population knew just how bad military mental health was, they would be outraged. Since the show's inception, there have been over 115 episodes, reaching thousands of listeners.

It was not until 2023 that I had the pleasure of connecting with Dr. Marietta because our missions had so much synergy. From the stories he heard and witnessed firsthand to the stories I personally experienced, everything that is said in this book, hands down, happens in real life. I can confidently say that because I saw the other side, the patient perspective where I was invalidated, unsupported, and made to feel as if my mental health did not matter. I say this not to put the blame on any one individual but to highlight the fact that the mental health system within the military is broken. And as you will read throughout this book, the hundreds of policies that exist throughout the branches do not solve the overarching problem—people are still dying.

This book is important whether you are a top leader of the United States Armed Forces, a politician, an active member of the military, a veteran, a military spouse, or a civilian. We cannot fully understand the scope of the problem until we know all sides of the problem. For far too long, we have been silenced, and it's time to bring these issues to the surface so that we can collectively move toward fixing and then healing.

Thank you, Dr. Marietta, for having the courage and bravery to talk about your experiences, and to you, the reader, I hope this book deepens your knowledge and understanding of what so many of today's service members experience throughout their service to this country. The battle is no longer only fought on the battlefield; it is in the hearts and minds of service members who raised their right hand to give their life. Thank you for being a part of the change.

> —Rachel Oswalt, host of *Your Story Doesn't End Here* and Navy AT2 (AW) veteran

INTRODUCTION

I AM A CAREER uniformed military psychiatrist, a medical doctor with a master's degree in public health. I graduated from medical school at Saint Louis University in St. Louis, Missouri, in 2000. In 2001 I completed an internship in internal medicine at what was then called National Naval Medical Center in Bethesda, Maryland. Following this, I completed a psychiatry residency at Naval Medical Center Portsmouth in 2004, where I was chief resident. As of this writing, I have over twenty years of uniformed service. I served in the Navy for eight years, completed a three-year tour with the Marine Corps in 2008, and achieved Fleet Marine Force officer qualification. I left the Navy, worked for the public/private sector, then achieved a commission with the Public Health Service (PHS) in 2011, where I have remained since. As a PHS officer, I completed tours of duty with the Air Force, Coast Guard, and Navy, and I continue to serve with Veterans Affairs.

Throughout my career in mental health, I have worked in many different settings and roles. I worked as a clinician, manager, and administrator. I have worked in the inpatient psychiatry unit, in the outpatient mental health clinic, in substance abuse programs, with the sexual assault program, and in family advocacy and other helping programs, including the Exceptional Family Member Program (EFMP), financial counseling, and employee assistance programs. I deployed on multiple occasions with the PHS and

Department of Defense (DoD) and am well acquainted with mental health in an operational setting. I worked in community mental health, engaging with people who were at their darkest hour, and helped them come back from the brink. I have spoken with tens of thousands of patients, authored more than 600 medical boards, talked to hundreds of senior military officials, and testified in military legal proceedings.

I served with the Navy twice in my career. After the Navy paid for medical school through the Health Professional Scholarship Program, I served as an active-duty Navy doctor from 2000–2008. Later, I completed another tour at Naval Medical Center Portsmouth from 2019–2022 as a PHS officer. During this time, the Navy experienced the widely publicized *USS George Washington* and Mid-Atlantic Regional Maintenance Center (MARMC) suicide clusters that involved my duty station. These crises were described by the commander of the US fleet forces command as a 9/11 event for the Navy. The publicly released formal investigation reports scratched the surface and hinted at deeper underlying issues that were described as a "vexing problem" by the chief of naval operations, Admiral Mike Gilday. The investigation and news reports lack the perspective of insiders who worked within the Navy's military health system. This was a familiar scenario I'd experienced throughout my career. Year after year, there are numerous news articles about military mental health. Hundreds of millions of dollars have been invested, but the reports, investigations, and efforts only scratch the surface.

Throughout my career as a military psychiatrist, I experienced a mental health system that was chaotic, crisis-driven, and patched with quick fixes. My colleagues and I were aware of chronic system problems, but the root causes and fixes were elusive. Every moment of our time was spent focused on getting the mission done, helping service members, and there was rarely time to pause, reflect, and engage in long-term planning, program improvement, and implemented course corrections.

After a certain point in my career, I started to take notes. Any time a patient told me a pearl of wisdom, something significant happened, or I remembered something important, I jotted it down. After many months and years, I had pages and pages of notes. Common themes and lessons were identified. These were formed into sections, then chapters. Soon, a book began to take shape. I wrote *Reflections of a Military Psychiatrist* to complete the reflection, the deep dive and longer look that was never done. I set out to communicate a deeper understanding and perspective of military mental health, to prepare future leaders to strengthen our military, to prepare service members for the battlefield, and to make recommendations for reform.

Military mental health is a difficult subject to write about. It is complex, and there are many different aspects. There are personal accounts about how it impacts service members, veterans, and their families. There are big news stories, including political wranglings. There is science and data, including numbers and rates. As you will soon see, military mental health is a complicated mess. It took quite a bit of time and effort to develop the best format to tell the story. What I settled on was a five-part journey. The first part of the book discusses the experiences I had serving with the Navy, Marine Corps, Air Force, Coast Guard, and Navy a second time through. I explore differences between the services. Then I delve into the Navy's highly publicized suicide clusters of 2022, offering an insider's perspective based on my firsthand experiences while serving at Naval Medical Center Portsmouth during that time. The middle part of the book takes you through the challenges my colleagues and I faced. Common issues service members face, lessons learned, and positive coping mechanisms are discussed. In the latter part of the book, I discuss provider burnout, how serving as a military psychiatrist personally impacted me, how I overcame it, and my work at Veterans Affairs. The book contains stories from veterans and lessons for recovery. The last part of the book features recommendations for improvement. This book has been a labor of love for me. I love the military, I believe in its mission, and helping service members and their families is my passion. I believe improving the military mental health system will strengthen the military.

I have worked in the realm of military mental health for many years and have been desensitized to what goes on. For some, the content in this book is upsetting and triggering, especially to those who have suffered from what is described here. I went back and forth when trying to find the best way to tell the story. I'm told some truths are hard to hear, but they need to be told, and the public needs to know. I did not want to do a disservice to those who have suffered. I recommend approaching this subject matter with a *how can we make things better* approach.

The accounts, opinions, and beliefs contained in this book are mine and do not represent and are not on behalf of any other entity. I did my best to get it right. Many individuals reviewed this book and provided feedback. I did my best to back up the contents with evidence and references. Ultimately, the contents of this book are my truth. I see it as both an academic and literary work. The book is an accomplishment and career goal to write about my life's work.

CHAPTER 1

Leyte

THE YEAR WAS 2006, and I was serving as the 3d Marine Division—colloquially referred to as third-psychiatrist at Camp Courtney in Okinawa, Japan, when the call came in. There was a large-scale disaster in the Southern Philippines that occurred in our AOR, area of responsibility. A catastrophic mudslide hit a rural village and buried an elementary school. The *USS Essex* and about 2,000 marines were in the area, and all available military personnel were redirected to assist. I was part of the "OSCAR team," short for Operational Stress Control and Readiness. We were an early implementation of an embedded operational military mental health team and part of the III Marine Expeditionary Force (MEF). III MEF included an infantry division, logistics group, and air wing. The 3d Marine Division was spread across Okinawa, Japan, and Kaneohe Bay, Hawaii. The size of III MEF and the division was in the thousands, but our team consisted of three individuals: myself, another psychiatrist, Lieutenant Commander Randolf Dipp, and a Navy psychiatric technician, HM2 (hospital corpsman second class) Travis Sells. At one point, we were assigned a marine Corps gunnery sergeant (GySgt) who himself was on limited duty. The math was simple. Due to the number of marines and sailors, geography, and our small size (two psychiatrists, a psychiatric technician, and a marine Corps GySgt on loan), we were outnumbered and had limited ability to do our jobs.

We were some of the first mental health providers embedded in operational Marine Corps units. We were also some of the first Navy medical officers to achieve Fleet Marine Force officer qualification. Except for the GySgt, we were all active-duty sailors. The Marine Corps did not have its own doctors, chaplains, or corpsmen, and we were on assignment from the Navy. There was no playbook or Marine Corps order explaining what we were to do or how to do it. Our job was unclear, undefined, and contentious. We were largely left on our own to develop our own program. There were widely divergent opinions as to what we were supposed to be doing and how to do it. There were those who even questioned the validity of our existence.

Since there was no standard operating procedure, we learned the hard way via trial and error and lessons learned passed down from our predecessors. When I first checked into the duty station, a story was told to me about how the previous 3d Marine Division psychiatrist gave a presentation to a Marine Corps general about PTSD. The psychiatrist was met with hostility and defensiveness. The Marine Corps general told him, "This is the United States Marine Corps. Marines don't have problems like that. Get out of my office and don't ever come back." The confrontation was seen as a setback for the advancement of operational mental health, and we had trouble even getting our foot in the door. The advice I was given was "be careful what you say to Marine Corps generals."

In the Navy, there were two communities affectionately referred to as the "blue side" and the "green side." The blue side was the big ships and the Navy's hospital-based medical system, while the green side referred to the Marine Corps. The blue side included the three large Navy hospitals: Bethesda (now Walter Reed), Portsmouth, and San Diego. The Navy hospitals featured graduate medical education training programs that trained future doctors. The blue side and green side were locked in a chronic battle for personnel, resources, policy decisions, and control. The Marine Corps prided itself on a history of valiant battles and performing on a shoestring budget. It was a huge transition going from the protected walls of the Navy hospital, where I was part of a large department, to an operational assignment, where I found myself on my own at an overseas location. On the ground, I observed a disparity of resources. One of the most striking examples of this was the Navy and Marine Corps medical facilities in Hawaii. On one side of the island of Oahu, the Pearl Harbor Navy base had a nice, clean, modern medical facility and mental health clinic. On the other side of the island, the 3d Marine Regiment in Kaneohe Bay had an operational medical clinic that was in disrepair, to put it kindly. The buildings were in a condemned state. The situation seemed like an injustice. The marines were the ones busting down doors, taking fire, and getting injured during combat in Iraq and Afghanistan, but the lion's share of the resources, money, and medical personnel were on the blue side.

The guidance received from senior Navy mental health providers on the green side was this: Our job was to be part of the Marine Corps operational units. We were discouraged from providing clinical care. We were to experience everything the marines experienced, including combat, and in doing so, the idea was that we could relate to them and be in a better position to assist with mental health issues. The role of a psychiatric technician also differed. At a Navy hospital, a psychiatric technician answered the phone, scheduled appointments, filed charts, and performed administrative tasks. In the field with the marines, our psychiatric technician was part of the team and provided psychological first aid and intervention.

The idea of embedding mental health providers in the Marine Corps was frowned upon by the senior blue-side Navy doctors and mental health providers. The blue-side Navy doctors preferred to be embedded within hospitals and clinic walls and would do anything to resist operational assignments and resource or policy requests from the green side. The blue side viewed the Marine Corps as taking away from resources. Once, I attended a presentation by the Navy psychiatry specialty leader. He said the entire Navy was 83 percent manned for psychiatry but effectively manned in the low 60 percent level because so many were deployed. The senior blue-side doctors felt our place was in the clinic seeing patients rather than in the field. We found ourselves in a crossfire. During my three-year tour with the marines, I witnessed blue-side Navy medical officials repeatedly trying to block and sabotage projects, programs, and resource requests from the marines. They argued this was the Marine Corps' problem, and they should pay and provide staffing. I witnessed Navy captains playing games with resource and staffing requests, such as claiming the requests weren't an official request or routed through the correct officials. They cited decreased clinical productivity data as an argument against increasing staffing for the OSCAR program. To be fair, there were some unanswered questions as to the overall premise of the OSCAR program. The OSCAR program managers recommended we needed to become marines to be successful, but we didn't feel that was the case. Our experience was that it wasn't an efficient use of resources to have medical personnel doing nonclinical work. Similarly, a mental health provider does not need to be assaulted to assist assault victims.

Around 2007, I participated in a conference where the role of OSCAR teams and Navy and Marine Corps operational and combat stress control programs were being discussed. The senior Navy mental health leaders argued mental health issues were a combat stress injury. The conference broke out into small group discussions. In my group, there were several marines and a Navy psychiatric technician. We came up with the idea that mental health issues could be both a combat stress reaction and an injury and proposed a color-coded continuum. The Navy and Marine Corps Combat Operational Stress Control (COSC) continuum was born that day, and the rest was history.

Over time, the OSCAR team evolved into a work routine that

was split into thirds. We invested a third of our time performing administrative functions, including attending meetings, program development, analyzing data, and performing special projects for leadership. The next third was conducting outreach. We traveled from unit to unit, providing briefings, networking, and conducting mental health skills training. The final third was conducting clinical care. When a marine was struggling with mental health issues, ranging from simple to complex, we were often the first point of contact and opportunity for intervention and assistance. The marines had a general distrust of Navy medicine and preferred to receive care from organic, embedded providers that were part of their units.

The needs of marines and sailors varied widely. On the blue side, military mental health providers were frequently asked to evaluate sailors or other service members who complained that they couldn't deploy or go back to the ship. The worst time to be on call was the night before an aircraft carrier deployed because, like clockwork, ten sailors would present to the emergency room, complaining they would kill themselves if they were returned to the ship. I had the opposite experience serving with the Marine Corps. Once, I was asked to conduct a mental health evaluation on a marine in the infantry who had volunteered for too many deployments. It was explained that he had been to the Middle East multiple times. The unit was concerned about his mental state because he had volunteered to go again. The command wanted me to make sure he wasn't suffering from a mental health disorder that was impacting his judgment. I spoke to the marine. He was a successful, strong, well-adjusted individual, dedicated to the Marine Corps and his country. It was inspiring and a privilege to talk to service members like this. My teammates and I felt we were able to conduct early mental health interventions to prevent problems down the road. I worked with a marine who served in a combat zone. His buddy was killed. He put him on his shoulder and carried him out. He suffered from PTSD and came to see me after suffering from marital problems. He was unable to open up to his wife about his experiences, although she desperately knew something was bothering him and wanted to help. I participated in a family session where he was finally able to discuss his combat trauma with his wife. She responded by being supportive and loving. I will never forget that moment. On that day, fighting PTSD became a couple's sport, and it demonstrated the power of the OSCAR team and early intervention. It was a watershed moment, and the burden he was carrying was lifted.

We were initially skeptical about having a limited duty marine on the OSCAR team, but the GySgt was a game changer. He was an actual career marine. He understood the culture, the language, and logistics of the Marines and became our guide. He became an integral and effective part of our team, connected us to marine units, and opened the door for outreach, education, and intervention. We discovered that having an actual marine on the team was more effective than for us to try to become marines, as suggested by the OSCAR program managers. He demonstrated the effectiveness of peer support. In addition to the above job responsibilities, we interfaced and created a support network with local resources, including Marine Corps Community Services and the Navy hospital located on Camp Lester. The result was that we established a web or small community that advocated and intervened on mental health issues for marines and sailors. We were a good team, but given our small size and geographic constraints, we had limited ability due to the work that needed to be done. We established collaborative alliances to get things done. Frequently, we had to beg, borrow, and steal.

I made it a habit to attend the annual Marine Corps ball. It was something else to put on a service dress uniform, watch the cake-cutting ceremony where the oldest and youngest marines cut the cake, and read from a scroll. The toast was even better. The marines toasted to famous battles and fallen marines throughout history. It was exciting to be part of something bigger and to serve with the marines who were highly professional and motivated.

On short notice, I boarded a KC-130 four-engine turboprop cargo plane at Futenma Marine Corps Air Station. The engines were loud, and we wore earplugs. The marines operating the plane affectionately handed everyone a plastic-wrapped chocolate chip cookie for a snack. I felt like I was in an Indiana Jones movie, with the black line moving across a map of the Pacific to music. We flew to Clark Air Force base near Manila and then Tacloban City in the Philippines. During a long layover, I got my hair cut. To my surprise, the barber used a straight razor, and I wasn't quite sure if that would have been permitted by USA health regulations. We had no food and ate dinner at a hole-in-the-wall restaurant in Tacloban City. It was a locally owned restaurant with a patio and a bar. There were lizards crawling all over the walls. We walked into the middle of karaoke night. None of the locals spoke English, but it was amazing to watch them sing. They sang karaoke in perfect English. Finally, I boarded a "53" Navy helicopter, and we headed for the *USS Essex*. The back end of the helicopter had a ramp that remained open the entire flight, and it was a beautiful view. The sky was clear, blue, there were palm trees everywhere, and the water was a pretty blue. In flight, it began to rain, and the helicopter was forced to set down at the disaster site until the weather improved. The site itself was impressive. The city had been in a valley under a mountain. The mudslide covered the city so well, you couldn't even tell that one existed.

When I arrived aboard the *USS Essex*, I was invited into the Marine Expeditionary Unit command center. I was introduced to a grumpy marine colonel with the familiar "Who are you?" and "Why are you here?" Meetings were conducted with key stakeholders, including Marine Corps officers, Navy line officers, medical officers, and chaplains. Many were supportive of the mission to provide operational stress control for marines and sailors to support the disaster relief efforts. The medical personnel, especially the corpsmen and chaplains, were supportive, but the war-fighting officers did not feel that mental health services were needed and felt "pressured" into requesting such services. I was pulled into a room and encouraged to keep a low profile to "avoid creating problems." This was consistent with stigma and leadership pushback and was like what we experienced on a regular basis, and the team discussed strategies to work around this. Junior marines were open and interested in mental health, but it was difficult, if not impossible, to access them due to lack of buy-in from the top. From a cultural perspective, the marines were afraid of appearing weak and did not trust Navy medicine. My green-side mentors explained that working with the marines was like peeling the layers of an onion and encouraged me to be patient.

I had never served on a Navy ship before. On my first night aboard the ship, I recall a memorable experience. There was a sailor caught smoking a cigarette on the ship. The ship's commanding officer boomed across the ship's public address system in an angry voice for the master-at-arms to arrest the sailor who was smoking on the ship's fantail. There was a lot of scrambling, but I'm pretty sure he got away.

The mission was a search and rescue operation to assist with disaster recovery. In the hours and days that quickly passed, weather conditions deteriorated due to rain. The safety of the disaster site was compromised, and ultimately, the rescue and recovery operations were terminated. The mudslide took the lives of an estimated 1,000 people, including approximately 200 children who were buried in an elementary school.

After the mission changed, I switched to plan B, which was to provide routine OSCAR services for Marines and Navy personnel, including mental health outreach, education, and sick call. I was able to connect with several corpsmen who were suffering from deployment related mental health issues. Each morning, there was a huddle with all the Navy medical personnel in the ship's medical section located on the bottom of the ship. Life on a Navy ship turned into *Groundhog Day*, doing the same thing day after day. I saw several junior enlisted sailors who struggled with mess cranking, a.k.a. dishwashing duties, and suicidal thoughts. Some were briefly hospitalized in the ship's medical section and benefited from taking a break.

While on the ship, I slept in a stateroom. The rooms were metallic, with a sink and four bunk beds. My room was below the flight deck, so I could hear chains being dragged, and I felt it when helicopters or the Harrier jets took off. We put our laundry in a bag with a large metal clip, and twice a week, the ship's crew would clean it and return it to us. All the officers ate in the wardroom. I met a lot of people and made a lot of friends there. I met a pilot named Rory Kipper who swam in high school with my brothers, Marshall and Jason, in Cape Girardeau, Missouri. One day while eating in the wardroom, a Naval officer refused to sit by me because he said he was fearful I would psychoanalyze him. At the time, I told him I wasn't, but it seems the psychoanalysis is complete, as evidenced by this book.

On Thursday nights, the ship had movie night. On Sundays, we had a special brunch. The ship had limited internet and payphones. I was able to keep in touch with my family most of the time. The *USS Essex* had a well-equipped gym. The ship would bob up and down with the waves. Working out under these conditions added an interesting twist. If you were doing push-ups when the ship hit a wave, all of a sudden, your weight increased dramatically. In college, I swam at Saint Louis University and worked out in the weight room with the Division I basketball and baseball players. Working out with the marines was similar. Whenever we had "green" hours in the gym, it was overflowing with marines lifting insane amounts of weight and driving the cardio machines at full blast.

One morning during the medical morning huddle, the team discussed the case of a female sailor who had severe anemia and kept passing out. She fainted in a ship's ladder well. The ship had red blood cells, but they couldn't transfuse the patient because of a problem with lab equipment. The general surgeon, OB-GYN, two family practice docs, and lab techs couldn't figure it out. During college, I worked in a research lab. Throughout my education, I participated in numerous science classes and worked with many different pieces of laboratory equipment. Operational tempo was slow, and I was determined to help. I walked back to the laboratory. It turned out that the device that was broken was a refractometer. This was a device containing a prism I used extensively to mix salt water for my aquarium back in Virginia. I calibrated the device, and the blood transfusion was completed. An emergency medical evacuation off the ship was averted. Serving with the Navy and Marine Corps as a psychiatrist felt like being an unsung hero at times. It was nice to make a tangible difference.

CHAPTER 2

Flagship

I JOINED THE NAVY through the Health Professionals Scholarship Program. The Navy paid for all four years of medical school, and in exchange I agreed to serve four years on active duty. After graduating medical school at Saint Louis University, I completed a one-year internship in internal medicine at what is now known as Walter Reed National Military Medical Center. When I trained there, the facility was known as the National Naval Medical Center. The old Walter Reed Army Medical Center closed in 2011 and merged with the Navy facility to establish the new Walter Reed.

The Navy had three large hospitals. These were in Bethesda, Maryland, Portsmouth, Virginia, and San Diego, California. These were affectionately referred to as the "flagship," "slave ship," and the "starship." The nicknames referred to the differences between the facilities. National Naval Medical Center in Washington, DC, was top heavy with a large contingency of senior and flag officers and had a politicized atmosphere. The facility catered to DoD flag officers and elected federal officials, including congressmen, senators, and the president. It had a VIP section, leather sofas on wheels, and a private galley that was utilized whenever a VIP was hospitalized there. In the DC area, and especially at National Naval Medical Center, the traffic and parking were horrendous, and there was a certain palpable tension in the air. During many clinical rotations, it was necessary and customary for physicians to wear scrubs throughout the day. I spent time at all three Navy hospitals, but the flagship was the only one where people would stop you in the hospital hallways, accuse you of being out of uniform, and demand to know why you were wearing scrubs. It was not uncommon to be stopped in the parking garage and confronted for wearing a white coat outside of the hospital. Out of all the Navy hospitals, Naval Medical Center Portsmouth in Portsmouth, Virginia, served the region with the largest fleet concentration, was the busiest hospital, and earned the name "slave ship." I completed my psychiatry residency there in 2004. There was so much clinical work to be done, there wasn't time for military games. This made for a more friendly, warm environment. Everyone was working together to serve the fleet. Naval Medical Center San Diego was the most desired Navy hospital to serve at due to its California location. The "starship" nickname referred to the West Coast lifestyle, the sun, surfing, lighter clinical workload, and the stars who worked there.

When you work as a doctor, there are certain cases that you remember forever. The National Naval Medical Center and National Institutes of Health had a prestigious hematology oncology fellowship. The Navy hospital had a cancer ward where doctors from NIH rotated and helped to provide treatment for hospitalized cancer patients. One night while I was on call, there was an older female struggling with cancer. One of the clinical labs we tracked was the complete blood cell count, which included white blood cells, hemoglobin, hematocrit, and platelets. To this day, she had the lowest lab values I had ever seen. Her immune system was weak, she lost a lot of blood, and her body wasn't producing enough blood cells or platelets to compensate. My colleagues and I worked tirelessly all night to keep her alive. I recall coordinating with the lab and asking for recommendations to safely administer blood cells, platelets, and fresh frozen plasma simultaneously. She survived that night and for months afterward. We saved her life that night, and I was proud of the work we did and of Navy medicine.

One of my first clinical rotations of my intern year was an internal medicine month at Washington Hospital Center located in Washington, DC. The patients were underserved and very sick, and the rotation was very busy. I remember vividly witnessing a patient with "coffee grounds emesis" I had read about in medical school textbooks. That patient was a severe alcoholic who vomited up blood due to a gastrointestinal bleed. I never witnessed anyone that ill at a Navy hospital and will never forget that sight. The atmosphere of Washington Hospital Center was very warm, collegial, and collaborative, and I felt supported by the attendings and residents I worked with.

My next rotation was in the Intensive Care Unit at the National Naval Medical Center. There was a Navy captain named Dr. Roberts who was a pulmonologist, and he had been a doctor for one of the presidents. He had a calm demeanor, was always kind and encouraging, and I really appreciated his leadership style. He had this wonderful prank where he would ask the junior doctors to interpret an X-ray. Everyone would stand there stammering. It turned out, the X-ray was of a pig, and he had a cheesy story about how he had obtained it. The ICU rotation was my first real introduction to Navy medicine and was a bit of a shock. Although the unit was an ICU, the patients were not so sick, and the workload was light. There weren't many medical procedures to go around, and there was always competition to get them. The attending, residents, and others referred to the patients as "chronically critically ill" and "subacute." The rotation lacked patient volume and acuity. The attending, resident, and training program made up for it with bullying and other toxic behavior.

"Pimping" is a historical teaching method in medical education where senior doctors put junior doctors on the spot and ask them probing, challenging, and intimidating questions. The questioning is done publicly, especially in front of peers. It is intended to prepare doctors to think on their feet and handle the real-world challenges of patient care. The practice is stressful, intimidating, and humiliating. It was more a tradition and a rite of passage. I recall a situation I encountered at my medical school in the neurosurgery department. The tradition was for medical students to wear short white coats while doctors who had graduated medical school wore long white coats. The neurosurgery program had a reputation for being malignant and required the first-year residents to wear short coats.

What I experienced at the Navy hospital ICU was a wake-up call. My attending was a pulmonologist and critical care specialist. He had roughly seven years more training than me. He had completed an internal residency and fellowship. He also had years of clinical experience. In addition, he wasn't just a doctor; he was a Navy captain, and he made it a point to make everyone aware of this fact. Our team would walk around the ICU during rounds, stopping at each patient's bed. He behaved like Darth Vader, and I felt gripped and choked. Together with his resident, they would pimp us mercilessly. He would ask us difficult questions and then criticize us for not knowing the answer. I refused to let this get me down.

My intern class was the last one before graduate medical education work-hour restrictions were implemented. It was not uncommon for us to work eighty to one hundred hours per week. As junior doctors, every morning, especially after working a twenty-four-hour shift, we would participate in a 7 a.m. internal medicine morning report. We would discuss the patients who were admitted overnight, the medical workup, the patients' clinical progress, and treatment plans. We were put on the spot and asked to interpret chest X-rays and discuss events that transpired overnight. There was a group of senior Capt./O6 doctors, with strong personalities, who were harsh and judgmental. There was another set of midcareer doctors, LCDR/O4 and Cmdr./O5, who would tiptoe around the senior Capt./O6 doctors. Graduate medical education was challenging, but the military system, rank structure, red tape, and culture added another dimension to the pain. I heard a story about an Air Force staff nephrologist, a senior kidney doctor, who had a reputation for being very cruel. In front of a nurse, he told a junior doctor she could have killed a patient, told her she was an idiot and incompetent, asked the nurse to assist him in placing a dialysis line, and kicked the junior doctor out of the room. I experienced a significant amount of this behavior, and after a certain point, my pain threshold increased, I better understood the game, and I developed thicker skin and more resilience.

In medical school, I loved physiology, the study of organ systems. On paper, I loved the heart, lungs, liver, and kidneys, their inner workings and how they worked together. The practice of internal medicine was frustrating and draining. Many patients had unhealthy lifestyles, were noncompliant, and presented to the hospital with frequent crises. Appointment times were short. It was difficult to get at the root causes of their issues. I saw many patients with severe diabetes who didn't take their insulin properly, suffered from the health consequences of the same, and would show up with blood glucose levels off the chart. One night when I was on call, I remember finding one of my patients with diabetes and pancreatitis in a hospital gown at 2 a.m. at the vending machine. He was supposed to be "NPO," which was short for a Latin medical term that meant "nothing by mouth." Instead, he was eating a massive 1,000-calorie cinnamon roll with a big smile on his face.

One day during internship, there was another doctor who appeared depressed and was struggling. I recognized this even before receiving any mental health training. I recall talking with her for a few minutes and offering her encouragement. Later that night, while she was on call, she made a suicide attempt in the call room. For sure she had her own internal issues, but medical training in general and the Navy medicine environment contributed to her decline.

While I did learn some valuable lessons and grew professionally, I was impacted by the toxicity I experienced during my internship, and so were others. Many of my professional colleagues were subjected to the same behaviors, didn't feel it was right, and made it a point not to do it to others. The behavior was demoralizing, and I learned it was okay, part of the Navy medicine culture, and necessary for survival. As my career progressed, I discovered that the "Navy doctor persona" was counterproductive, and it took me years to unlearn this mindset.

CHAPTER 3

Slave Ship

UPON GRADUATING FROM medical school, one earns the title of doctor. After successfully completing residency training, one becomes a full-fledged doctor. The military, and especially the Navy, had a practice of utilizing so-called general medical officers (GMO). These were licensed doctors who completed only the first year of their residency training, also called internship or post graduate year-1 (PGY-1). The GMO system was unpopular. Many states wouldn't grant licensure for doctors who had completed a single year of training, and there were issues with patient safety because of the big difference in training and clinical experience between a doctor who completed a PGY-1 and those who had successfully completed a multiyear residency training program. On the other hand, service members tended to be young and healthy, with straightforward, uncomplicated issues that didn't require much training or experience to manage. Due to the GMO system, all Navy doctors had to apply for a PGY-2 position. I applied for various positions. I was a competitive swimmer in college, loved the water, and applied for an undersea medical officer GMO position. I also applied for a PGY-2 position in internal medicine and psychiatry. At the time I really wanted to go into undersea medicine. The Navy had this way of always giving people what they didn't want. I was accepted to the psychiatry residency program at Naval Medical Center Portsmouth.

Naval Medical Center Portsmouth was a bustling and vibrant military hospital. It was open to active duty, family members, and retirees. The halls were filled with subspeciality clinics and the doctors to staff them. As a PGY-2, I worked thirty-six-hour shifts every fourth night. I would get to work around 7 a.m., provide care on the inpatient unit, carry a call pager all night, and work until lunchtime the next day. The emergency room at Naval Medical Center Portsmouth was busy, and sometimes I would conduct as many as ten psychiatric consultations per night, especially when ships were deploying the next day. Sailors from a deploying ship would show up in the emergency room saying they were suicidal and refused to go back to the ship. Some would make statements like they wanted to serve in the Navy but not be on a ship. Others would threaten to kill themselves unless they were discharged. A small number of sailors confessed to being coached on the internet to make suicidal statements to facilitate discharge. The stakes were high, and my colleagues and I faced high pressure to filter out the true positives from the false positives and preserve military readiness.

As the on-call resident, I could independently evaluate patients and had the authority to admit any service member, family member, or retiree I chose. On my first call night, I evaluated an older woman in a wheelchair. By the book, she met criteria for severe recurrent major depression and was expressing suicidal thoughts. I made the decision to admit her and called the on-call staff backup to ask a question about the admissions process. I was caught off guard when the attending was dismissive of the woman's concerns, called her "a borderline," and expressed disappointment with my decision to admit her. It was a red flag. I felt pressured to make certain diagnoses and not to admit patients from many different levels. In the emergency room, we were trained and encouraged to ask sailors if they just wanted to get out of the Navy and if discharging them from the Navy would solve their problems. We were taught to provide sailors memos documenting that they were incompatible with military life, suffered from suicidal thoughts, and were recommended for expeditious release from military service. The practice was largely effective, at least on the surface. When offered a way out, their demeanor changed, the suicidal thoughts resolved, they said, "Yes," took the memo, and went home. I would estimate that a third of sailors complaining of suicidal thoughts wanted to get out of the Navy. We were trained that this was a curative treatment called "ad sepamine." Sailors struggled with the unique stresses of military life. The treatment was administrative discharge from the Navy, and they would be expected to return to baseline levels of functioning after discharge.

The people and the environment of Naval Medical Center Portsmouth and the psychiatry residency training program were warmer and more positive compared to internal medicine at National Naval Medical Center. One day I remarked to the attending doctor I was working with that I was having a bad day. Much to my surprise, she whisked me off to a private room and asked me what was going on in a caring way. This was a far cry from getting pimped and choked by Darth Vader.

Deciding to become a psychiatrist was the best career decision I made. It is a humanistic field. We are able to sit and talk with patients for a reasonable length of time, get to know them, and assist them. Sometimes the practice of psychiatry went too far in the wrong direction. There was an older Navy psychiatrist in his late fifties, possibly early sixties. He had a computer in his office, but he never used it. Sometimes we had to use his office, and the computer had been used so infrequently, the Windows login screen had been burned into the old cathode-ray tube monitor. We had case conferences where we would discuss a patient in depth. One day there was a sailor who had shot himself, and this doctor offered a psychodynamic case formulation that he tried to "impregnate himself with a bullet." My colleagues and I rolled our eyes at that.

One night on call, I was called by a nurse and requested to come speak with an agitated female dependent who had been admitted to the psychiatry unit. Earlier in the evening, she had a positive urine drug test for cocaine. When I spoke to her, she was agitated and argued with the unit staff and myself, demanding another test. We were at our wits end trying to help her to calm down. I ordered another drug test, hoping it would help her calm down, and it worked. About an hour later, the lab called me with an urgent result. The second urine drug screen was positive for Kool-Aid! The patient had put fruit punch in the urine sample cup.

I will never forget September 11, 2001. I was a second-year psychiatry resident and working on the psychiatry emergency room service. My friend, Jerry Schmuker, was also a second-year psychiatry resident. We watched the twin towers collapse on a clinic TV. The hospital commander announced what was going on, and we were put on alert. I was on call that night and had no idea what to expect. I thought things were going to get very busy, but the opposite happened. Everything went on lockdown, almost no one came into the hospital, and the facility became a ghost town. Days later, the Navy surgeon general came to the hospital and gave a speech in the auditorium about how he had witnessed the Pentagon burn.

The first time I met a Navy admiral was in the hospital cafeteria. I had no idea who or what he was. He sat down next to me in the galley, was kind, asked me questions, and offered encouragement. He talked about "customer delight." As I recall, sometime later, the hospital experienced a multimillion-dollar budget shortfall, and he left the facility. The next admiral had a reputation for being very harsh and was focused on cost savings. When a patient couldn't be seen in a timely manner at the Navy hospital, a network deferral was submitted. In our department, if we could not see an active-duty patient within a specific time frame, we would submit a network deferral so the patient could be seen by an off-base provider through the TRICARE network. When the new admiral took over, there was a halt to network deferrals. We were told the admiral personally reviewed any such requests for off-base services and anyone making such a request risked facing his wrath. Everyone was terrified. When a network deferral was requested, the naval officer reviewing the consult would kick it back with the verbiage, "No network deferral per the admiral." We were told there was no need for a network deferral because personnel could work longer hours to meet the clinical need. We were told the clinic could stay open into the evening or through the weekend. Each resident was assigned a senior psychiatrist mentor. My mentor, a Navy Capt./ O6, told me the admiral referred to the Navy's substance abuse residential treatment program facility located on the Norfolk Naval Base as "an expensive hotel" and tried to pressure him to agree to closing it down. Fortunately, my mentor convinced him of the importance of the facility, and he agreed to let it remain open. It was reported that the hospital achieved a multimillion budget dollar surplus, and the admiral soon achieved a second star.

Today, no one would ever question the utility and benefit of clinical social workers. They play a critical, versatile role in every mental health program everywhere. At some point in my residency during 2001–2004, the Navy came close to eliminating social workers, but at the last minute, this effort was canceled. Navy medicine was a very dynamic environment and could experience drastic changes at a moment's notice. It was an atmosphere where anyone and everyone was on the chopping block at any time, and this contributed to anxiety and stress.

When I was a second-year psychiatry resident, I experienced the loss of a patient for the first time. A sailor who suffered from depression and alcoholism went home and committed suicide by proxy. He called the police to his house and shot at them with the intent to draw them into a gunfight and be killed. He killed a police officer and then was killed by law enforcement. I had seen the sailor earlier, and it was a very difficult situation to process. The experience was devastating. I called the patient's mother and spoke to her. The experience helped me understand how serious the job of being a military mental health provider was. As a result of that situation, I learned there are three kinds of psychiatrists: those who have experienced patient suicide, those who will, and those who were not psychiatrists.

One night while on call, around 2 a.m., I was called into the ICU. The senior doctor explained that a young sailor in his early twenties was suffering from pneumonia and his death was imminent. The parties involved said they were trying to race against the clock to facilitate an emergency medical discharge prior to his death to optimize benefits for his family. The process involved a psychiatrist signing off on it. I remember trying to talk to the sailor at bedside with a junior resident who was on call with me. There wasn't much we could do since he was unconscious, on a ventilator, and unable to speak. We reviewed the medical records and documented a note. I signed off on the paperwork and was told it was forwarded up to Washington, DC, for processing. About a week later, I came across the sailor in the hospital. He was walking, talking, and appeared healthy. Miraculously, he survived that night and went on to make a full recovery. He wanted to remain on active duty and was searching for ways to undo the medical discharge, but there was no way to do it. The situation was something straight out of the novel *Catch-22*. He had been medically discharged. I remember telling him he did everything he could to reverse it, it was the Navy's mistake, and I suggested he enjoy the lifetime disability pension that came with it.

Psychiatry was a four-year residency training program: one year of internship and three additional years of training. During my fourth year, it became time to pick my assignment. All my mentors talked about being assigned a "utilization tour." This is where you would pay back the service commitment to the scholarship I had received. In addition, the most junior service members picked from the bottom of the barrel. I called the detailer and was offered San Diego. In a heartbeat, I agreed to the assignment and was issued orders. About a month before I was to undergo permanent change of station (PCS), I logged onto a Navy website called BUPERS Online and was shocked to see my orders were canceled about a month before. During this time, I signed a contract to purchase a house, and the house I was living in was under contract to be sold. The Navy psychiatry specialty leader and the detailer had canceled my orders without telling me. It was very poor leadership, organization, and planning, an underhanded move that damaged my relationship with and trust in the Navy. The feedback I received was that I should have waited until I arrived at the next duty station before buying a new house, and it was a slap in the face. It was also poor advice for a young professional with small children. In the end, I was able to sell my house in San Diego right before the 2008 market crash, make a little money, stay an extra year at Portsmouth, and then PCS to the 3d Marine Division in Okinawa, Japan. In retrospect, everything worked out for me for the better. The assignment with the Marine Corps was a much better and fulfilling assignment.

CHAPTER 4

Air Force

WHILE SERVING WITH the Navy and Marine Corps, I had limited dealings with the Air Force in Hawaii and Okinawa. I observed that in Oahu, the Air Force and Navy had modern, clean, and well-staffed mental health clinics, while there was a disparity of resources with the Marines on the other side of the island at Kaneohe Bay. The same applied to the barracks in Hawaii. The Navy and Air Force had nicer accommodations for their service members. The Marine Corps buildings, medical clinics, and barracks were in disrepair.

After working in community mental health for a few years, I was offered a commission in the PHS as a psychiatrist. My first assignment was 2011 at Langley Air Force Base in Hampton, Virginia. The Air Force's mental health and medical systems were a surprise and a breath of fresh air. The Air Force Medical System leadership was very different from the strong, harsh personalities I experienced in the Navy. The senior officers had a calm demeanor, were methodical and well organized, and frequently referred to and followed policies.

The Air Force had an Air Force Instruction (AFI 44-172) for mental health that went into excruciating detail about how the clinic was to be run. It was a difficult adjustment for me coming from the Navy, where there wasn't much organization or direction, and the culture was to go it on your own. The document was comprehensive, thorough, and well balanced. When I served with the Marine Corps, it was frustrating and disappointing that our program was unclear, undefined, and lacked a policy. At one point, LCDR Randolf Dipp and I, the OSCAR psychiatrists, were tasked with writing a MEF or division order for the OSCAR program. In retrospect, we were asked to do the job that the headquarters element had failed. The Air Force had effectively accomplished what we set out to do. They had a policy document that was cohesive, logical, and functional and had been signed by senior leadership.

When I first experienced how the Air Force approached the issue of diagnosing personality disorder, I was skeptical because it was radically different from how the Navy handled things. In the Navy's mental health system, the threshold to diagnose a personality disorder and recommend administrative separation was low. If an airman was suspected of having personality disorder, a command-directed evaluation (CDE) was conducted. The airman was presented with specific concerns, in writing, about their behaviors, and it was a wake-up call. If the member continued with the same behaviors, they were processed for separation. A lot of times, the Navy got it right, but there were times when the separation recommendation was premature or wrong. Sailors complained that they went to mental health, were diagnosed with personality disorder, were recommended for discharge, and had little recourse. There was a situation where that exact scenario played out on the *USS Abraham Lincoln* when a sailor was recommended for separation prematurely and he successfully fought it (Ziczulewicz 2022). This didn't happen in the Air Force system. The Air Force was much more cautious about recommending mental health administrative discharges for airmen. The CDE added protection for the service member and resulted in better outcomes. I observed that the Air Force had fewer personality disorder discharges and retained more airmen because of this approach.

Another best practice was the Air Force high interest list. This was, in effect, an involuntary outpatient commitment program. When Air Force mental health providers identified a service member as high risk, they would enter them into a roster and direct weekly face-to-face mental health sessions with the service member. Upon enrollment into the program, a face-to-face meeting was conducted with the service member, mental health provider, senior commander, and senior enlisted. The service members were tracked on a spreadsheet, and if they didn't show up for an appointment, the patient's senior commander was called within an hour of the no-show. Each week there was a multidisciplinary team meeting to discuss the cases on the list and strategies to assist them. A consensus of mental health providers, in coordination with the command, decided when the patients were appropriate to leave the list.

The way that the Air Force chain of command interacted with mental health and how they supported their airmen was refreshing. Air Force leadership was frequently in tune with mental health issues and would often be the first to contact mental health and make a referral. Anytime a service member was in trouble, the senior commander and senior enlisted were often the first to call mental health and would readily come to the clinic for team meetings to discuss efforts to support their airmen. Air Force commands had a first sergeant, also known as "first shirt," whose job it was to assist airmen. I witnessed firsthand the power of collaboration with commands. In the Air Force system, there was positive command involvement, even for service members who were facing prosecution in the military justice system. I recall an Air Force Col/O6 telling an airmen he had to be held accountable for something he had done but that he cared for him and wanted to help him. Positive involvement and influence from the command greatly improved the outcomes of cases.

The Air Force had another unique program called the Limited Privilege Suicide Prevention Program. If a service member was considered a suicide risk, a lockbox could be put on the patient's medical record to provide increased confidentiality and protection from prosecution. This way, a patient who was being accused of criminal acts could discuss their thoughts and stresses in a safe place. The paper records and notes protected by this program were sandwiched between two colored sheets. When notes went electronic, the top of each note indicated that the information was protected by the program and could not be disclosed. The airmen could discuss issues without fear of its use as evidence in the military justice system.

What I had experienced in the Navy was considerably different from the Air Force. In the Navy, high-risk sailors would frequently present in crisis then disappear. Sometimes they would say they were feeling better but then return in crisis weeks or months later. Commands were detached, at times disinterested in the welfare of their sailors, and it wasn't uncommon for them to add to a sailor's distress. The idea of tracking high-risk sailors was discussed by Navy mental health providers, but it was frowned upon. Sailors would present to the emergency department with a chief complaint that they were suffering from maltreatment from the command and wanted to kill their chief. I spoke to a sailor once who was so desperate to get off the ship, he drank motor oil. There were disgruntled airmen too, but those types of complaints were much less common. I evaluated thousands of airmen, and I don't think I ever saw a single one complain that they wanted to kill their supervisor. In the Navy mental health system, I witnessed several situations where a sailor's medical records were scrubbed and information was used for adverse personnel actions and military justice proceedings. Protected health information grabs were less frequent in the Air Force system.

The way the Air Force managed limited duty was computerized, organized, accurate, and effective. There was a website that accurately tracked limited duty. The chief of aerospace medicine had a list of airmen on limited duty, including the total number of limited-duty days. We had a monthly meeting where we would run the list and discuss the clinical progress of each airman. Representatives from the medical boards office were also present. The indications and triggers for initiating a medical board were clearly defined in policy. If an airman had a catastrophic condition, a medical board would be initiated promptly. In the Navy system, there were lengthy delays, sometimes a year or longer in initiating a medical board. Sailors would frequently get lost and drop out of treatment during this time. There were sailors I saw one time who would return six months later after their period of limited duty expired.

Patients who dropped out of treatment and had not returned for an appointment were identified, and intervention was conducted in the Air Force mental health system. A psychiatric technician would scrub clinic records for airmen who hadn't returned to the clinic and reach out to the patients to make sure they were doing okay. Some left the Air Force, and others had moved to a new base, but it wasn't uncommon to discover a patient was struggling, and the phone call reconnected them to care. The Air Force mental health system had an inspection system with some teeth. The items in the policy were granular and inspectable, and the Air Force was serious about conducting inspections and implementing corrective actions.

A memorable case from my time serving in the Air Force mental health system was a highly successful senior enlisted patient who suffered from renal cancer, chronic pain, and PTSD-like issues. He had surgery to remove a mass from his kidney. In the recovery room, he woke up to find his doctors panicking that he was losing blood. He was taken back to surgery, and his entire kidney was removed. In the months that followed, he developed debilitating anxiety and chronic pain. One day, he sent an email to many senior military leaders and me:

> *All,*
>
> *Sorry for the email but wasn't sure who would be the proper office to speak with. Also, wanted to ensure everyone involved in my care was in the loop.*

> *After a long, hard battle with daily, crippling foot pain for the past year-plus, I have decided I am ready to pursue total/ partial amputation. No other treatment has been effective, and I am not able to cope effectively any longer.*
>
> *Please place a referral to the appropriate office to begin the consultation process...*

The military health system was flooded with emails, but to this day, I've never read an email that made an impression on me like that one. The email captured the extent of his distress and suffering. I felt great empathy and compassion for his situation. We tried to no end to alleviate his suffering, but he had chronic treatment-resistant symptoms and ended up being medically retired through the medical boards process.

A colleague described the culture and approach of the Air Force in a way that has stuck with me today. The screws on an aircraft had marks that lined up with marks on the fuselage. During a preflight check, if the marks didn't line up, the implication was that the screw had moved. After discovering this, personnel went through a comprehensive checklist to ensure safety, and there was a low threshold to scrub the flight. The Air Force was the most organized and had the best planning of all the services I served with, and this was reflected in the outcomes they achieved. The Air Force consistently had the lowest suicide rate of all the services. Some would argue this is because the Air Force had better resources and lacked infantry and combat exposure the Army and Marine Corps had. I suspect it had more to do with organized, careful, and methodical planning. Such an approach would have greatly helped the Navy and Marine Corps.

CHAPTER 5

Coast Guard

THE COAST GUARD had roughly 50,000 active-duty service members. The eleven missions of the Coast Guard were very broad and included drug interdiction, migrant interdiction, ice operations, and search and rescue. The entire size of the Coast Guard was equivalent to the size of one large DoD installation, but it was spread across smaller bases across nine distinct geographic districts. The Coast Guard was considered "military" and an "armed service," but it was part of the Department of Homeland Security. There was a technicality that the Coast Guard could become part of the DoD during times of war. Active-duty Coast Guard affectionately referred to themselves as "coasties." They deployed anywhere at any time. I deployed many times as a PHS officer. Frequently, when I arrived at the deployment site, the Coast Guard was part of the mission and already on the scene. I encountered coasties at a border patrol mission in Texas and at an Army camp for Afghan refugees in Texas.

The Coast Guard was at the mercy of language in federal law, including the annual National Defense Authorization Act that determined budgeting. If a law or funding source referred specifically to DoD, Coast Guard was excluded. Any time a new law came out, for example, referencing sexual assault or other military programs, headquarters would comb through the regulations to see if they applied to the Coast Guard. Sometimes I wondered if the legislators were fully aware of the implications of the different terminology. I was a doctor in the Public Health Service. The PHS and National Oceanic and Atmospheric Administration (NOAA) suffered a similar stepchild plight. PHS and NOAA were "uniformed services" but were not "military" or "armed services." Once, while serving as a PHS officer with the Coast Guard, I was at the airport ticket counter with my children and asked for the military baggage fee discount. The airline employee looked at my DoD ID card that documented me as serving in the PHS and told me I wasn't in the military. It was insulting and a slap in the face. There was a *Washington Post* article that captured the plight officers in the sister services faced (Davidson 2018). We ran into similar issues with the uniformed services organization (USO). The USO airport lounges serve "Armed Forces" but not PHS or NOAA.

The Coast Guard strived to provide similar services to what the DoD had but lacked resources. The Coast Guard did not have its own family service centers and relied on resource-sharing agreements. Sometimes the agreements were informal, based on a handshake, and on occasion, coasties were turned away. There were Coast Guard bases like Seattle that were closer to an Army base and others like Portsmouth that were closer to Navy installations. The Coast Guard bases relied on the DoD installation in the closest geographic proximity for support, irrespective of service branch. The DoD had the Military OneSource program, where service members received confidential counseling from a community mental health provider. The Coast Guard was not included in Military OneSource and had to create and fund a contract for a similar program called CG SUPRT. The Coast Guard's sexual assault program was tightly tied into the DoD's program and was able to access DoD electronic systems, but the Family Advocacy Program (FAP) was a different story.

The Coast Guard was like the Marine Corps in many ways. They prided themselves on getting the mission done on a shoestring budget. I visited a helicopter maintenance service center located in

Elizabeth City, North Carolina. A lot of the aircraft the coasties used were hand-me-downs from other services. The helicopter service center took the helicopters apart piece by piece, reassembled them, recertified them, and returned them to the field. The Coast Guard had its own medical corpsmen but, like the Marine Corps, did not have its own doctors. The Coast Guard utilized PHS physicians and had a close relationship with the PHS since the days of the Revenue Cutter Service in the 1800s.

Every service had elite members. The Navy had SEALS, the Army had Green Berets and rangers, the Marine Corps had Force Recon, and the Air Force had pararescuemen. The Coast Guard had rescue swimmers, and their training facility was in Elizabeth City, North Carolina. I was a competitive swimmer in high school and swam on a Division I swim team at Saint Louis University during college. There were times in my athletic career when I swam before and after school. We would swim for an hour in the morning and two hours in the evening, for a total of 10,000 meters per day. The discipline and dedication needed to become a doctor were the same as what was needed to be a competitive swimmer, and the sport helped me become who I am today. For a swimmer like me, the Coast Guard rescue swimmer training facility was like something out of a wild dream. It had ropes that hung down from the ceiling over the swimming pool where the rescue swimmers would climb out of the water. Once in the air, they would cross the ropes like something out of a Donkey Kong video game. There was a movie about Coast Guard rescue swimmers called *The Guardian*, starring Kevin Coster, that was released in 2006. I always had an itch to get back in the pool with the Coast Guard but was never able to do it.

Every service had a culture of how they treated service members and their families. On one of my first days serving with the Coast Guard, my commanding officer sat me down and explained that the Coast Guard takes good care of its people and has high retention, and coasties tend to stay lifelong. The Coast Guard treated their active duty and family members well. When a family had special needs, such as a child with autism, the Coast Guard went out of their way to modify orders and relocate them more so than I had experienced with other services. When a hurricane was coming, the Coast Guard would evacuate families in advance. In Kodiak, Alaska, the Coast Guard would routinely fly service and family members out for routine medical care.

The Coast Guard utilized what they referred to as the mission support business model. This is where headquarters wrote the policies, service centers conducted middle management, and personnel in the field completed operational work. It was great on paper, but in practice, it didn't work so well, at least on the medical side. Frequently, personnel in the field spoke directly to headquarters, bypassing middle management, and this contributed to confusion and chaos. Inside the Coast Guard medical enterprise, there were different divisions and bureaucratic lines, including Operational Medicine ("Op Med") and Work-Life. Work-Life had "nonclinical" mental health providers, and Op Med had clinical ones such as psychiatrists and psychologists.

Early on in my career, while serving with the Navy, I encountered Critical Incident Stress Management (CISM). This was a practice of "debriefing" service members who had experienced trauma, such as combat, to try to mitigate its effects and prevent PTSD. There was some research that suggested the practice made things worse, and the practice was discontinued. CISM lived on in some form in the Coast Guard. CISM was intended for post-trauma, post-disaster mental health intervention, but the Work-Life team would frequently say they were going to conduct a CISM for almost any situation. Once, a Work-Life employee said they were going to conduct a CISM after a coastie threatened suicide. The mental health providers in Op Med were in favor of replacing the practice with psychological first aid, but the Work-Life employees were reluctant to do so. It was an uphill battle to accomplish this, but I was told it did get done. The employees felt their job security was threatened and would do everything in their power to resist or block policy updates.

During my tour with the Coast Guard, I was sent to the Coast Guard boot camp in Cape May, New Jersey, after they lost a mental health provider. I spent months at the facility assisting recruits. It was magic watching the bus filled with recruits pull up to the barracks, watching the company commanders walk on the bus, engage the new recruits, and witness the birth of their military careers. Some of the boot camp recruits I spoke with were afraid, fearing they made the wrong choice in joining the military, and I delicately offered them hope and encouragement. The Coast Guard Training Center Cape May had an amazing galley with custom china. Every morning, I looked forward to getting up, exercising, and ordering made-to-order eggs served on nice dishes. The gym at Cape May was the most spotless gym I ever worked out in. It had the flags of the fifty states around the ceiling. Every evening, the recruits perfectly aligned the machines, wiped them down, and swept the floors.

The Coast Guard managed substance use disorders differently compared to the DoD. The Coast Guard had a system where the primary care manager diagnosed and managed substance use disorders. The Coast Guard had its own on-the-job training program where primary care providers went to the Hazelden Betty Ford Center in Minnesota to learn how to diagnose and manage substance use disorders. For a while, the DoD/Veterans Affairs clinical practice guidelines specified that a subspecialty mental health provider was to diagnose and manage substance use disorders. That was updated to include primary care providers, and I'm confident the Coast Guard successfully lobbied for the change.

While I was serving with the Coast Guard, the longest US government shutdown in history began on December 22, 2018, and ended thirty-five days later on January 25, 2019. Active-duty members and their families missed paychecks. PHS officers were impacted too because our paychecks were funded by the Coast Guard. We were told to prepare to miss our next paycheck. The situation was horrific and stressful. Some of the junior enlisted stayed home because they didn't have enough money to pay for gasoline. My pay cycle was monthly. I think I was paid on time, but it was a close call. Halfway into the shutdown, I contacted my part-time job and asked for more hours in anticipation of lost income. An entrepreneurial coastie created a "shutdown coin" that captured the situation. The coin featured a Monopoly-looking man, dejected, with his pants pockets turned inside out and his hands gesturing down. The coin read *United States Coast Guard* at the top and *Essential Personnel* at the bottom. A flier with tips for coping with a furlough from one of the programs I had a hand in was somehow featured on *Jimmy Kimmel Live!* He said, "Not only is the shutdown affecting current members of the Coast Guard, it's affecting recruitment to the Coast Guard too." The narrator read: "At the US Coast Guard, we're working hard, protecting our ports, defending our borders, driving our Ubers, babysitting, walking dogs, delivering Postmates, and selling pot." He joked, "Why not sell a kidney while you are at it?" The act closed with the slogan, "The Coast Guard. Can we please get back in our [bleep]ing boats now?"

CHAPTER 6

Navy a Second Time Through

BY 2019 I MADE the decision to make a change and try the Navy again, this time as a PHS officer. At this point in my career, I was a captain/O6, more experienced, mature, and ready for the challenge. I returned to the place where I graduated residency, Naval Medical Center Portsmouth, over a decade after I left the Navy and began working in the outpatient mental health clinic. The hospital was known as the "first and finest." Building 1, where the commanding officer's suite was located, was a historic building that had been the original naval hospital and had been around since the early 1800s. The building was made of stone and had a dome on top, where it was said early Navy surgeons performed their work under sunlight. Outside of Building 1 was the hospital point. Every morning at 0800, the flag was raised. It was said that this ceremony had been consistently performed for 200 years regardless of weather conditions. There was nothing like walking up the stone steps of Building 1 and entering the massive foyer.

When I arrived at the facility, the Defense Health Agency (DHA) was in the process of taking over all military medicine, and there were DHA signs everywhere. There had been many changes since I left the facility in 2005. Recognition and demand for mental health increased, and the directorate grew. When I served as a Navy psychiatrist from 2004 to 2008, there was a palpable disparity of resources between the operational community and hospital system. A 180-degree had transpired. The Navy had taken many doctors and reassigned them to operational units. The last time I served at the hospital, the halls were bustling with family members, retirees, active duty, and busy subspecialty medical clinics, but it felt like a ghost town. The halls and clinic waiting rooms were empty. The facility had a parking garage with six floors, including the rooftop. When I served at the facility in the early 2000s, the parking garage was full by 0800, but by that time the second time around, I could still park on the third floor. It was bittersweet. It was great to see operational units had been beefed up with medical providers, but it was sad to see that Naval Medical Center Portsmouth was a fraction of what it once was. The name was even changed to Naval Medical and Reserve Training Center Portsmouth; however, everyone continued to refer to it as Naval Medical Center Portsmouth.

There were rumors and conspiracy theories about the fate of the military health system and facility. The former dean of the Uniformed Services University of Health Sciences wrote an opinion piece about the degradation of the military health system (Kellerman 2023). He wrote that families and retirees were sent elsewhere, and this deprived military healthcare professionals, especially those in training, of the complex patients they needed to treat to acquire and sustain their skills. Kellerman shared a graph of the military medical budget that remained flat and advocated for a funding increase and for the military health system to be rebuilt. I found what Kellerman wrote to be true. The mental health directorate was closed to family members and retirees, except for child mental health. When I was a psychiatry resident, our clinic was open to family members and retirees. I learned a lot from them, including valuable life lessons and about the cycle of the disease process. From the perspective of a military mental health provider, it was educational to provide care to veterans and the families of service members, to appreciate and understand the impact military service had on them. I recall a specific case where a service member, his wife, and their child were all receiving care in our clinic. My colleagues and I worked together to assist them and strengthen their family. Our clinic was closed to family members, and we lost the ability to provide that type of service. The inability to serve family members and retirees negatively impacted medical training and clinical practice. It was also mundane to work with young, healthy active-duty service members all the time.

The lack of retirees and family members impacted the care of sailors too. The substance abuse treatment program was closed to them, and it impacted care and training. A critical part of substance abuse treatment was for the active-duty sailors to be taught life lessons from that old Navy chief who struggled with chronic alcoholism. That piece was missing. The sailors didn't hear that story about the mistakes he had made.

I had fond memories of eating at a hole-in-the-wall restaurant, the Dancing Goat Café, with my colleagues when I was a resident. Thankfully, it was still there. The same pleasant woman was still running the place, albeit with some gray hair. She remembered me, and I was able to enjoy the same chicken parmesan sandwich and french fries I enjoyed a decade earlier.

When I served at Naval Medical Center Portsmouth the first time, in the early 2000s, our directorate had about five or more active-duty Navy Capt./O6. Serving in a leadership position at one of the big three naval hospitals was a stepping stone to promotion for a senior rank. I was caught off guard this time around to find that personnel were much more junior, fresh out of training, less experienced, with lower ranks. There was only a single Capt./O6 psychiatrist.

The Navy had always been a gruff place. It had a get-back-to-work, back-to-the-ship mentality that permeated and trumped everything. The Navy had a cultural tradition of being hard on sailors, turning issues around on them and looking at problems through a disciplinary lens. When I was a resident, I recall one specific case where a sailor threatened suicide, a senior officer in his chain of command handed him a knife and told him to do it, and he cut himself. The sailor was flown off the ship and admitted to our inpatient psychiatry unit. Mental health providers were harsh too. I recall during residency training, my attendings, the full-fledged doctors who were my supervisors, would guilt-trip sailors. They told them they signed a contract, made a choice not to go back to the ship, and would pressure them to return. Once, a Navy psychiatrist told a patient he could start medication for depression, but it would likely cause impotence, hoping it would discourage him from doing so. Another psychiatrist diagnosed a sailor with malingering and had the sailor escorted off the psychiatry unit by military police.

The climate was such, I rarely advocated for a sailor when I was a resident. I recall a specific case where a sailor's wife left him and their child with autism, and he was struggling with depressed mood and suicidal thoughts. He had pending orders to report to a ship. I decided on what I thought would be a simple phone call with the detailer. Instead, it turned into an argument. The detailer explained to me that he heard sob stories every day and the sailor's wife "didn't come in his seabag." As a result, I put the sailor on limited duty.

A Navy veteran shared a progress note written by an active-duty mental health provider that captured the lack of compassion, empathy, and harshness he experienced:

> *Service member showed up to his appt 25 mins late in an improper uniform. He was wearing his Navy Working Uniform Type 3 pants and an untucked brown undershirt without a blouse or belt. He stated he was rushing to come to his appt which is why he was not properly dressed.... Service member was asked to return to his car and put on the rest of his uniform. When he returned, this provider spoke with him briefly to see if there were any acute issues. He stated he was just feeling very anxious today and did not report any safety concerns. He did not need a medication refill and stated he was "giving up" on sleep.*

The sailor was really struggling and needed a Navy mental health provider to listen to him, help him, and not be judgmental about his uniform and situation. He told me after this experience that he gave up and stopped going to Navy mental health appointments.

The second time around with the Navy, I found myself busy again, providing full-time outpatient clinical care for many sailors. Many complained that after they were put on limited duty, members in their chain of command pulled them into an office and berated them. The sailors told me they were accused of being a "deployment dodger" and of violating the Ship, Shipmate, and Self code. Their transfers off the ship were discouraged and delayed, and security clearances and other administrative actions were taken against them. I talked to one sailor who couldn't work on limited duty after he left his ship because his previous command had caused his security clearance to be suspended after a suicide attempt. Without the security clearance, he was unable to access a computer and thus unable to do work.

At this point in my career, I served with the Air Force and Coast Guard and was accustomed to service members being treated more positively. What I experienced serving with the Navy a second time was shocking and disappointing. Airmen and coasties rarely complained about those sorts of issues. I remember one case of a sailor whose mother was suffering from terminal cancer, and her request for humanitarian reassignment was not proactively dealt with during the overseas screening process. They had identified the issue, but it wasn't dealt with. A week after she arrived at her overseas duty station, she predictably fell apart. Promptly afterward, she was sent to our facility at Naval Medical Center Portsmouth via the medical evacuation process. To add to her problems, her mother was terminally ill in California. She had been placed on limited duty on the East Coast, and the Navy would not permit her to complete the limited duty on the West Coast. She needed to be near her dying mother. Her command was understanding and granted her liberal leave, and she was able to spend a significant amount of time with her mother before her death. I saw a number of these types of situations at Naval Medical Center Portsmouth. Several sailors had family on the West Coast but were forced to stay in Virginia, away from their support system. It was like the system was engineered to add to stress and make situations worse. Once sailors were placed on limited duty, it was impossible for them to move to the opposite coast.

Sailors complained that they faced real-life consequences for receiving help. "Nuke" was a term used to refer to a sailor who specialized in nuclear engineering. I worked with a Navy nuke who was disqualified after requesting assistance with mental health and alcohol issues. Despite struggling with issues for years, he was able to perform his duties. He introduced me to a colloquial expression for getting blackballed at the command due to mental health issues. He said this was "being sadded out" and explained it was exactly what happened to him. He had issues for years, including hardcore alcohol use, and was able to satisfactorily function in his job. His performance improved after getting help. Losing his qualification made no sense and resulted in a moral injury. Patients would complain about these types of situations to us mental health providers. We did not have the ability to fix chronic systemic problems or change the culture of the Navy. It contributed to a feeling of burnout.

Patients would languish in the Navy limited-duty system and weren't actively managed. When I arrived at Naval Medical Center Portsmouth, I inherited many patients from another mental health provider who left the facility. He put sailors on extended periods of limited duty and renewed them for a second term even when it was clear initiation of a medical board was indicated. It was disappointing because the Air Force system would readily identify airmen in need of medical boards and promptly initiate them. Sailors would be placed on limited duty and then drop out of the system. We had an electronic system, LIMDU Smart, that was intended to track and coordinate limited duty and medical boards, but it was nothing like the system the Air Force had. It took me a good while to write a bunch of medical boards to get caught up. I'm sure my colleagues would argue that understaffing contributed to these issues, but so did the lack of well-thought-out, organized, effective strategy, and modern information technology I experienced with the Air Force.

There were a couple mental health providers in the department, so-called "convening authorities" who reviewed medical boards, limited-duty requests, and administrative separation recommendations. I suspect they had these roles because they didn't like to see patients or were burned out. They documented brief five-line notes stating the record was reviewed, the sailor didn't have a boardable condition (frequently they did!), and they recommended the sailor be separated or returned to duty. At times, I wondered if they even reviewed the records. Once, it was announced there were too many sailors on limited duty at MARMC and the threshold and level of scrutiny for limited duty was arbitrarily increased. I was at a social function, and a discussion with a well-seasoned, experienced mental health provider who had begun working at the Naval Medical Center Portsmouth captured it all. He was working with a sailor who had extensive trauma documented in the medical record, he clearly met all criteria for PTSD, but none of his previous mental health providers documented the diagnosis in the chart. He said his experience was that the medical board reviewers were laser-focused on discharging sailors via personnel actions. One of the convening authorities called him on the phone and chewed him out for thirty minutes for diagnosing and initiating treatment for PTSD.

When I arrived at the hospital, the mental health director was a psychiatrist, but he was replaced by a psychologist. A Navy psychiatrist pulled me aside and explained that the Navy psychologists had a reputation for undermining psychiatrists and encouraged me to watch my back. Navy psychologists were part of the Medical Service Corps, while psychiatrists were part of the Medical

Corps. Psychiatrists complete medical school, achieve an MD, complete a residency training program, and prescribe medications. Psychologists complete graduate school, achieve a PhD, complete a postdoctoral fellowship, and conduct psychotherapy. Both are valuable mental health team members. I have enjoyed positive collaborative relationships with psychologists, but the hierarchy and rank structure of the Navy added a twist to the dynamic. There was palpable tension between different mental health disciplines in the Navy. I had a conversation with a Navy LCDR/O4 about it. He and I got along great. He explained that there were those who had a reputation for not "playing nice in the sandbox." In my experience, the retention rate for psychiatrists was lower compared with Navy psychologists, and this compounded the problem. I suspected some of the tension might have been due to different treatment approaches, differences in pay, or higher promotion rates for psychiatrists. I was told Navy psychologists were under even more pressure to focus on career progression over patient care compared with psychiatrists.

At Naval Medical Center Portsmouth, there was a high turnover rate, we were short-staffed, and there were policy gaps. Frequently, our department heads rotated or deployed, and this contributed to chaos. At its worst, I experienced department head changes every six months. Similar to what happened when the director changed, every time someone in a leadership role changed, it shook up the system. The education, training, opinions, preferences, and personalities of whomever was in charge filled gaps in policy. The system was overwhelmed, sailors complained they had difficulty accessing care, they looked to us to help them with work environment issues, and they directed their frustrations out on us. Sailors experienced lengthy delays in the medical boards process. Many sailors working at the facility resented the DHA and rallied against the DHA's involvement in Navy medicine. The outgoing director explained that he and his staff worked tirelessly to improve mental health provider contracts, but their compensation recommendations were disregarded by the DHA. One day I went to work, and a number of mental health providers abruptly left the facility due to contracting issues. I spoke to a psychiatrist who left the facility. She said the contractor changed, she was threatened with a significant pay cut, and she quit. It was a slap in the face for healthcare professionals who were working to get sailors' needs taken care of and accomplish the mission despite many obstacles. Many quit and moved on to greener pastures, disrupting the care of many sailors. The contract changes might have resulted in short-term savings but increased long-term costs and negatively impacted clinical outcomes for the Navy. Later I found a DoD inspector general report that put it into perspective. The report documented that Naval Medical Center Portsmouth had 357 unfilled MTF contractor positions, and this number was the highest number of unfilled positions across the entire military health system (DoD Inspector General 2023).

Most of the active-duty Navy providers were focused on career progression and were not in a good position to advocate for change. Many providers showed signs of burnout, struggled with compassion and empathy, made invalidating statements to sailors, and were in cahoots with the command regarding negative administrative and personnel actions. I overheard the director telling a colleague a sailor was going to "get some bad news," and he seemed to be delighted.

The COVID-19 pandemic was declared a national emergency on March 13, 2020, during my time at Naval Medical Center Portsmouth. It was a crazy time. My son was a sophomore in high school. He made the varsity soccer team, but the entire season was canceled after the first week of practice. The next year, when the soccer season resumed, a new rule was implemented that the coaches had to wipe down the game balls at halftime with bleach wipes. My daughter had just started her sophomore year at Virginia Tech during the fall of 2020. The school closed the dorms, and students returned home to take online classes. I don't think it was fair that my daughter had to take organic chemistry through Zoom meetings. At Naval Medical Center Portsmouth, face-to-face visits were canceled, and appointments were changed to telephone only. The medical providers were given the option to remain home and telework to communicate with patients. During the first week of April 2020, an email was sent out by the DHA, authorizing the use of Apple FaceTime, Google Duo, and Microsoft Skype for clinical care. The situation was unprecedented. Normal bureaucracy was suspended, and we were suddenly able to use modern technological solutions.

I had an old iPhone, added a line with my carrier, and used it for patient care. Initially, I was apprehensive about doing this, but it turned out to be incredibly helpful. I quickly discovered sailors enjoyed the convenience of being able to participate in mental health treatment remotely. Many I worked with had anxiety around people, and technology reduced barriers for care. The downside of this from a selfish perspective was that my workload increased because my no-show rate markedly decreased. I was afraid technology was going to be abused, but it never happened. From time to time, a patient texted me for a refill or something else, but it was never an issue. At some point, the special authorization was rescinded, and we were transitioned to an official DHA telehealth platform, but for a small moment in time, using FaceTime for clinical care was a best practice.

There were many success stories when I served at Naval Medical Center Portsmouth. I helped many patients. Many recovered from limited duty and continued in the Navy. Their mental health symptoms improved, they slept better, they learned to use alcohol in a healthy way, and they improved relationships. I remember one sailor who suffered from abuse and assault issues. While on limited duty, she decided she wanted to become a nurse after being pulled off a ship. There were so many sailors on limited duty, and it was easy to get lost in the system. This sailor was highly motivated. Somehow, she found a way to work on a medical unit during her limited duty assignment to advance her career.

CHAPTER 7

USS George Washington and MARMC Suicide Clusters

I SERVED AT Naval Medical Center Portsmouth from 2019 to 2022, during which time the Navy experienced two widely publicized suicide clusters onboard the *USS George Washington* and at the MARMC, pronounced "mar-mack"). Naval Medical Center Portsmouth was historically one of the premier three naval hospitals and was the hub of the Navy's mental health system for the area. Our hospital served many ships and operational units. Naval Medical Center Portsmouth had an emergency room where sailors frequently presented in crisis, an inpatient psychiatric ward, a partial hospitalization program, an outpatient mental health clinic, and a thirty-day residential treatment program for substance use disorders. We also had a program called "PCaT," Psychiatry Continuity and Transition Team, that managed sailors who were on limited duty and undergoing the medical boards process for mental health conditions. Naval Medical Center Portsmouth managed limited duty and medical boards for all the sailors in the region and managed the care at the branch health clinics in the area. The care and management within the facility directly and indirectly impacted the outcomes of the sailors. MARMC was known as a holding command for sailors on limited duty and had the highest concentration of sailors on limited duty and undergoing medical boards in the area.

USS George Washington

In mid-April 2022, three sailors aboard the *USS George Washington* died by suicide within one week. Even more had died by suicide in the past year, and there was an estimate that ten sailors died over the course of ten months (Toropin 2022). The master chief of the Navy gave a speech to the ship's crew that was received as tone deaf with a "suck it up" message. He said things could be worse, and they should be thankful they were not sleeping in a foxhole (Martin and Watson 2022). The story broke, and his comments were featured all over the national news.

The *USS George Washington* was an aircraft carrier undergoing major maintenance in the yards. There were issues with the environment of the ship, including the living spaces, and pictures were published in the news reports. There were issues with electricity, air-conditioning, plumbing, food service, and parking. A news report described the ship as uninhabitable (Lieberman and Klapper 2022). Some of the sailors were described as sleeping in their cars to avoid conditions on the ship. Leadership and work schedule issues varied. Some sailors reported that they were underutilized, and others felt overworked. Sailors reported a mix of leadership issues. The sailors complained that they could ask for help but had difficulty accessing care and the culture of the ship was to suck it up. Many of them felt they had to "do something stupid" to get help. I recall a specific situation from earlier in my career when a Navy officer LT/O3 cut his neck out of desperation to get out of a toxic shipboard environment. At the time, in the early 2000s, I was a junior doctor, just starting out. I thought it was a shame that a service member would have to resort to such extreme measures to have his issues addressed. The issues described above were consistent with what I experienced both times serving with the Navy.

Several sailors spoke out and were interviewed by national news outlets. One sailor described the situation as trying to live in a construction zone (*NBC Nightly News* 2022). Another struggling with mental health issues said she asked for help, felt she spoke into thin air, and ended up having a suicide attempt. She felt she was dying, sad, and tired of being on the ship and dealing with the situation. She complained that no one from the chain of command cared, and requests for help were not met with necessary resources. The service members were reported as being fearful of the consequences of speaking out and were reluctant to speak without anonymity. They said they brought the issues up to the chain of command, and rarely were any of the issues addressed.

I spoke to a sailor from the *USS George Washington*. His comments echoed what was said in news reports. The ship was his first assignment in the Navy, and he hit a breaking point after one year of service. He completed A School and C School to become an electronics technician but was given duties outside the job he signed up for. He felt he was forced to work outside his career field and wasn't permitted to do his job. He painted, needle gunned, and performed cable inspections. He complained that it was depressing and discouraging because his ship was unable to deploy or participate in military operations. He felt the overall situation was a negative environment. The living conditions were poor. He turned to the bottle to cope. After work, he would go to bars and drink a dozen drinks per night. The drinking progressively worsened over time. He tried to self-refer to the command Drug and Alcohol Program Adviser (DAPA) multiple times but felt pushed to the back burner, and no appointments were made. It wasn't until he disclosed suicidal thoughts to the chain of command that he was able to receive a screening from the ship's psychiatric technician. He was then referred to the emergency room for admission to the hospital. He told me the operational mental health section on the ship had a terrible reputation. He said sailors waited months to get an appointment, couldn't get help, and received a message that they were insignificant, and many stopped trying. He stated that the history of deaths by suicide on the ship spoke volumes to the situation.

One of the sailors interviewed about the *USS George Washington* described the situation as "a bunch of small stuff that adds up and adds up and adds up but never goes away." Another told *CBS News*, "It feels like Big Navy has left us out to dry. Nobody cares" (Martin and Watson 2022).

The stresses and problems described onboard the *USS George Washington* were common across other Navy ships too. A retired Navy veteran told me sailors were under intense pressure to get ships ready for deployment and inspections, dealing with a broken personnel system and coping with an unfair promotion system. She said to thrive in the Navy, sailors had to cope with the impact military life had on mental health and family life.

One sailor who served on an aircraft carrier explained that there were thousands of service members on a ship, and an estimated 15-30 percent were seeking mental health treatment. He said the process for making an appointment was going to the ship's Medical and being placed on the ship's psychologist's schedule. He complained that there was only "one psych," it could take one to three months for an appointment, and a lot of sailors were sent to the TRICARE network to experience lengthy wait times. I was told the ship's psychologist was too busy and not involved in prevention and advocacy.

I spoke to a Navy veteran in her late twenties who had served on the *USS Gerald Ford*, another aircraft carrier. She said the ship was under extreme pressure to become operational. She had anxiety on the ship and was accused of faking it when she asked for help. She felt there was an overall atmosphere, no one cared, and no one mattered. She felt the environment was such that everyone stepped all over each other to get promoted. She said a shipmate asked for help repeatedly and was dismissed. Instead of helping, the chain of command tried to get him in trouble, and this contributed to his death by suicide. She was negatively impacted by everything that happened and suffered a psychological injury. It took her several years to recover.

Another Navy veteran I spoke to was thirty-six years old. He told me how he mentored two junior sailors while serving on a ship. He felt the Navy was overly focused on output and getting qualifications done, and the Navy didn't focus enough on the sailor as a person. He told me anyone who had issues was forced to work more. He said he tried to advocate for one of his sailors when the sailor was struggling, but he wasn't successful. A week later the sailor died by suicide. This sailor suffered a psychological injury and was adversely impacted by everything that happened. He became depressed, shut down, and left the Navy. He struggled with layers and layers of depression and false guilt issues.

Another Navy veteran described similar challenges the *USS George Washington* sailors faced. He told me about the challenges of life on a ship and how a suicide impacted him. He worked twelve-hour days. If the command was unhappy with work output, sailors were forced to perform extra work. He struggled with depression and anxiety and felt he was punished and made to work harder. He said anyone who had issues was told to work more. In the military, requesting time off for vacation is *requesting leave*. A sailor on the ship died by suicide after he was denied leave. After the death, the Navy veteran snapped, acted out against the command, and faced possible disciplinary action, but this was dismissed. He told me how he struggled with a drinking problem, shame, and false guilt issues years after these events transpired.

MARMC

About six months after the *USS George Washington* suicide cluster, a similar suicide cluster occurred at MARMC. Naval Medical Center Portsmouth, where I served, provided mental health clinical services and managed limited duty and medical boards for sailors in the region. MARMC was the largest holding command for sailors on limited duty and undergoing the medical boards process. It was reported that four sailors at MARMC died by suicide within a span of a month in late 2022 (Ziezulewicz 2023). The story documented that all the sailors had been on a limited-duty status, and there was a lack of communication between MARMC coordinators and the military treatment facilities. It was reported that limited-duty sailors were not properly managed or monitored within the command. Firearms were also a factor in the deaths.

In my experience and from my patient reports, a Navy ship was a challenging environment, with high operational tempo, stress levels, and increased means for suicide. Onboard a ship, a sailor could jump off the side of a ship and had increased access to weapons. There were occasions when sailors had to be pulled from the ship for their own safety, to facilitate recovery, and to ensure mission success. During the early part of my career with the Navy, the higher-ups referred to this as a "rescue board." Placing a sailor on limited duty would remove them from a challenging environment, give them some breathing room, and provide time to recover and improve coping mechanisms. After a period of limited duty, they would be reassigned to a new command and different work environment. I was trained to contact a command prior to removing a sailor from a ship to give the command an opportunity to try to salvage the situation and prevent personnel loss. It was challenging and draining to assist sailors who reached a breaking point while on shipboard duty. My colleagues and I were always under constant pressure to reduce personnel loss and keep sailors in an active-duty status.

A senior Navy Cmdr./O5 operational-embedded psychiatrist talked with me about removal and attrition of sailors from ships and other operational units. She told me her opinion was that operational demands were so high, they were driving mental health issues and breaking people. Commands were undermanned, nothing was removed from operational requirements, and demands to do more with less people kept adding on. She described a vicious cycle—manning issues increase operational stress, resulting in psychological injury and increased personnel loss. The operational mental health provider stated that administrative separations were viewed as service members taking themselves out of the cycle. "I quit. I don't want to do this anymore." The idea that leaving the command was "quitting" applied to sailors who were placed on limited duty too. Sailors complained to me that they were caught up in a nasty web of stigma, scorn, and retaliation for "quitting" shipboard duty. Their struggle was challenging enough, but on top of that, they were accused of letting their shipmates down and felt psychologically injured.

The operational mental health provider stated that she briefed her two-star admiral that until operational stress decreases, high numbers of unplanned losses would continue and the cycle would perpetuate. She felt helpless that anything could be done about the situation, and that contributed to her own provider burnout issues.

When a sailor was assigned to limited duty, Naval Medical Center Portsmouth would process the paperwork, and the sailor was transferred to a limited duty command such as MARMC. It was discussed within our mental health directorate that there were too many sailors on limited duty, possibly 1,000 or more, and the threshold for limited duty and efforts to return them to full duty would be arbitrarily increased. I received similar feedback from the sailors under my care. Service members complained that there were too many in the limited duty pool, the limited duty section was understaffed, and service members got lost in the system. Service members lost their job when they were reassigned from operational units, lost purpose, and felt underutilized. Many were not able to work within their career field, the limited duty environment was unstructured, and the command wasn't invested in their recovery. They found themselves in a suboptimal recovery environment, and this added to their psychological distress. The sailors struggled with bitterness toward their prior commands and the Navy for how they were treated. I observed a rotten-apple-in-a-barrel effect, where service members fed off and negatively impacted each other.

The story of a coworker captured the struggle of the limited duty sailors at MARMC. One day I came into work and a sailor who worked in a nonmedical career field joined our mental health office staff. She was in a limited-duty status, going through a medical board for cancer. Prior to joining our office, she felt underutilized, complained the environment was toxic, felt negatively impacted by other service members who were frustrated with the military, and felt she was stuck. She requested to be transferred to a different recovery environment and felt relief after she was reassigned to our office. She had no medical training. I was concerned about the appropriateness of her working in a medical setting, but the situation worked out well for everyone. She was highly motivated and thankful to be in a healthier environment.

Investigation Reports

There were three investigation reports that were published. There were two reports concerning the *USS George Washington*. The first was an investigation into the deaths (Caudle 2022). The second was an investigation into the command climate and quality of life for sailors (Caudle 2023). The third was an investigation report concerning the deaths at MARMC (Galinis 2023). Across all documents, there were over 350 pages. The names of the deceased were published in the reports and are referenced in this discussion.

The admiral who oversaw much of the Navy's East Coast fleet was quoted as describing the situation with the *USS George Washington* as a "9/11 like event" (Toropin 2023). The article detailed that the ship was understaffed and lacked senior leadership, and Navy surveys documented widespread thoughts of suicide among the crew.

Another news story discussed the findings of the MARMC suicide cluster investigation (Toropin 2023). The sailors were at various stages of the disability evaluation process and suffered from a confluence of external stresses, and the command was not well suited to manage the sailors. All four of the sailors had unrestricted access to personally owned firearms. Communication between the doctors, who were regularly seeing the sailors and leadership at the command, was fractured. There was noted to be only one command deployability coordinator who was tasked with accurate accounting and tracking of medical treatment and expeditious movement of sailors on medical restrictions.

Discussion of Investigation Reports

The overall finding of the reports was that there was no "direct correlation" that the suicides were linked, but there were common themes, issues, and problems that impacted those sailors and were prevalent in the Navy. Sailors onboard the *USS George Washington* served in a harsh environment where, like most other Navy ships, leaving the ship was perceived as a personal failure and quitting. The sailors worked outside of their career field and were functioning under severe resource constraints. They faced pervasive manning issues. There were barriers to getting help and access-to-care issues. The sailors did not trust the Navy's mental health system or mental health providers. They faced stigma and consequences for getting help. The ship's mental health team was under pressure to keep sailors on the ship and reduce personnel losses. There were issues with the command DAPA who was a peer volunteer. There was only one full-time primary duty DAPA for approximately 2,700 sailors. The report documented that sailors were referred for substance abuse issues, did not follow through, and slipped through the cracks. Some of the sailors suffered from severe marital problems, there were domestic violence allegations, but there was no mention of FAP involvement. The sailors at MARMC were all on limited duty, lacked positive command involvement, lacked purpose, and struggled with feeling underutilized. There were issues with limited duty and medical board tracking, coordination with command, and delays resulting in sailors finding themselves in prolonged limbo status. How sailors from the *USS George Washington* and MARMC were treated and managed and issues with the mental health system were a common theme. The sailors felt the Navy was not fully invested in their health and well-being. How the sailors felt or perceived they were valued by their leadership, command, and the Navy as an organization was a critical factor.

Another overarching theme was that the sailors who died by suicide made permanent decisions to deal with temporary problems. Someone told me when something bad happens, it is like all the holes on the Swiss cheese line up. Still, I could not help but wonder if the sailors could have been assisted with their struggles if a different outcome could have been achieved.

Organizational Issues in the Navy's Medical System

I spoke with a retired senior Navy psychiatrist and Cdr./O5, Dr. Greg Henderson. He spent time with the Air Force and Army during his career and developed an appreciation for their medical systems. He explained that the Air Force and Army were more collaborative and had a more unified medical system with the same mission and set of rules. He explained that the Air Force and Army had more predictable outcomes and consistent results because of the way their medical systems were organized. He observed that the Air Force and Army had a more standardized approach and consistent application of policy. He described a situation where he received care from an Air Force flight surgeon and how the Air Force flight medicine clinic was an extension of the hospital. The Navy system is organized differently. There is an organizational split between operational medicine and the hospital. Operational medicine providers are under a different set of rules, depending on leadership influence, the command, and coast. This results in tension and conflict between the Navy's hospital system and medical providers embedded in operational units. I experienced this firsthand when I served with the Marine Corps when I found myself in the middle of a battle between the blue side and the green side.

In an operational unit, the thought processes that drive decision-making are frequently focused on the best interests of the Navy, not the individual sailor. Medical officers on a Navy ship tend to be more junior, report to their commanding officers, and are under pressure to satisfy their requests even if it isn't medically the right thing to do. Junior medical officers face stigma and scorn if they are perceived as contributing to unplanned personnel losses. They can quickly find themselves in situations where their careers can end in a heartbeat. Operational medical providers face pressure to underdiagnose and keep sailors on ships to prevent unplanned personnel losses. They are also pressured to remove perceived problem sailors via the limited-duty process. Having a low threshold to put a sailor on limited duty can be advantageous for commands because it triggers what was referred to as a "hot fill" personnel action.

The investigation reports documented how MARMC and the Navy's medical system were overwhelmed with limited-duty sailors. The naval hospital tried to push back on this. I was passed on an account from a fleet surgical team psychiatrist that it was difficult and there was a ton of resistance to place a sailor on limited duty even when it was clearly indicated. The sailors who were struggling found themselves in the middle of this mess. For certain, the organization of the Navy's medical system, how limited duty was managed, and how sailors were treated contributed to the outcomes that occurred.

I spoke to a Navy Capt./O6 who was involved in making recommendations in the aftermath of the *USS George Washington* and MARMC suicide clusters. He described a dysfunctional organization where there were too many stakeholders and felt his recommendations went nowhere. His experiences captured the frustration, dysfunction, and organizational problems in the Navy and military's mental health system I experienced.

Consequences for Getting Help and Stigma

One of the findings in the investigation report that touched me most was that 58 percent of sailors aboard the *USS George Washington* did not trust military mental health providers. A Naval Health Research Center rapid response surveillance survey found that sailors reported discouragement, shame, and stigma for seeking both mental and physical health care.

After I left Naval Medical Center Portsmouth, I began to serve at a Veterans Affairs Medical Center. A sailor I worked with was diagnosed with recurrent major depressive disorder just a few months after a Navy mental health provider documented that he had adjustment disorder, "no boardable condition," and facilitated his discharge. The sailor was underdiagnosed and felt harmed by the Navy's mental health system. Another day, a former Navy nuke came to see me. He told me how he avoided getting help for years to prevent loss of his nuke status. Finally, a senior Navy officer, a former aircraft carrier commanding officer, came to see me. He told me how his mental health issues would have been career-ending, how he compartmentalized them, barely made it across the finish line to retirement, and was now ready to address his issues. None of those sailors trusted the Navy's mental health system or its mental health providers.

Leadership Involvement

In the MARMC report, a finding was that the command master chief wasn't readily available to sailors. A common theme with the patients I treated at Naval Medical Center Portsmouth and with both the MARMC and *USS George Washington* reports was a lack of positive leadership involvement in sailors who were struggling. There wasn't much in the reports about leadership identifying mental health issues, proactively meeting with mental health, having passion about the welfare of their sailors, and trying to improve things. It was particularly difficult for me after having witnessed firsthand the power of positive involvement from senior officers and enlisted leadership in the Air Force and Marine Corps. Air Force leadership was frequently the first to refer an airman who was in distress and to be positively involved in their care. The marines looked out for the needs of their subordinates. They had a value system to "Know your marines" and "Look out for their welfare." I read that a major part of Army leadership was "continuous social work," including helping soldiers with significant personal problems, including family, financial, and health issues (Martin 2023). Reading between the lines of all these reports, there was a missing human factor. Struggling sailors needed positive senior personnel to take them under their wing, mentor them, and be invested in their success. One of the sailors who died by suicide in the *USS George Washington* report was described as possibly having benefited from disciplinary counseling. I had a different take on the situation. He would have benefited from a positive nondisciplinary leadership approach focused on mentorship and his personal well-being. Disciplinary action should have been a last resort.

In 2024 NBC published a follow-on investigation of emails obtained via a FOIA request of those involved in the *USS George Washington* suicide clusters (Chan 2024). The news report documented that leadership responded with denial and anger. A common theme I heard from sailors who were struggling was that they felt leadership lacked empathy and compassion and made their lives more difficult instead of assisting them with their struggles. To a certain extent, I experienced this while serving with the Air Force, Marine Corps, and Coast Guard, but it was far worse in the Navy.

Recovery Environment

For a brief time, being off a ship and on limited duty was therapeutic. Sailors got a breather and a break from stress, but long-term, it made things worse. Limited duty was unstructured, and sailors lacked purpose, felt underutilized, and lost competency in their career field, which contributed to mental and physical health decline. The result was increased attrition from the Navy. I frequently worked with sailors for whom being in a prolonged limbo or limited-duty status away from their support systems made their situations worse. From the report, it appeared one of the sailor's situations dragged on for several years or more. He was quoted as saying the Navy was holding his life back. The prolonged limbo status he suffered from contributed to the issues he was having.

Underdiagnosing and Conflicting Diagnoses

The *USS George Washington* report (Caudle 2022) discussed a sailor with bipolar disorder whose diagnosis was changed to adjustment disorder and personality disorder by a Navy psychiatrist at Naval Medical Center Portsmouth. The report suggested that this impacted the sailors medical boards process, and transition between providers was a factor. That was putting it kindly. The Navy's mental health system was infamous for underdiagnosing sailors, undertreating them, and getting them out via administrative personnel actions. I witnessed this behavior from my colleagues from the inside and had issues trusting some of them too. The report documented that 99.7 percent of administrative separations of carrier sailors over the past five years related to a behavioral health issue and that the number of separations had increased by 120 percent. The Navy had effectively made wanting to quit a mental health disorder.

One of the sailors from MARMC in the report, ETSN Armstrong, was diagnosed with "morbid obesity due to excessive calories." He felt ashamed and ridiculed. He complained that physical health issues negatively impacted his ability to exercise. The Navy had a cultural tradition of turning things around on sailors. The diagnosis basically accused the sailor of being fat. The exact details of the case are unknown. In my experience, providers outside the Navy system would have likely diagnosed binge eating disorder or something nonstigmatizing. Obesity is a treatable condition. These include diet and exercise, medications (especially GLP-1 agonists and stimulants), and surgical procedures such as gastric banding. A military medical provider working with ETSN Armstrong documented that active-duty members received bariatric surgery at other commands. However, a bariatric surgery consult that was submitted was canceled because "bariatric surgery was not authorized for active-duty service members."

ETSN Armstrong's story reminded me of a Navy veteran I spoke with who had served on active duty for seventeen years starting in the mid-1990s. He had back surgery on active duty and suffered from chronic pain but was unexpectedly found fit for full duty during the medical boards process. His ability to exercise decreased due to back pain. He gained a lot of weight and ended up getting discharged due to body weight issues. By the time I had seen him, he had a second back surgery and continued to struggle with obesity. The Navy had this way of unexpectedly returning service members back to full duty and turning situations around on them. Thankfully, he received benefits and care from Veterans Affairs. The patient felt that what happened was not right and made his problems worse. I couldn't help but wonder if ETSN Armstrong suffered a similar plight.

The story of Brandon Caserta, a Navy sailor who died by suicide, was widely publicized in the media (Kime 2019). Had he been evaluated by a mental health provider at Naval Medical Center Portsmouth, there is a reasonable probability that Brandon Caserta would have been diagnosed with failure to adapt to military life and personality issues and recommended for administrative separation. The truth was, he suffered from psychological injury and significant mental and physical health issues.

The way the Navy mental health system diagnosed and managed mental health issues was different and more stigmatizing compared with the other services and agencies I had served with. I was told a lot of this had to do with thought processes that emphasize the needs of the Navy instead of the individual sailor. My experience was that an airman was more likely to be diagnosed with major depression and referred for medical board compared with a sailor who was more likely to be diagnosed with adjustment disorder and referred for separation. I've observed the consequences of this at Veterans Affairs. A sailor who was diagnosed with adjustment disorder and processed out for separation by the Navy would present to the Veterans Affairs Hospital and be accurately diagnosed with a more severe problem sometimes months after discharge. They would also complain of feeling harmed by the Navy's mental health system.

In the Navy system, there was an unwritten rule or belief that if a sailor could not serve on a ship, they had some sort of personal failing. They were incompatible with military life, and discharge was warranted. It felt like the diagnosing patterns reflected that belief system. Some of it makes sense. A sailor who cannot perform their duties should not be in an operational environment, but approaching everything as a personal failing or disciplinary problem adds to stigma and psychological distress.

Limited Duty and Medical Board Management

The MARMC report discussed issues with limited duty, medical boards, lack of coordination with the Navy medical system, and command involvement. Sailors on limited duty were affectionately referred to as on "LIMDU," and MARMC was overwhelmed with them and other sailors undergoing the medical boards process. The report documented a recommendation for monthly meetings between Naval Medical Center Portsmouth and the command to review and discuss limited-duty cases and concerns. This was comparable with the best practice I experienced in the Air Force system. There were significant issues with how sailors were managed in the limited-duty system. The mental health clinic generated and reviewed a list of limited-duty sailors weekly. There were many sailors who were under the radar and didn't show up on the list. The processes never fully worked. The report hinted that the LIMDU

Smart system used to manage sailors on limited duty was broken. Many sailors were lost to follow-up after the limited-duty process was initiated. The Navy lacked a sufficient mechanism to track and prioritize high-risk sailors. I worked with a patient who waited two years for a medical board, even though one had been directed by higher headquarters, and the delay contributed to her distress and work issues. One of the sailors in the MARMC report suffered from seizures. There was a high likelihood that delays in the medical boards process for this sailor contributed to the outcome. In my experience with the Air Force system, the need for a medical board would have been identified much earlier. I couldn't help but wonder if the sailor would have been home much sooner and the death by suicide would have been prevented if his medical board had been processed in the Air Force system.

There were sailors who needed to be on limited duty who weren't. Sailors would frequently find themselves in Catch-22 situations, where they were suffering from real problems and had significant boardable conditions but were fit for duty on paper. For example, one Navy mental health provider wrote, "No limited duty is warranted at this time; however, the service member is not worldwide assignable, should not carry a weapon, and is not deployable."

The verbiage effectively put the sailor on limited duty and not on limited duty at the same time.

Similarly, there were sailors who needed to be medically boarded, and there were extensive delays both with the recognition a board needed to be initiated and with processing time once the decision to proceed with a board was made. There were issues with board results. A small percentage of medical boards came back unexpectedly with return to full duty recommendations that didn't make sense. I participated in a meeting at Naval Medical Center Portsmouth where the department head for medical boards said the Navy had the highest return to duty of all the services, and they were looking to make changes to fix it.

Need to Fast-Track Medical Boards

One of the roles I had at Naval Medical Center Portsmouth was to be a psychiatrist for sailors who suffered from severe mental illness, including schizophrenia, schizoaffective disorder, and bipolar disorder. Some of them were fragile, required constant intervention, and had recurrent behavioral incidents, including suicide attempts. These were high-risk individuals. After a certain point, they were stabilized, and remaining on active duty exacerbated their conditions. They needed to return home to be near their support system. We consulted with our directorate and medical boards office. We asked if we could have a monthly meeting with the medical boards office to discuss the status of the cases, but this was declined. We were told there was no way to expedite a sailor with severe or catastrophic health issues. If there had been a way to fast-track the needs of sailors with severe mental illness, epilepsy, or other severe conditions, they could have been processed more rapidly through the medical board system and returned home to their support systems sooner to achieve better outcomes.

Aircraft Carrier Mental Health Provider Issues

The first "battlefield psychiatrist" was Dr. Thomas Salmon for the US Army in World War I (Warner, et al. 2011). Across my career, there was an increasing trend of embedding mental health providers in operational units. Mental health providers were placed in Army, Navy, Marine Corps, and Air Force units and are referred to as operational mental health providers throughout this book. Placing mental providers closer to service members at the ground level increases access to care and provides opportunity for early intervention so that problems are addressed before they hit a crisis point. An embedded operational mental health provider is in a better position to work with command to conduct organizational interventions. When I served with the Air Force, there was an operational psychologist who was embedded in an intelligence squadron. The airmen watched live execution of missions on the operations floor and witnessed significant carnage. The psychologist was a resource to turn to for help and coping. The unit had a tradition of ringing a bell every time a target was hit. The Air Force psychologist observed that the bell contributed to airmen's distress levels and worked with the command to change the practice.

The Army has behavioral health officers assigned to brigades under a division. They see patients but also serve as consultants to the brigade commanders. There is a division psychiatrist who oversees the brigade behavioral health officers, serves as consultant to the commanding general of the division, and sees patients. The Army has COSC units that assist with behavioral health. These units typically deploy with combat support hospitals and can provide area support for behavioral health. They have a mix of providers, including behavioral health technicians, social workers, psychologists, psychiatrist nurse practitioners, and psychiatrists. Chaplains and chaplain assistants also serve with Army COSC units.

My wife is a psychiatric nurse practitioner who served on an Army base in a mental health clinic and as an embedded behavioral health provider in a mortuary affairs unit. The company commander and 1SG/E8 had her personal cell phone number and would contact her at any hour of the day when soldiers needed assistance or had questions about mental health. The commander, an Army LTC/O5, and mental health providers observed an increasing trend of mental health situations in the unit. The commander was very interested, involved, and had passion for the welfare of his soldiers. The mental health clinic, embedded behavioral health, and commander worked collaboratively to identify issues that were driving the trend. They were able to successfully make changes to the unit to improve stress levels and mental health issues, and it was a win for everyone.

The Golden Gate Bridge was a popular spot for suicide attempts. There were thirty confirmed suicides occurring annually. Coast Guard sailors assigned to Coast Guard Station Golden Gate near San

Francisco, California, utilized lifeboats to race to the scene, rescue, and recover the jumpers. I spoke to the sailors performing this mission. They saw a lot of death, and it was a difficult job. The entire Coast Guard had a single behavioral health technician assigned to the station. He worked with the sailors to successfully provide intervention. When I left the Coast Guard in 2019, the program was considered a success, and they were looking to expand the program and increase the number of behavioral health technicians.

Historically, the Navy had embedded mental health providers on aircraft carriers and in Marine Corps infantry divisions, but the practice expanded to other units. Navy aircraft carriers and operational psychologists have received a lot of bad press in recent years. A sailor onboard the *USS Nimitz*, an aircraft carrier, died by suicide in 2019. News reports suggested the command viewed his problems through a disciplinary lens, and there were concerns about care rendered by the ship's psychologist. The sailor's family submitted a malpractice claim, but it was denied because the care was not rendered in a covered military treatment facility (Ziezulewicz 2021). In 2020 there was an active-duty sailor who was underdiagnosed by an operational Navy psychologist in Hawaii. The sailor fatally shot two Pearl Harbor naval shipyard workers and injured another before shooting himself (Ziezulewicz 2020). During 2021, a workgroup report (Mental Health Informed Consent Working Group 2021) from the Navy about the situation was published during the time I served at Naval Medical Center Portsmouth. There was some discussion of the incident and report inside our directorate, but no real changes occurred.

The *USS George Washington* report hinted at issues within the aircraft carrier psychology program. Issues with operational mental health providers, such as aircraft carrier psychologists, were not uncommon. Their role wasn't clearly defined. The ideal or maximum patient panel size for the ship's psychologist and Navy embedded mental health providers was not well defined. The report documented that the psychologist and behavioral health technician were overwhelmed, and there was an appointment backlog. Sailors presenting to Naval Medical Center Portsmouth's emergency room were recommended to follow up with the ship's psychologist. This raises the question of how sailors would follow up given appointment availability issues.

Most carrier psychologists were fresh out of training and lacked experience. I worked with sailors under my care who received care from a ship's psychologist. It was not uncommon for their visits to be undocumented. When documentation was present, frequently, sailors were underdiagnosed with "emotional distress in the context of occupational stress," "occupational problem," or "other problem related to employment" when it was clear they suffered more severe conditions. I worked with a sailor whose ship's psychologist accused him of malingering and participated in his prosecution. This increased his psychological distress and suicide risk.

Several times during my career, I observed situations where the Navy asked psychiatrists to serve on aircraft carriers. I'm confident it would have been a great practice, contributing to mission success, but the senior Navy psychiatrists were terrified of this possibility and did everything in their power to stay in the hospital and avoid demonstrating that psychiatrists on aircraft carriers was an effective and best practice. It was explained to me that this would set the precedent they would need to do it again.

Substance Issues

Issues with substance abuse treatment and command DAPAs were mentioned in the report. The MARMC report specifically documented that sailors referred for alcohol issues did not report to the command DAPA and were lost to follow-up. The *USS George Washington* quality of life report (Caudle 2023) found issues with command DAPA availability and with bed dates for residential treatment. Around the time the news surrounding the *USS George*

Washington broke, I reviewed two substance abuse evaluations and referrals for service members from the *USS George Washington*. The referrals documented alcohol use disorder and were made during the summer of 2021 but didn't reach the Navy's Substance Abuse and Rehabilitation Program (SARP) program until May 2022, over nine months later. The patients had no documented follow-up and were not tracked to ensure program enrollment and completion. We were told the Navy was one of the only uniformed services that utilized a peer volunteer system to manage substance issues. The term co-occurring disorders refers to the situation when both mental health and substance use disorders are present simultaneously. Frequently, Navy substance abuse evaluations did not address co-occurring disorders. The sailors' alcoholism was addressed but not the PTSD and other conditions that were driving alcohol use. There were gaps in mental health policies, especially regarding substance abuse. The substance abuse policy did not clearly define time deadlines from diagnosis to treatment start date.

Domestic Violence

The reports documented that sailors struggled with severe marital problems and there were alleged domestic violence incidents that resulted in police involvement. Domestic violence incidents are considered a mandatory report to Family Advocacy. There wasn't any mention of Family Advocacy in the reports. The way the Navy and other services approached Family Advocacy differed, and this could have impacted the outcomes. I spoke to a veteran who served as an active-duty Army Family Advocacy clinician. After leaving the Army, she took a job working for the Navy in the same role as a civilian. She said the Army FAP had a stronger multidisciplinary approach. She said commands, law enforcement, and medical were more involved and invested in success. She observed that the Navy FAP lacked buy-in from commands. They had a tendency not to be responsive or follow through with recommendations, and the outcomes weren't as positive compared with her experiences in the Army. In the Air Force and Army, Family Advocacy fell under the medical department. The Army and Air Force FAP shared office space with the mental health clinic. If there was a concern about domestic violence, I could walk down the hall and make a face-to-face referral to a Family Advocacy clinician. There was also significant cross talk. We had multidisciplinary team meetings where mental health, Family Advocacy, and substance abuse were all present in the same room. We put our minds together to achieve better outcomes. I never saw much cross talk in the Navy's mental health system. In the Navy, Family Advocacy fell under the community services umbrella. If a sailor had domestic violence issues, we had little or no visibility about the services they received, and making a referral was like sending information down a black hole.

Firearms

Firearms were a common issue in the reports and military mental health. If a service member reported struggling with thoughts of hurting themselves or others, we would inquire about access to weapons, especially firearms. If a service member had access to firearms, we would take steps to try to remove them. We would also try to reduce the number of pills to prevent stockpiling of medication that could be utilized for overdose. A common practice was to communicate with command and request guns be secured. It worked best when the senior officers and enlisted in the command were positive, supportive, and invested in a service member's well-being. I'd seen many situations with positive outcomes where a senior service member went to someone's home, conducted a welfare check, and secured firearms. The best outcome for firearms was when the service member willingly relinquished firearms to command, a family member, or a friend. I encountered situations where the command was not invested or a service member refused to give up personal firearms, especially if they lived off base. Those situations were challenging. I never saw a policy or formal legal ability for commands to compel a service member to relinquish personal firearms. Having the legal ability to secure personal firearms for at-risk individuals would reduce future deaths.

CHAPTER 8

Navy Mental Health Case Examples

THE USS GEORGE WASHINGTON and MARMC discussion and investigation reports hinted at common issues sailors faced, including harsh treatment, leadership issues, a culture of turning things around on sailors, feeling undervalued, issues with limited duty, medical boards, the substance abuse program, and access to care. Those issues were not uncommon for the sailors who were under my care. What follows are case examples that further illustrate these issues and the impact they had on sailors.

Alcohol, Trauma Issues, and Lost to Follow-up

The sailor was a thirty-two-year-old male, chief/E7, with twelve years military service. In the past, he had treatment for depression, including a previous inpatient psychiatric hospitalization at a prior duty station. In May 2021 he hit a breaking point, experienced suicidal thoughts, and was hospitalized on the psychiatry unit at Naval Medical Center Portsmouth for care. After several days, he was discharged. He rapidly decompensated and was readmitted to the psychiatry unit a week later. During the first hospitalization, he was diagnosed with major depressive disorder, recurrent. After the second hospitalization, a diagnosis of alcohol use disorder, severe, was added. The member indicated that he had difficulty opening up about his problems during the first hospitalization and during the second revealed he was using alcohol to self-treat depression. He was recommended to begin residential treatment for alcoholism immediately after discharge from the hospital but declined and requested the treatment to be scheduled at a future date. He was recommended to follow-up with the command DAPA for scheduling.

The inpatient psychiatry team initiated a six-month period of limited duty. Most services, even Veterans Affairs, had a best practice that a patient discharging from inpatient care would have a post-discharge appointment with a mental health provider within a week after discharge, but the Navy substituted this with a discharge group. The sailor was recommended to follow up with the outpatient mental health clinic's inpatient discharge bridge group a week after discharge, but this did not occur. After he missed the appointment, there was no command notification or wellness check documented. He was checked into the PCaT program that assisted with the tracking and management of service members on limited duty for mental health issues. The substance misuse portion of the PCaT program documentation was blank, although he was documented as struggling with alcoholism and had been recommended for residential treatment. He was scheduled for a psychiatry intake evaluation during July 2021, but this did not occur. Throughout the spring and summer of 2021, the PCaT program documented record reviews. There was no coordination of care with the substance abuse treatment program or the command regarding treatment dropout.

From the spring to the fall of 2021, the service member remained lost to follow-up. He later explained that during this time, he was receiving counseling from the Fleet and Family Service Center, although he had a history of recurrent major depression and severe alcoholism and the services offered by the Family Service Center were limited to nonmedical clinical counseling, a type of counseling limited to brief problem and solution focused counseling. The service member felt the counseling he received helped his mood and assisted him in maintaining sobriety. There was no coordination of care between the mental health clinic, including the PCaT program, the Fleet and Family Service Center, and the substance abuse treatment program.

His first outpatient mental health appointment was in September 2021, four months after he was placed on limited duty. He was evaluated by a clinical social worker at the military hospital who documented that he was doing better, removed the major depression diagnosis from his record without explanation, and wrote he was noncompliant with his substance abuse treatment. The service member had three visits with the social worker. He was never re-referred to the substance abuse treatment program, and there was no coordination with command regarding the treatment recommendations. Prior to the expiration of his limited duty, it was documented he was doing better and recommended to be returned to full duty.

A psychologist conducted a review of the recommendation to return to duty. The review consisted of a five-line note in the medical record saying the review had been conducted, the service member's primary issue was alcoholism, which was not a ratable or referable condition, and he was recommended for return to duty. The note did not address the incompletion of substance use treatment or why the major depressive disorder was removed. The well-documented history of recurrent major depression contradicted the brief note as it was a ratable and referable condition, especially when there was a history of recurrent hospitalizations.

In March 2022, eleven months after he was diagnosed with alcoholism during his inpatient psychiatric hospitalization in 2021, the service member presented to the command DAPA complaining of continued struggles with alcohol and was scheduled for residential treatment of alcoholism. When the service member was reassessed, he said his understanding of his mental health conditions was depression and alcoholism. He stated that when he was participating in therapy, he did well, but when he "stopped talking," he "started bottling." He used alcohol intermittently during the time he was on limited duty. He felt like he was in a good place when he talked to the clinic social worker. He said his pattern was to have two or three good months, relapse, then have a bad month. He never went back to the command DAPA despite the treatment recommendation because he felt his alcohol use was in control. Concerning his lack of participation in his care, he complained that it was difficult to access care, he changed his phone number, and the limited duty process was fragmented. He stated that he was unaware of some of the communications, and his limited duty coordinator never reached out to him to inform him of a problem.

The service member finally made it to residential treatment for alcoholism in May 2022. Within the first week of his participation, he opened up about how he had been a victim of male-on-male sexual assault, was ashamed, and struggled to come to terms with it. It was clear his diagnosis was PTSD, as the trauma was underlying all his issues, including alcoholism. He began therapy and medication and was finally able to begin recovering from what happened to him.

Overall, the situation was a mess and captured many of the issues discussed in this book. A service member who was discharged from the hospital due to suicidal thoughts didn't have adequate follow-up. Instead of a one-on-one appointment, he was placed into a discharge follow-up group. He remained in a limited-duty status for an extended period and was put in a situation where he wasn't actively managed and slipped through the cracks. The service members' recommendation for residential treatment of alcoholism wasn't tracked. There was a lack of meaningful care coordination and cross talk between programs and the command. The sailor's care lacked oversight and wasn't well managed. He was signed off as good to go even though he had not completed the alcohol treatment program requirements, and his needs weren't addressed.

It is setting up the military and the service member for failure to place an untreated service member who can't control their drinking to return to or serve in an operational environment. The situation of having a service member with untreated mental health and substance use disorders for an extended period was in and of itself a risk to the mission. There have been fatalities where service members who were identified as having drinking problems suffered a motor vehicle accident under the influence that resulted in fatality before they were able to start treatment.

Prosecuted for Malingering for Vague Suicidal Threats

The sailor was a twenty-year-old male assigned to a Navy aircraft carrier. He had one year of military service. He presented to the ship's psychologist during the late summer of 2019 complaining of difficulty coping with Navy life, depression, suicidal thoughts, a back injury, and chronic back pain. During his first ever mental health appointment, the operational mental health providers, including a psychologist and psychiatric technician, documented a clinical suspicion that his primary problem was malingering, intentionally feigning illness to get off the ship.

The psychologist wrote, "Since the spring of 2019, seven physicians/providers have conducted several physical examinations/assessments on patients consistently resulting in no clinical findings and lack of clinical explanation regarding patient's ongoing reports of pain." The psychologist wrote that the patient's depression was fueled by the patient's dissatisfaction with being onboard the ship and concluded he wanted to get out of the military.

About a month later, the sailor presented to the emergency room complaining of suicidal thoughts and was admitted to Naval Medical Center Portsmouth's inpatient psychiatry unit for a week, where he was diagnosed with *other problem related to employment*.

After discharge from the psychiatry unit, the patient's back pain was assessed by a primary care provider. The primary care provider was concerned about the patient's mental health and lack of post-hospitalization discharge follow-up and contacted the hospital's psychiatry duty pager.

Soon after this, the patient was referred to me. He told me he had been struggling, unable to adapt to the Navy, and the shipboard environment was stressful and harsh. He said he had difficulty tolerating getting yelled at and suffered from depression and anxiety associated with this. He described a trapped or boxed-in feeling. He said he had fought impulses to cut himself. He tried to hang himself, but the knot slipped. He telephoned his mother for help and ended up on the inpatient psychiatry unit. He told me he felt better than before but was still struggling with suicidal thoughts and saw getting out of the Navy as the solution to his problems. He was having difficulty coping with leaving home and unresolved family problems that predated military service.

I contacted the ship's psychologist and was told the suicidal threats he made prompted the command to conduct a preliminary investigation into whether a malingering charge was warranted. The ship's psychologist indicated that he was talking to the command about possible legal charges and had not disclosed this to the service member.

The patient continued to struggle and was referred to a five-day partial hospitalization program. He had difficulty participating in the program. The patient told me he didn't feel mentally well, felt he was breaking down, wasn't in the mood to open up and talk about his issues. He left the program early and returned home.

Months later during the early fall of 2019, the patient complained he felt worse and continued to struggle with suicidal thoughts. He reported that his girlfriend back home broke up with him, and he had a breakdown on the ship where he cried in the bathroom. He was on the verge of being readmitted to the hospital. He did complete the partial hospitalization program. The psychologist who treated him documented this: "The patient expressed concerns about returning to his ship. He stated that being on a ship is too stressful for him, and that he fears that he will experience another suicidal attempt in that environment," and "There are no acute safety concerns at this time; however, he expressed chronic emotional distress and thoughts of death related to remaining in the Navy."

By the late fall of 2019, he began receiving individual therapy from a seasoned member of our department. She and I discussed the case. We felt the patient was immature, had coping skill deficits, was desperate to get out of the Navy, and was not malingering. The patient called us both in a panic, saying he was being threatened with going underway on the ship again, although we were told he would be removed from the ship, placed on a beach detachment, and processed for separation. We felt the patient was at increased risk for suicide and communicated our concerns to the ship's psychologist, and he was dismissive of the levels of risk. We observed that the operational mental health provider was uncaring and unempathetic, making harsh, superficial judgments about the patient, and was part of his criminal prosecution. Further, it appeared his command and operational mental health provider were egging the patient on and making his situation worse. For example, they were toying with him, telling him he was going to be taken underway. The ship's psychologist expressed frustration that the patient was communicating with us and not working through the ship's medical department, although the patient was complaining to us that the ship's medical department was not responsive to his needs and had no appointment availability.

Six months went by, and the patient remained in a military limbo situation. We were later told that the decision to separate him was made in December 2019, but an investigation determined that the patient was malingering and being processed for nonjudicial punishment, captain's mast, and separation. It was interesting to note that the outcome of the captain's mast was apparently predetermined prior to the actual proceeding occurring. The patient did later follow up with me. He explained that he went to the captain's mast, was given sixty days restriction for malingering, and was recommended for separation. He felt depressed, upset, and betrayed by the operational psychologist and command. He felt that no one listened to him. He did feel relief that he was finally getting out of the Navy.

The patient was evaluated by pain management. The physician who evaluated him noted that he had an abnormal magnetic resonance imaging (MRI) during the summer of 2019, showing a lumbar disc protrusion, mild to moderate degenerative changes, and a minimal posterior bulge in this thoracic spine. The abnormal findings could have played a role in his back pain. The patient received an epidural steroid injection in December 2019 and reported significant improvement in his pain.

From the time the patient first presented and asked to be discharged from the Navy, eight months elapsed. He was evaluated by the ship's psychologist thirteen times and Naval Medical Center Portsmouth mental health providers fifteen times, and he had six days of inpatient psychiatric hospitalization, five days of partial hospitalization, three emergency room visits, and roughly a dozen crisis telephone calls.

A best practice for military mental health was that the diagnosis of malingering was not made unless there was substantial and definitive evidence. This included collateral and objective sources that false or grossly exaggerated symptoms were intentionally produced for external incentives (Weiss and Van Dell 2017). The hospital psychologist and I, who both had many more decades of experience compared with the operational mental health provider, did not feel malingering was an appropriate diagnosis. The operational mental health provider's conduct in the case was concerning. Instead of caring for the patient, he facilitated the prosecution of the service member. The diagnosis and mere suggestion of malingering had devastating consequences for the sailor. It influenced the medical providers who worked with him regarding his back issues. He was prosecuted, and it delayed his discharge from the military.

There was a similar situation that occurred around the same time frame, involving ASAN Michael Gregg onboard the *USS Dwight D. Eisenhower*, that was reported in the *Federal Way Mirror* (Sullivan 2021). The article described the sailor as being forced to return to the ship despite it being a "trigger point" for his suicidal thoughts. Despite being provided a medical excuse from work by non-Navy providers, he lost rank and was punished for unauthorized absence during captain's mast. The article documented later that his rank was restored, and the punishments were reversed. The ordeal was described as "nine weeks and three days of twenty-four seven hell" by the sailor's family. The sailor received conflicting evaluations and care from the ship's psychologist, non-Navy mental health providers in the community, and three inpatient psychiatric hospitalizations before he was finally separated in December 2021.

My Coworker, A Domestic Violence Victim

I worked with a woman in her early twenties who went through a messy divorce. She explained that she had been in a dual military relationship. She and her husband were married about two years and geographically separated for most of the marriage. She felt he was controlling, lying, and verbally and physically abusive, and it got worse when she became pregnant and had a baby. One night during September 2020, she stayed up all night taking care of the baby. She asked her husband for help, and he yelled at her and refused. She hit a breaking point, came to the realization that the relationship needed to end for her own health and well-being, and communicated her desire for divorce. Her husband responded by threatening to harm himself and her family. She alerted her chain of command and her husband's chain of command and felt nothing was done to address the immediate safety concerns.

Shortly after this, her chief/E7 directed her to come to work in a dress uniform. She was escorted to an office where her soon-to-be-ex (STBX) and his chief were present. Her chief told her each of them had conflicting stories about the situation and recommended marital counseling. My coworker told her STBX he was abusive, there was no fixing the relationship, and she wanted a divorce. In the weeks that followed, her STBX's behaviors escalated. She felt stalked at work, received threatening text messages, and complained that her STBX also made suicidal threats. Eventually, she requested a military protective order (MPO). She complained that her chief did not support her, made harsh judgmental statements about her, took her STBX's side of the story, and made her situation worse. After two junior sailors advocated for her, an MPO was put in place. In the days that followed, the command coordinated her move out of the apartment. Her STBX destroyed her personal property and stole her possessions. A Family Advocacy victim advocate got involved and witnessed the destruction and abusive text messages, but she felt nothing was done about the situation. A month had elapsed since her separation initiated, and with the mounting stress, she had an emotional breakdown at work.

During December 2020, my coworker received a memo from Family Advocacy stating the abuse allegations were unsubstantiated despite irrefutable evidence of abuse, including text messages and pictures of destruction of property. She told me she had never heard the name of the Family Advocacy clinician in the letter and had never met with her. No Family Advocacy clinician ever met with her, conducted an interview about her side of the story, conducted a risk assessment, or helped formulate a treatment plan.

My coworker felt the chief failed her as a person, violated her rights, and made her situation worse. She felt her chain of command didn't believe her, took her husband's side in the divorce, and put her safety at risk when there was a forced interaction between herself and her STBX. In 2021 she was downgraded on her annual performance review from *Must Promote* to *Promotable* without explanation. The message she received was that her evaluation was downgraded due to circumstances surrounding her divorce, and her chain of command wanted to get rid of her. It worked. She planned to leave the military at the end of her service obligation. This was consistent with the accounts of many sailors who faced real-world consequences for mental health issues. She felt she was in a vulnerable position while serving in the military. She experienced loss of control over her life, and the chain of command had too much power and wasn't looking out for her best interests. She vowed never to be in a situation like that again.

From Migraine Headaches to Court-Martial to PTSD

A twenty-nine-year-old female sailor came to see me during early 2020. She had been suffering from migraine headaches for the past several years. Around 2017, she was serving overseas and suffered from migraine headaches. She was placed on limited duty, her overseas tour was curtailed, and her care was transferred to Naval Medical Center Portsmouth. By the time I had seen her, she had completed two periods of limited duty throughout all of 2018 and some of early January 2019. She was recommended for a third period of limited duty by neurology, but this was denied.

She complained that she received an unexpected disciplinary action that shocked her. She was accused of unauthorized absence, did not feel the process was fair, and was recommended for captain's mast. I had spoken with many service members who had been accused of unauthorized absence, and what she described didn't fit the usual picture. She was being charged with minor things like missing a training and a meeting. In discussing the issue with her, I felt many of her issues were due to migraine headaches. For example, she would suffer from a migraine headache at work and retreat to a dark room. She requested court-martial, and the command opted not to pursue further charges. Even though the captain's mast and court-martial were dropped, she received an adverse performance evaluation, lost eligibility for a commissioning program, and suffered a moral injury. The patient had always been an *Early Promote* sailor, but all that changed with the situation. She felt depressed, was having crying spells, felt anxious, was having trouble sleeping, and dreaded coming into work. She felt hypervigilant and under constant threat by her chain of command. She told me she felt the relationship with her command had been burned, she couldn't trust anyone, and she didn't feel comfortable speaking to anyone or seeking mentorship inside the chain of command about her issues. She had a therapist she was talking to about her issues. I started her on medication for depression. She felt better but was continuing to struggle with migraine headaches and had another emergency room visit for the same.

Several months later, she called me, upset. She was doing well but walked into work and was informed she was under investigation again, this time for creating a hostile work environment. She was fired from her job in the medical clinic and was made a patient greeter. The patient stated that she was forced to sit around and do nothing. She felt persecuted, punished, attacked, embarrassed, isolated, and humiliated. I was scratching my head about the whole thing. If she had served with another uniformed service, a medical board would have already been initiated. I didn't hear stories like this from marines, airmen, or coasties. I attempted to conduct a command intervention by talking to her master chief/E9. We discussed her history of migraine headaches, the level of distress she was suffering from, the suicide risk, and the possibility that she could be moved to a different workspace since it didn't seem to be working out for any party. I was shocked by the response from the master chief. He was blaming, made harsh, judgmental statements, was dismissive about the concerns, and lacked any compassion or empathy concerning the situation. He promised to meet with the service member but never did. I complained to my department head and director about the master chief's behavior. There was a face-to-face meeting with myself, her therapist, and our department head, and concerns that she was suffering from hostile workplace issues were discussed. The director provided feedback that he suspected personality disorder, although her records did not support this. We discussed the possibility of placing the patient on limited duty. We felt the hostile workplace environment concerns were primary and recommended that the patient consult with the Command Managed Equal Opportunity (CMEO) program, IG (inspector general), or other legal/occupational support programs to address toxic workplace issues and that limited duty was not a substitute for this.

As the crisis unfolded, I took a deeper look at her records. She had seen mental health in the past, but her treatment was focused on dealing with chronic pain from migraine headaches and other low-grade issues. Her mental health records were clean. There wasn't any record of personality disorder. Her mental health issues were few and far between up until late 2019 and early 2020. Her records revealed that she had chronic intractable impairing headaches that were negatively impacted by chronic sinusitis, with a history of two ear, nose, and throat surgeries. I was surprised to learn, during the spring of 2020, the Navy personnel command directed the patient to undergo a medical board for migraine headaches. The medical boards office told me neurology refused to author a medical board. Despite being returned to duty, she continued to have migraine headaches and received Botox injections.

I talked to neurology to coordinate care. The nurse practitioner, who was managing the case, stated that the patient had not responded to multiple medications and was recommended for a third period of limited duty. However, this was denied. The patient had also obtained two second opinions from neurology for her persistent headaches, as her condition showed little and unsustained improvement. I discussed concerns that her headaches were contributing to the situation at her command. We discussed that the patient clearly met criteria for the medical board. I inquired about a reference from the DoD instruction that her specific type of migraine headaches were grounds for a medical board, but neurology did not want to initiate a medical board.

By late 2020, she complained of continued depression and anxiety and felt her main issue was being unfairly treated by the command. At some point, she did end up taking three-to-four weeks of leave. She said her anxiety improved away from the work environment but returned when she came back. She told me she filed a CMEO complaint, but it was returned because she wasn't discriminated against. She ended up filing a congressional complaint. She felt the results were mixed. She said the complaint was turned around on her because she didn't speak with the commanding officer, but she was allowed to change work sections and, ultimately, PCS to a new command in Feb 2021. She stated that the congressional complaint also found that the CMEO did not document her concerns.

The patient felt her chief and master chief colluded against her. She said their opinion was that she was faking, malingering, and trying to get out of trouble. She said she was counseled by her internist and neurologist that the chain of command had spoken with them and told them not to put her on limited duty or give a sick-in-quarters chit unless it was absolutely necessary. During 2021, her chief was replaced. The patient stated that her new chief was much more understanding and was able to intervene in her situation. She stated that her chain of command greatly exacerbated her stress by prosecuting her for malingering. She said this made her pain and anxiety worse, and their actions caused her to miss more work. She felt the military as an organization, especially the Navy, had a bias against service members. She felt that her situation was perceived as her trying to take advantage and get out of work and trouble, which was not the case.

The service member ended up receiving a PCS to a new command at a different duty station. She was reevaluated by mental health. She was documented as continuing to struggle with significant mental health symptoms, and her self-reported ratings scales were off the chart. Her mental health providers documented that she was struggling from distrust of Navy chiefs. She was diagnosed with "reaction to severe stress." The mental health provider documented that she suffered from all the classic symptoms of PTSD except criteria A, witnessing or experiencing a life-threatening situation. After arriving at her new duty station, medical providers identified the need for a medical board but gave her time to recover and determine the impact the stress had on her health. A medical board was later initiated in December 2021 for migraine headaches and fibromyalgia.

This situation was disappointing. The patient started off with chronic treatment-resistant migraine headaches that resulted in an overseas tour curtailment. Her headaches caused impairment and disability and contributed to the conflict with her chain of command. The patient was in a difficult situation. She was having difficulty functioning yet was being told she was fit for duty. A medical board was indicated at multiple points and was even service directed, but it was never done. My impression working with neurology is that they didn't want to deal with her. Her command was frustrated that she was having issues doing her job and viewed her issues through a disciplinary lens. Trying to get help from my chain of command, including my department and director, didn't help. The hospital was political, they were ladder climbers, and it was difficult for them to do the right thing. The patient's problems got worse and worse until they escalated into a PTSD-type situation and she ended up with a medical board.

The patient felt that being a corpsman at a military medical center made her situation worse. She felt her leadership all served in the medical career field and abused their authority to review her medical records and speak with her medical providers.

There were mental health patients where a medical board

was indicated, but it wasn't done or there were extensive delays in the initiation of a board. Everyone, including the medical board's office, was overwhelmed and felt short-staffed, and patients slipped through the cracks. Sometimes it took years for a board to occur. Policy did not clearly define how communication with command should occur or how commands would communicate with service members who were struggling. Far too often, service members were perceived as malingering or taking advantage of the system. A disciplinary approach was utilized, and it worsened the outcomes of situations.

A Navy Nurse Is a Navy Nurse

A Navy nurse, a LCDR/O4, who had over twenty-six years of military service, came to see me. She was enlisted for about eight years prior to becoming a nurse and officer. She had subspecialty certification in several areas of nursing. She came to see me because she was in a crisis, was stressed out, and complained of a toxic work environment. The nurse complained that she was recovering from the aftermath of being accepted and promised the opportunity of going to nurse practitioner school, but the funding and training opportunity was canceled, and she received a military change of station. Shortly after arriving at our command, she complained that she was forced to work on the labor and delivery unit. She had achieved subspeciality certifications in other areas she excelled at and asked to be reassigned. Her friend had died while giving birth about five years ago, and all these factors contributed to her anxiety.

She tried to talk to her chain of command, but they doubled down. She complained that the culture was horrible, and nursing retention was terrible. She felt they didn't care, and they didn't want or let people be happy. The hospital had several units where she could have worked, doing what she was good at and felt comfortable with, but this was not allowed. She told me the command put her in orientation on labor and delivery for eight months. During this time, she had four different preceptors and was never allowed to leave orientation. The nurse felt she was bullied and everyone else was bullied too. The message she received was that she had to pay her dues. She told me she hated every minute of it and began to hate being a nurse in general. In the end, she was moved to the medical surgery unit. She told me she received a red flag on her clinical credentials, saying she couldn't work in labor and delivery. She felt retaliated against by her command as she was given a job for a junior nurse and was threatened with a deployment after that fell through.

I tried to advocate on the patient's behalf with mixed results. My observation was that the command had the mentality that a nurse was a nurse. It didn't matter if she had subspeciality training. Her duty was to go where they sent her. It was as if they wanted to make a public example out of her. She felt she was being targeted, tortured, hazed, and publicly humiliated by her chain of command. She was failing clinical orientation and felt threatened by possible adverse action against her clinical privileges that would negatively impact her nursing career. The patient felt that the command was driving her mental health issues and forcing her into the mental health system. The command suggested that she get on limited duty and be removed from her assignment, although that was clearly a leadership call, not a medical call. From the patient's perspective, she felt the command wanted to push her to a breaking point and either make her comply or get rid of her. The military had this toxic cultural tradition that the more a service member wanted to go somewhere or do something, the less likely it was allowed to happen, but this situation took it to another level. As the situation unfolded, I found myself thinking, *What is wrong with these people?*

The patient ended up retiring from the Navy. She said the main reason was because of what happened to her. After leaving military service, she got a job in the private sector, worked in the intensive care unit, treated sicker patients, felt more part of a team, and felt appreciated. She told me on the way out, despite her twenty-nine total years of service, the command told her she was deserving of a Navy Achievement Medal but promised an upgrade to a Navy Commendation Medal. This was a slap in the face on her way out. She told me she felt the command were "vindictive assholes."

The military needs a nurse who can do anything, anywhere, at any time. Still, it was unnecessary and not a good risk management strategy to force someone to do something they don't feel comfortable doing. It was also different how other services or agencies would have handled the situation. I deployed to Africa and worked on an Ebola treatment unit in the field. One of the nurses didn't feel comfortable working in the hot zone, so she was reassigned to monitor the health of the officers deployed. She did a great job, made significant contributions to the mission, and felt valued. The situation raises questions about patient safety. My youngest son, Robert Jr., was born in Naval Medical Center Portsmouth's labor and delivery unit. Thankfully, he came into this world healthy, and he and my wife received good care. I would not want anyone to receive medical care in a unit where nurses are working outside of their comfort zone. The command was so determined to teach this nurse a lesson, they were willing to put her in a patient care area where she had anxiety and didn't feel comfortable.

While serving at Veterans Affairs, I spoke with a similar patient, a thirty-seven-year-old female who served in the Navy as a hospital corpsman for thirteen years. She suffered PTSD and depression after a stillbirth that occurred at Naval Medical Center Portsmouth. In the last weeks of her pregnancy, she didn't feel right, went in to get checked, and the baby was found not to have a heartbeat. She struggled with nightmares, false guilt, and sadness. She ended up going to cardiovascular technician school. After graduating, she was forced to return to Naval Medical Center Portsmouth despite her trauma and requests for reassignment. She felt extreme discomfort returning to the facility where she lost her baby. She got pregnant again, became depressed, and had a suicide attempt.

She was considered a high-risk pregnancy and recommended for medical limitations not to work nights. She felt the command was toxic and hostile and forced her to work nights. She ended up leaving the Navy via the medical boards process. To this day, she feels retaliated against by the Navy and feels she is a basket case around the anniversary of her baby's death.

Daniel "Doc" Jacobs

Daniel "Doc" Jacobs is a Fleet Marine Force corpsman and Navy wounded warrior who was hit by an intermittent explosive device while on deployment in Iraq in 2006. He wrote a 300-page book describing what happened to him, his recovery, and his efforts to remain on active duty (Jacobs 2020). He spent a third of the book describing in painful detail how he felt his chain of command openly played games with him, including telling him they would make sure he would "never go on a deployment out of this command." He described how he felt they gaslighted him and thwarted his career progression and assignments process. He wrote about how he spoke to a Navy admiral who supported him and as a result how a bogus page-thirteen counseling sheet was placed in his service record for jumping the chain of command. He discussed how this was repeatedly held over his head, how he was told not to seek assistance outside the chain of command and how he was threatened with more legal action and loss of Veterans Affairs benefits. Doc Jacobs wrote that he was told he shouldn't talk about what happened to him because he didn't have an award to back it up. He wrote about how the command scrutinized his medical appointments, accused him of missing medical appointments, and interfered with his medical care. He felt openly and relentlessly persecuted by his chain of command. He wrote about how he was reassigned from his duties when he was undergoing the medical boards process and a chief physically assaulted him and told him to sit at the front desk "like a good little broken sailor and not do anything else." Doc Jacobs's experiences were eerily similar to the sailor with the migraine headaches who faced legal persecution and humiliation before being reassigned as a clinic greeter.

Doc Jacobs wrote about how the Navy medical board system found him fit for duty, yet he was repeatedly found to be not medically cleared, and his chief gave him a piece of paper that said *Not Medically Ready*. He described how he felt subjective decision-making and political factors were utilized to disqualify him, including a situation where his command influenced a medical provider. He provided a scanned document showing where the medical provider reversed a medical clearance determination. The sailor described the impact of suffering from a limbo status where he couldn't do his job and there was conflicting guidance about his duty status.

Doc Jacobs described how this took a toll on his mental and physical health. He felt blacklisted and discriminated against. He wrote that the Navy stressed him out to the point of a heart attack or stroke. He described how he went on a rampage of taking it out on other people and had a brief stint of unhealthy alcohol use. He wrote about how he reached a point where he had enough, sought help from a Marine Corps psychiatrist, and was recommended for a medical board.

There was a silver lining to Daniel Jacobs's story. He achieved a promotion to HM2/E5. After he left the Navy, he had many widely publicized Major League Baseball tryouts. He demonstrated that he could perform at a level comparable to other candidates despite having an amputation. Six years after he left the Navy, he was awarded a Bronze Star for Valor and wrote that this gave him closure. He recovered and thrived after leaving the Navy, even becoming a successful author.

CHAPTER 9

Fight to Deliver Mental Health Services

I SPOKE WITH a retired Navy captain, John Cordle, who has written about and advocated for mental health in the Navy. We discussed his experiences with the Navy and military's mental health system. He felt there were many hurdles that had to be crossed for a sailor to get help. The first hurdle was finding courage to work through all the obstacles to ask for help, including career repercussions, and then to receive the help. He described a peer who made it through the first part but then had difficulty accessing care and the frustration that followed.

Numerous service members and veterans have shared their experiences regarding the challenges of dealing with mental health issues in the military. There isn't much about what it is like serving as a military mental health provider. In the next few chapters, I will pull back the curtain and shed light on the inner workings of the military's mental health system. The next part of the book will explore issues with the military's mental health system.

Wild West Approach to Mental Health

Conventional wisdom was, and medical research showed, for mental health treatment to have a meaningful effect and positive outcomes, weekly or biweekly mental health appointments were necessary. If an appointment was less than monthly, the therapeutic relationship between the patient and mental health provider was negatively impacted and the relationship had to be restarted.

At Naval Medical Center Portsmouth, our outpatient mental health next available appointments were one to three months out. Everyone agreed it was an issue. Sometimes patients were observed to get discouraged waiting for an appointment and dropped out of treatment. Solving the problem was an insurmountable challenge.

While working at a residential treatment program for substance abuse disorders, our team coordinated care with the patient's outpatient mental health provider regarding a complicated patient. His email captured appointment availability challenges we faced:

> *Thanks to the team for the consistently great work. I'm open to recommendations regarding planning for the next steps of clinical focus in therapy. If you think a change of providers is in the patient's best interest, let me know. At this point I am concerned my appointment availability is not helpful for most patients, except where every 4 weeks is good enough.*

A colleague on an Army base told me that within twenty-four hours after discharge from an inpatient psychiatric hospital, a soldier would receive a comprehensive face-to-face evaluation to ensure their needs were being met and to reduce suicide risk. That was a best practice and what I was accustomed to when working with the Air Force. Naval Medical Center Portsmouth had a busy inpatient psychiatry unit. We didn't have enough outpatient appointment availability, so patients were placed in a post-hospitalization discharge group or provided a telephone phone check. The MARMC investigation discussed the practice of utilizing "bridging group sessions" that were also referred to as "discharge groups." The *USS George Washington* investigation report documented that the ship's psychologist considered switching to group therapy from individual therapy due to access-to-care issues but didn't do it because the practice hadn't worked in the past. It's possible if the Naval Medical Center Portsmouth mental health clinic conducted face-to-face post-discharge follow-up appointments, outcomes would have been improved.

Sometimes patients were fortunate to receive a comprehensive evaluation one month after discharge. Our clinic offered a lot of do-it-yourself group classes like depression, anxiety, and insomnia workshops. We had case management services where a military treatment facility mental health provider would send sailors to the TRICARE network for care. Through this process, the patient would receive treatment from an off-base provider and would receive a telephone call every one to three months from our facility to ensure their needs and readiness requirements were being met. Our clinic offered acupuncture and transcranial magnetic stimulation. Several of the mental health providers had part of their schedules blocked so they could provide patients with these treatments, although there were questions about whether the time would have been better invested in delivering routine mental health care. Some of the providers I worked with were adept at adjusting their work hours and optimizing their appointments and billing codes to minimize their workload. One provider showed me a professional-looking template for a pre-appointment record review they would document the day before an appointment to count toward their workload. I didn't agree with the practice, but I can't necessarily blame them. Optimizing workload was like trying to minimize tax liability.

In the absence of clear policy, frequently, it was up to the person in charge to make judgment calls. It wasn't clearly defined what services we could or could not offer, how many patients a mental health provider would see in a day, or even the hours of operation. Appointment times differed from location to location. One facility where I worked had sixty-minute intake appointments, another had ninety, and yet another had two-hour intake appointments. The minimal manning needed for operations was undefined. There was no guidance for optimal or maximum patient panel size for each healthcare provider. If a provider hit a maximum panel size, new intakes could be frozen to focus care on existing patients. Access-to-care standards weren't clearly laid out. We had an emergency room that was open twenty-four seven. Technically, we always had immediate availability because a patient could go to the emergency room.

Unnecessary appointments took away from those who needed them more. There were patients who had trouble sleeping in the absence of any other mental health disorder, those who just wanted a network deferral, or those who needed a simple blessing to return to work. There were a lot of simple, straightforward mental health issues that could have been addressed in primary care, but there was a low threshold for primary care providers to refer to subspeciality mental health. I suspect some of it was because there was so much scrutiny, rules, and regulations pertaining to mental health that the primary care providers were apprehensive.

Over the course of my career, the number of consults from the emergency room and other sources increased. The threshold to request a psychiatrist and other mental health providers to come into the emergency department after hours and on weekends to assist in the evaluation and management of cases decreased over time. In the private sector, the emergency department handled most mental health, sometimes with the assistance of an in-house licensed clinical social worker or telehealth provider. The private sector emergency department only consulted psychiatry when there was a management problem. The overutilization of emergency department psychiatric consults drained and taxed military mental health providers. The issues were all related, and patients resorted to going to the emergency department due to difficulty accessing outpatient mental health appointments.

The DHA had an online secure messaging and appointment scheduling tool where patients could contact their provider, but it wasn't utilized for mental health. There were concerns about the electronic phone reminder system. Specifically, a high-risk patient could cancel their appointment by phone or text message and slip through the cracks. If a high-risk patient requested a cancellation, it was desired for there to be communication between them and a live person to ensure they were okay and their needs were met. There wasn't a clear mechanism for tracking patients who dropped out of treatment. The Air Force clinic I worked at scrubbed a list of patients to see when their last appointment was. If they hadn't come for an appointment in three months, they would have received a phone call. It wasn't spelled out what to do if someone missed an appointment. I would try to telephone the patient and ask them how they were doing, but it wasn't in policy. It was challenging to book a patient for a month's worth of weekly consecutive appointments. Operational mental health providers used Microsoft Outlook for scheduling, which was more flexible and effective compared with the DHA electronic appointment scheduling software.

Another best practice I'd experienced was for the mental health clinic to contact military law enforcement weekly, review a list of behavioral health-related incidents, and call service members who were involved to offer appointments. That was a good organizational risk management best practice, but it wasn't in policy either. There wasn't a policy for how to transfer cases between duty stations. One clinic where I worked had a practice for the provider to call the gaining clinic and document a note in the electronic health system. Sometimes patients were told to just follow up with mental health at their next duty station. They wouldn't, and they slipped through the cracks.

The no-show rate was an issue that was discussed. Our no-show rate was higher compared to private sector clinics. The private sector clinics charged patients an appointment cancellation fee, but we could not. Once, I spoke to a patient who was receiving care outside of the system. He explained that he wanted to come back because he was charged a $100 appointment no-show fee. If we could have charged a $50 to $100 no-show fee, that would have been a game changer. Our no-show rate would have drastically declined, and our clinic would have made a lot of money.

There were various efforts to combat missed appointments over the years, including repeat offenders being referred for disciplinary action, but there were concerns that this would increase stigma, and I don't think it ever happened. I saw a note template that contained the verbiage that something like this could happen: "Service member advised any no-show appointments would be reported to Command through an automatic notification system."

The issue of documentation standards or templates came up too. Some providers copied and pasted canned narratives into notes. The narratives tended to be lengthy and vague. There weren't clear standards of how mental health providers embedded in operational units would document the services they provided. It was not uncommon for a patient to show up, discuss having multiple encounters with their operational mental health provider, and find no mental health encounters in the system. Not documenting encounters seemed like a recipe for disaster and subpar care.

We would have benefited from having a business manual and DHA practice manager to lay out how the day-to-day operations would proceed. It would have been helpful to have all these processes the same at every duty station in the DoD to standardize care and reduce chaos and confusion.

In 2020 there was a DoD Inspector General Report that addressed access to mental health care issues and captured many of the issues discussed here (DoD Inspector General 2020). The report found that the DHA published inconsistent and unclear access to mental healthcare policies and lacked a Military Health System-wide model to identify appropriate levels of staffing in direct and purchased care. It also found that the DoD did not consistently meet outpatient mental health access-to-care standards for active-duty service members and their families. A subsequent DoD Inspector General Report documented that the issues remained unresolved several years later (DoD Inspector General 2023).

A senior Navy psychiatrist told me that programs and initiatives were often based on leadership calls and were personality driven. The mentality was to decide what needs to happen or, if someone says no, to find a way around it. He explained that instructions say what you *cannot* do, not what you *can* do. Lack of clear direction and policy resulted in a situation that was ripe for abuse and manipulation. Individuals would engage in regulation and "commanding officer shopping" to get things done. This occurred when individuals would pitch the same issue to multiple senior officers until one was found to sign off on the initiative. Sometimes programs and initiatives were successful, but sometimes they backfired in a big way.

I was told a story about a Navy psychiatrist who set up a concierge clinic for a regional submarine force. He was readily accessible for mental health issues, therapy, and rapid intervention. He would take referrals from sailors, commands, and other medical and mental health providers. The initiative had some success. Unplanned personnel losses decreased drastically, but there were mixed results. There were concerns about underdiagnosing and overemphasis on outcomes (retention of submariners on the boats). The program was changed after there was a bad outcome. The initiative would have benefited from a more organized, structured, and standardized approach.

From a certain perspective, not having policy was great. No one could be held accountable because there was no policy defining what needed to be done. There were no tracking mechanisms, so it was difficult to conduct or enforce any type of quality measure. It was like the Wild West. An operational mental health concierge clinic, post-hospitalization discharge group, or telephone phone check wasn't optimal, but these were innovative solutions, and something was better than nothing. On the other hand, it was stressful. Things were poorly defined, chaotic, and risky. It felt as if 30 percent of our attention and resources were spent spinning our wheels, and we were constantly flying by the seat of our pants. It was stressful and contributed to burnout and attrition.

Manpower Issues and the Churn Rate

Major issues we faced were staffing shortages and the personnel churn rate. In every review or discussion of military mental health, a common theme is increasing the number of mental health providers and recommendations for improving recruiting and retention. The patient load, or demand, always outstripped the number of mental health providers available to provide the services. Manpower issues affected everyone at every level. In the military health system, people, resources, and programs were shifting all over the place, all the time. Every time there was turnover, there was chaos. Working in the military mental health system felt like musical chairs. On a regular basis, providers were deployed, changed duty stations, or quit disrupting the care for thousands of people. It took two to three years for a mental health provider to master their job, and at that point, it was almost always time for them to receive a permanent change-of-station move. One day the department head for Mental Health, who oversaw multiple divisions and a large number of personnel, sent an email saying she was going to be deployed to Cuba for six months. It was frustrating and stressful because she was a lynchpin, holding together multiple divisions, and she had done a great job putting everything back together that the previous department head had screwed up. Thankfully, the deployment didn't pan out. However, within weeks, it was announced that the department head for the SARP was going to be deployed to Africa for several months. Within days, he was gone, and the program was disrupted. The acting department head remarked that the last time the department head deployed, there was a wave of personnel who turned in their resignations and quit.

At Naval Medical Center Portsmouth, leadership turned over multiple times in a three-year period. Programs changed, depending on who was in charge. Gaps in policy were left to interpretation to whoever was in a leadership role. Every time leadership changed, lessons learned were lost, and the same mistakes were made over and over. Employees got frustrated and banded together, and there was increased tension with leadership. All this contributed to a feeling of chaos and burnout, and we felt like we were suffering from organizational attention-deficit hyperactivity disorder (ADHD). One of the most senior doctors in the DoD, Vice Admiral Raquel Bono, described similar challenges. She said the biggest issues she faced in her position were politics and leadership turnover (Shane III 2019): "I'm on my sixth acting leader right now . . . and we're coming up on another election year. . . . The turnover within military leadership ranks has complicated that process, requiring a significant amount of remedial explaining as new officials come in."

The military treatment facility and operational forces seemed locked in competition for personnel. In my career field, there were not enough psychiatrists to go around. The hospital and operational forces both wanted psychiatrists. It was in the hands of senior Navy officials to determine which positions would be filled and which would go unfilled. From a broader perspective, both the operational units and military treatment facilities had staffing issues. Anytime a military contingency occurred, such as a real-world event or military exercise, operational needs took precedent. Personnel were taken from the military treatment facility. Logically, it made sense that real-world operational issues took priority. The remaining personnel would be tasked to find a way to get the mission done regardless of the circumstances.

Manpower issues impacted service members and mental health providers. Military personnel were active duty, civilian employees, contractors, and volunteers. Compared with the private sector, it was difficult to obtain civil service employment with the military. The personnel system was bureaucratic, slow, and unresponsive. Whenever there were budget issues, civilian employee positions were low-hanging fruit. Once, a substance abuse counselor got frustrated and quit abruptly. We were told his position, along with twenty other vacant federal service positions from our directorate, were "sucked up into an administrative black hole" and lost due to funding issues. Periodically, there were civilian employee hiring freezes for months on end. Once, a clinic where I worked interviewed a psychiatric nurse practitioner for a job. She was an ideal candidate. She had worked as a psychiatric nurse on an inpatient psychiatry unit, then went back to school and became a nurse practitioner. She waited months, only to be offered a salary that was 50 percent lower than what she could make elsewhere. The Human Resources department said there were issues with the classification and coding of her position and struggled to make the necessary adjustments. A colleague of mine, a psychiatric nurse practitioner, had an interview and was told she was accepted for a position in February, but the paperwork wasn't completed until August, six months later. By that time, she had found a better job elsewhere.

At two separate duty stations where I served on short notice, the contracting companies who employed the doctoral-level psychologists and psychiatrists changed. The healthcare professionals were told they could keep their job but would have to take significant pay cuts. The experience was like a corporate shakedown for money. At one duty station, after a couple weeks of wrangling, the healthcare providers were allowed to continue employment at their same rate of pay. At Naval Medical Center Portsmouth, medical providers were unsuccessful in renegotiating their pay contracts, and they quit. Both situations caused quite a stir, were unnecessarily stressful, and disrupted care. The loss of the mental health providers was a devastating loss to patient care. The contracting companies were like a placeholder and payment source for the employee. They added little or no value to our mission or day-to-day operations.

The DHA instruction for substance abuse (J-9 Research and Development 2019) directed "a data-driven, risk adjustment model to set staffing levels for trained professionals, treatment personnel, and support staff required to ensure program effectiveness," but this never happened at the Navy SARP program where I served. There was always talk about using an objective algorithm to set mental health staffing levels, but I never witnessed this. The issue became relevant when personnel filed a grievance complaining that staffing levels were inadequate. The language in the policy was vague, and it was impossible to comply with or enforce staffing standards that weren't spelled out.

While serving as an operational mental health provider, a policy came out that directed thousands of active duty to receive an automated neuropsychological assessment. This was computerized testing designed to evaluate baseline brain functioning as part of an initiative to address military traumatic brain injury. The policy was a mandate that lacked both funding and resources. The personnel, means, resources, and methods needed to conduct the testing were not provided. We didn't have the physical space, computers, or personnel needed to execute the initiative. We didn't have the time or energy to invest in developing and maintaining an implementation strategy. When the issue was reviewed, everyone raised their hands, shrugged, and said there was no way to do it.

Another issue we faced was supervision and management of personnel. Even if the people were on hand, sometimes it was difficult to manage them or get them to perform the work. At one point in my career, I was aware of a situation where Navy surgical technicians were accused of trying to delay and/or cancel surgical cases to get out of work. From a selfish perspective, it was advantageous for them. If they succeeded, the case would be pushed to the next shift. They still received the same amount of pay, whether they completed the work or not. I was at a meeting where the issues were discussed. Patients were frustrated, and the surgeons complained. Federal employees were known to engage in bureaucratic guerrilla warfare and were resistant to change, and leadership lacked the authority to make it happen.

Disagreements Regarding Staffing and Deployments

During my career, I witnessed frequent disagreements and conflict over staffing issues and deployments. A deployment tasking or some other staffing request would come in, and everyone would fight about it. The staffing and deployment issues were stressful because the overarching issue was that there weren't enough personnel to begin with, and the disruptions caused by staffing changes impacted the lives of people and patients.

Consider this scenario. There was a high-profile behavioral health episode on a small base. The base commander, who was highly successful, well-known, and liked, demanded more resources and longer working hours for the mental health clinic. There were no objective access-to-care standards, working hours, or staffing standards. As a result of the pressure, another base was directed to loan a mental health provider to provide temporary additional duty support. A potential telehealth solution was discussed. Although it was a best practice and the most logical and cost-effective solution, the base commander refused to allow telehealth and demanded a mental health provider be physically present on-site. The base commander had a close relationship with a senior flag officer and had political leverage to get what he wanted. The individuals involved in the dispute invested hours preparing briefings and other information, only to have a flag officer make a unilateral decision to back the base commander's requests. The result was that we were tasked with providing frequent temporary duty trips to the smaller base.

Around 2008, when I was serving with the Navy in Japan, an

Army deployment tasking for a psychologist came in. The Navy argued about it internally, and the tasking was given to a Navy psychologist in Okinawa, Japan. From an organizational standpoint, it didn't seem logical to deploy someone from Japan since there was no TRICARE network for patients to fall back on. The psychologist who was tagged for the deployment was new to the Navy and hadn't completed her psychology licensing. She was deployed and sent to operational training for weeks. Her deployment disrupted operations and care for hundreds of patients. When she arrived in the Middle East, no one met her at the airport, and the Army had no record of her deployment. When the Army learned she wasn't licensed, they put her on a plane and sent her home.

In a similar situation, the Army deployed a psychiatric nurse practitioner from the Midwest to Texas. He arrived on-site, and a day later the hospital commander on the other side of the United States threw a fit, claimed the hospital couldn't function without his presence, and successfully facilitated his immediate demobilization.

During my career, fighting for staffing and resources felt like *Hunger Games*, where the characters fought each other to the death. In the absence of policy and staffing guidance, everyone fought for resources. There were always situations, staffing shortfalls, and gapped positions that were out of everyone's control. A standardized staffing configuration, footprint for operational mental health billets, and mental health clinics with set working hours would have gone a long way to prevent and alleviate these situations.

Resource Disparity Between Locations

When I served as a Navy psychiatrist with the Marine Corps in Okinawa, Japan, my first experience with resource disparity between the services was on the island of Oahu in Hawaii. The Army had a beautiful coral-colored and well-resourced Army hospital on a hill. This was Tripler Army Medical Center. It was located on a joint campus with a Veterans Affairs Medical Center. I recall touring the facility and meeting with an Army mental health provider. He was a COL/O6 who bragged about having a conference room with a $50,000 big-screen television. The Army also had a clean, modern, and well-staffed mental health clinic at Schofield Barracks. The Air Force had a similar clean and well-staffed mental health clinic at Hickam Air Force Base. During the fall of 2006, a congressionally mandated DoD mental health task force traveled to Honolulu, Hawaii, and Okinawa, Japan, to study military mental health. One of the task force members asked me why the Army and Air Force had better facilities and resources compared with the Navy and Marine Corps. The Navy's mental health resources at Pearl Harbor and especially at Kaneohe Bay weren't on par with what the Army and Air Force had. To be fair, I observed that the Army and Air Force were better at organization and planning for medical programs and facilities. The Army was more organized and had a team that prepared mental health provider contracts and were better able to get it done. The Army was better supported and had a better support infrastructure in place to make things happen. In the Navy system, everything seemed to fall on the backs of the mental health providers to make things happen.

I served in the SARP program at Naval Medical Center Portsmouth from 2021 to 2022. The SARP building was on the campus of Naval Medical Center Portsmouth and badly needed renovation, possibly to be demolished and rebuilt. At one point, the building suffered from a rat infestation. A SARP counselor told me she was teaching a group when a rat fell from the ceiling and startled everyone. There was also a viral video showing someone walking down the hall, a rat the size of a shoe running out from under a door, and an individual being startled and jumping back.

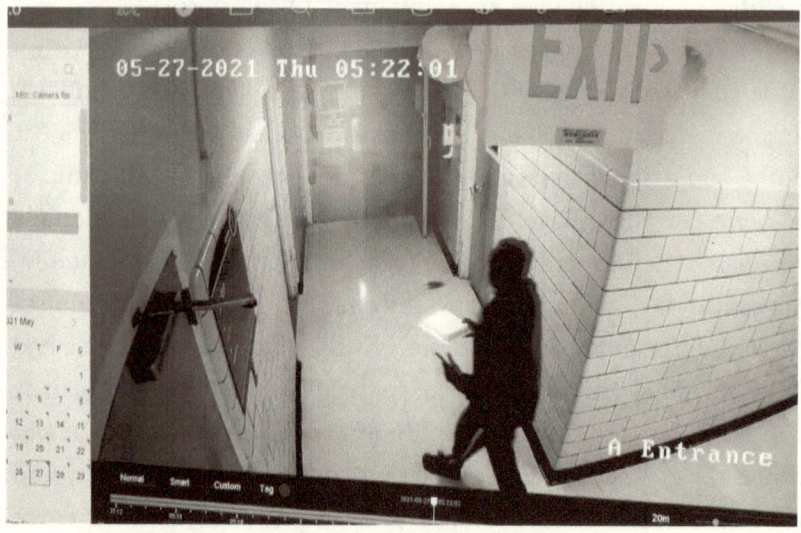

A frame from the viral rat video taken in May 2021 at Naval Medical Center Portsmouth's SARP Building

Another SARP counselor told me he saw many roaches, windows without seals, and mold around the windows that irritated sailors' sinuses.

The history of the building went back decades. At one point, the Navy SARP building was located at Naval Station Norfolk. I mentioned how a Navy admiral referred to it as an expensive hotel and lobbied for it to be closed in the early aughts. The SARP building was moved to an old school house located on the campus of Naval Medical Center Portsmouth in 2012 due to issues with mold (Simmons 2012). In March 2022, the SARP building reached a critical mass again, and the west wing of the building was closed due to facility issues, including a leaking roof. The sailors participating in the program were moved from the west wing of the building to the base barracks. The possibility of SARP being moved to Langley Air Force Base was briefly entertained. In late 2024, the SARP program was in the news again after its residential treatment program was shut down because of staffing shortages (Kime 2024).

The Navy had a West Coast SARP program located at Naval Base Point Loma in San Diego, California. We were told there was resource disparity between the two programs on multiple levels. Not only was our building falling down around us, but there was also a shortage of active-duty substance abuse counselors. We were told the West Coast SARP program had a better building, more active-duty substance abuse counselors, and a better mix of staff, including federal employees and contractors. Not surprisingly, the East Coast SARP program struggled with retention of personnel. From my perspective, the state of the SARP program, the building, and the disparity of resources symbolized the Navy's mental health system.

I was told in recent years that Walter Reed National Medical Center was in a healthier state than Naval Medical Center Portsmouth. I spoke with a colleague who was a mental health provider embedded in a primary care clinic at Walter Reed. Many of Naval Medical Center Portsmouth's primary care, behavioral health, mental health, and nursing primary care positions were unfilled. The Army was the biggest service and had a heavy presence at Walter Reed, and it's possible the Army's influence had a hand in securing more resources. Walter Reed was in the heart of the nation's capital, and maybe having more resources was a capital beltway thing.

White Space and Attitudes Toward Nonmilitary Providers

The Coast Guard coined a term "white space" that had broad applicability. The Coast Guard had small bases all over the United States where it was impractical to have a medical clinic. At these locations, coasties and their families were sent to white space. This meant the service members and their families received care through the TRICARE network. White space wasn't optimal because service members fell off the radar. It was hard to track whether service members were meeting readiness standards and if they were getting good, quality care when they were getting care outside of the system.

The *USS George Washington* investigation report discussed a sailor who was receiving care from a nonmilitary provider, and the medical records were not available for review. That sailor fell off into white space. Some service members sought out and took advantage of white space. They could receive treatment outside of the military health system without having to worry about the negative impact on their careers. A service member told me, in white space, he could receive treatment for his PTSD and bipolar disorder and remain on active duty without his command finding out.

Our mental health clinic struggled with white space issues. Due to a backlog of patients, we sent many patients to the TRICARE network. We tried to follow up with them, but the fact of the matter was, they were in white space. Records from clinical services delivered in the TRICARE network were supposed to be scanned and uploaded into a computer system called HAIMS as part of the billing process, but this rarely occurred, resulting in decreased visibility about their care. Mental health providers or patients typically had to request these. Often, patients had to carry them in for scanning.

When I worked in the military mental health clinic, the term "civilian provider" frequently had a negative connotation. These were TRICARE network white space mental health providers. The professional opinions and treatment recommendations of civilian providers were given less weight.

From time to time, I spoke with white space providers to coordinate care, and it went very well. Many of them were more seasoned, more mature, and experienced compared with the active-duty providers inside the military treatment facility. I found that they frequently wanted to be part of the team, share information, and coordinate care but didn't know how to accomplish this. There was no shared electronic medical records system, and they didn't know who to call.

Issues with Diagnosing

While serving with the Navy, I observed the diagnoses of adjustment and personality disorder to be overutilized. In my experience, adjustment disorder and personality disorder were more frequently diagnosed in military mental health, especially in the Navy's mental health system compared with any other clinical practice setting.

Most mental health providers were well intentioned. We went with the least restrictive or most conservative diagnosis during the first several visits. Often, patients presented in crisis, and it took time for them to come out of that state. It took time for the patient-doctor relationship to gel and for the patient to open up and discuss their issues. Sometimes it was difficult to get a solid diagnosis, and the process could take a few months or longer. Patients were sometimes caught in a limbo-type situation, where they couldn't get a stable provider due to the high churn rate. A lot of times, the diagnosis the last provider recommended was continued. Some patients were never able to work with a consistent provider, and the least restrictive diagnoses stuck over time.

Patients were underdiagnosed to protect or do the right thing for the patient. Mental health providers were apprehensive about the consequences of diagnosing someone with significant mental health problems. A mental health provider approached me and said, "I almost diagnosed PTSD right off the bat, but I didn't want to affect his career." A Navy psychiatrist told me she avoided certain diagnoses to prevent school disqualification.

Mental health providers are reluctant to diagnose a major diagnosis such as bipolar disorder in a career service member because, according to DoD policy, it was grounds for a medical board. General Gregg Martin was a retired two-star Army general who was diagnosed with bipolar disorder. He wrote about how he struggled to get a proper diagnosis. Army doctors initially determined he had no mental health problems. He wrote in his book later that an Army mental health provider counseled him to keep his diagnosis under the radar to avoid triggering a medical board or security clearance issues (Martin 2023).

I spoke to a forty-three-year-old Navy veteran who served twenty years in the Navy on submarines. He suffered from bipolar disorder. The condition wasn't diagnosed until after he left active duty. He explained that he was in a hypomanic state most of his career, with high energy and motivation levels, and he didn't need as much sleep as others. He felt that bipolar disorder enhanced his performance, and the structure of the Navy helped him control his moods. After he left active duty, he went through a divorce, suffered other major life stresses, and experienced a full-blown manic episode, and the diagnosis became apparent. If he had been identified as having bipolar disorder on active duty, that would have been a career killer.

Another scenario I encountered occurred when the patient and the command were desperate to facilitate release from the military as quickly as possible. The mental health provider felt pressure to underdiagnose or misdiagnose the patient to facilitate an administrative discharge. I remember when one of my attendings during residency convinced patients that a medical board was disadvantageous. She told them a medical board would take longer to get out of the Navy and prolong their misery and discharge. She told them they could get out faster via administrative separation and then pursue benefits from Veterans Affairs. When a boardable condition was present, administrative options were reduced, and it could take a year or longer for medical board processing. For the two-star Army general or a sailor who works on a submarine, if they had a record of good functioning, it doesn't make sense to disqualify them due to asking for help and receiving treatment, including taking commonly prescribed medications. The Army general must have performed at a very high level to achieve promotion to O8. With appropriate mental health treatment, he would be expected to perform at an even higher level.

Once, I worked with a conscientious objector in the Marine Corps who requested a discharge. The administrative requirements needed to make this happen were off the chart. As I recall, the chaplain and even the general provided an endorsement for discharge, but Marine Corps headquarters returned it without action. It was frustrating, and the situation resulted in a moral and ethical dilemma (Moldavsky 2006). The marine refused to serve and was incompatible with military life. In the end, he was discharged via a mental health pathway.

The process of diagnosing and determining military disposition was impacted by what was perceived as in the best interests of the Navy or the military and command influence rather than the individual's needs. The Navy had the ability to turn a blind eye to anybody they didn't want to see a problem in. Sometimes there was direct command influence and mental health providers were pressured and manipulated to change diagnoses. A service member might have PTSD or some other boardable condition, but the command didn't want to deal with the member who was perceived as difficult and pressured the mental health provider directly and indirectly through the chain of command for administrative action instead. I was sitting in a meeting, and the department head, a Navy LCDR/O4 psychologist, recommended to a room full of mental health providers that they avoid higher diagnoses that warrant a medical board. He explained that there were ramifications for certain diagnoses and the participants should avoid more severe diagnoses that remove administrative options for dealing with service members. Shortly after that meeting, I discussed a case with a mental health provider. She said the patient we were discussing clearly had PTSD, but "you heard the department head. I shouldn't put it in" the patient's medical record.

A senior Navy psychiatrist told me about a challenging situation and ethical dilemma he found himself in. There was a female sailor hospitalized in the inpatient psychiatry unit. A Navy ship pressured the hospital through multiple channels, including through the chain of command, personal connections with the command leadership, and directly to the psychiatry team. The senior medical officer, affectionately referred to as "SMO," met with the psychiatry team and confronted them. For sure, the SMO was under pressure from his leadership regarding the situation. The SMO argued about the PTSD diagnosis and sexual assault. The SMO pressured the psychiatry team to discharge the sailor so the command could initiate adverse personnel actions. The SMO said, "How do you know she was sexually assaulted? How do you know it really happened? How can you write a medical board if you don't know it really happened?" The psychiatry team felt their job was to support the fleet and felt under pressure to do what the fleet wanted, but in this situation, they said no. It may not have been what the ship wanted, but it was in the best interests of the organization and for the individual sailor. When I served with the Air Force, our hospital had a medical legal consultant who was good about getting involved in situations like this and setting limits with commands. Dealing with these situations was very stressful and contributed to burnout. Our commands didn't always back us, legal help wasn't readily available, and at times we were left to navigate these situations on our own and felt thrown under the bus.

Mental health providers, especially those embedded in operational units, face pressure not to create unplanned personnel losses. In the textbook *Combat and Operational Behavioral Health*, it is documented that in the Navy, a key aspect of the shipboard psychologist's job was to return sailors to duty to save money (Koffman, et al. 2011). The authors wrote that by preventing dozens of medical evacuations during a six-month deployment, the program was estimated to have saved $110,000. Sometimes the command influence was more direct. Commanders would lobby mental health providers or their superiors directly to remove or retain perceived problem service members. It was a compromising situation when a commander who bottom lined your annual performance review was pressuring you to perform certain actions.

Mental health providers were people too, and personal feelings and biases contributed to differences in diagnoses among providers. If a patient was perceived as refusing to return to work and being difficult, it was challenging to find empathy. Some mental health providers struggled with biases and negative feelings toward patients, and it clouded their judgment. It was easy for some to diagnose a difficult patient with personality disorder and make them disappear through the administrative separation process. Sometimes the mental health providers were vocal in that they felt a patient didn't deserve a medical board or it was their job to block a medical board or personnel action to safeguard government resources. Some colleagues told me, "The military was not a welfare system" and felt specific service members should not be entitled to certain benefits. "The government shouldn't pay for that," they would say. Others felt they had a personal duty to protect the operational forces by cleansing psychopathology from the military and referring service members with the slightest hints of personality disorder for separation.

Underdiagnosing and misdiagnosing were an easy way out. I reviewed a case of a service member who suffered from anxiety and substance use issues. A previous mental health provider documented only concerns about the substance use disorder. The patient was recommended to follow-up with the substance abuse program but not for mental health treatment. If a patient suffered from five years of intractable treatment-resistant anxiety symptoms and suffered from panic disorder or generalized anxiety disorder, a medical board was warranted. Once, I reviewed a case of a patient who had severe depressive symptoms for an extended period. Although the patient clearly met criteria for major depression, a senior mental health provider explained that the depression was primarily due to stress, the patient felt better on the weekend away from the stress, and they argued the diagnosis was most appropriately adjustment disorder.

A psychologist pulled me aside once and explained that she avoided documenting certain diagnoses because this evaded an electronic monitoring system. She avoided diagnoses of depression or PTSD because the computer system would start tracking the number of visits per month and start the clock ticking on required treatments once these diagnoses were made. Another explained that she avoided documenting the Columbia suicide severity rating scale so she wouldn't have to complete the risk evaluation and subsequent safety planning forms. There were occasions when mental health providers underdiagnosed to avoid having to author a medical board. If a service member or the mental health provider was up for orders, it was easy to punt the situation to the gaining command or next provider.

Underdiagnosing and misdiagnosing were significant issues that impacted military readiness and contributed to stigma. Individuals who weren't ready were returned to duty. It contributed to the problem of sailors mistrusting Navy mental health providers. Service members were reluctant to consult with a Navy mental health provider due to the fear that they would be deemed unfit and processed for separation. Receiving the wrong diagnosis could be a black mark in a service member's records and start them on a downward path of being rendered incompatible with military life. On some occasions, the practice impacted service members' ability to receive benefits. Joshua Kors described these issues in depth, including the negative impact that misdiagnosing in the Army had on soldiers in a three-part series (Kors 2007; Kors 2007; Kors 2010).

Gaps in policy, lack of oversight, accountability, and quality controls contributed to the situation. If a provider diagnosed personality disorder or recommended separation on the first or second visit, it was a red flag. Establishing a solid diagnosis took months, plus collateral information from command and possibly family members, yet there were no clear practice standards. Policies, procedures, and documentation standards for operational mental health providers were not clearly defined.

Clinical Skills Atrophy

Eric Elster, the dean of USUHS (Uniformed Services University of Health Sciences) School of Medicine, gave a grand rounds presentation about surgical skills atrophy. He talked about the Clinical Readiness Program (Holt, et al. 2021), an initiative to assess the knowledge, skills, and abilities of military surgeons to combat skill atrophy. He opined that military medical treatment facilities did not provide enough demand for general surgery services to achieve readiness. Another way of looking at this was that surgeons in the private sector performed more surgeries than their military surgeon peers who struggled to find balance between operating room time and competing priorities. He discussed a desire for the military medical system to expand access to care, partner with civilian institutions to address these issues, and recapture high knowledge, skills, and ability value procedures. The Air Force referred to this as maintaining provider currency and competency.

Promotion and career progression was weighted toward things outside of the clinical arena, outside of the operating room. Surgeons didn't get promoted for doing surgery. Career progression was more weighted toward "officership." If the emphasis on a surgeon's career progression was focused more on maintaining their skillset, it would be simpler, less stressful, and more rewarding to gain advancement and achieve career satisfaction.

Once, I flew from Hawaii to Okinawa, Japan, after a temporary duty trip with the Marines. The flight was about twelve hours, and there was a significant time difference. I pulled into our home at the Sunabe Seawall outside Gate 1 of Kadena Air Force Base. I was jet-lagged and exhausted. As soon as I got home, my now ex-wife, who was pregnant with our son Billy, was complaining of severe abdominal pain. She was in her early thirties, and never in my wildest dreams did I think she had a serious medical problem. She drove herself to the emergency room at Naval Hospital Okinawa. An hour or two later, I got a call that she had a twisted ovary that was necrotic and needed emergency surgery to remove it. I did make it to the hospital and fell asleep in the waiting room, and a Navy obstetrics and gynecology surgeon, Dr. Arfaa, saved the life of my ex-wife and unborn son.

Dr. Elster has a good point: There is surgical skill atrophy, but there is also skill atrophy across all medical professionals, especially with most medical facilities being closed to family members and retirees.

Sick Role Incentive

My wife and I were sitting at a high school soccer game, watching our son play and talking to the guy next to us who was retired military. He talked about how he served twenty years on active duty, including participating in combat. He started opening up and talked about his coworker, who served on active duty for just two years, who was going to the Veterans Affairs medical center and embellishing his issues to achieve a 100 percent disability rating, even though he appeared perfectly healthy. He remarked, "Hate the game, not the player."

There was a saying in the military health system: "You don't find a medical board; a medical board finds you." Most of the time, it worked out that way, but there were individuals who engaged in disability-seeking behaviors. Some of them were struggling with legitimate issues but were perceived as trying to optimize their disability benefits. A PHS colleague, a Cdr./O5 physical therapist who worked in the brain injury clinic at the Naval Medical Center, told me about how service members presented to appointments requesting "to get things documented" in anticipation of a future Veterans Affairs claim. It was frustrating. Patients suffering from real functional impairment needed those appointments and had difficulty accessing care. These types of behaviors contributed to provider burnout. We went to medical school to help patients, not pad disability claims. These visits were stressful, and patients would get frustrated when they weren't given what they wanted. Thankfully, the number of appointments where the primary purpose was focused on disability was low.

One day I was walking down the hall in my uniform at work. I passed by a gentleman who was bright and cheerful. He thanked me for my service. He stopped me for a second and said, "Stay connected and remember to document everything so you can get your one hundred percent." On another occasion, I was participating in training. The facilitator advocated joining the P&T club. I scratched my head. I had never heard that term before. She explained that it referred to permanent and total disability. She said join the club, don't pay property tax, and get college tuition benefits for your children. A well-known psychiatrist stated that malingering was the easiest diagnosis to understand and the hardest one to diagnose. It really was true. A small number of patients researched mental health disorders, were influenced by social media, and presented to mental health with classic symptoms of a disorder. I was told about so-called barracks lawyers who coached their peers on how to maximize sick role incentives, including money, missed work, canceled deployments, and medical board benefits. It was not always possible to identify if symptoms were being exaggerated. I would conduct a sixty-minute session with a patient, and then, right at the tail end, they would comment about a pending disability claim and ask me to document things in a certain way. The experience left me wondering about the validity of what they told me.

The Navy system pushed sailors on a path to disability. Many sailors worked long hours on ships, were treated harshly, felt unappreciated, and were underpaid. I talked to a sailor who quit a job working for Amazon, took a 50 percent pay cut, worked longer hours as a sailor, and was struggling. He experienced a mental health breakdown and had little motivation or incentive to return to work on a Navy ship. Sailors on ships were an at-risk population for mental health and chronic pain issues. A significant number of them were placed on limited duty. MARMC was well documented as a limited-duty command not conducive to healing and recovery. The choice to return to work wasn't appealing. Sailors could choose to go back to a work environment that had a negative impact on their health and wellness, where they had little chance of success or career progression. Alternatively, they could get out, blame the Navy, and pursue financial incentives for not recovering. A sailor could receive a medical board and disability compensation. There were sailors who were determined to make it back to the ship and continue in the Navy. In my experience, there was an equal number of sailors who lacked motivation or incentive to return to work.

My colleagues and I observed that service members would fall into a hole after suffering from mental health issues. They disconnected from others, isolated socially, lost motivation, lost purpose, stopped working, and used substances, especially alcohol and cannabis. Their identities became centered around being "disabled." It wasn't a full-on choice. Blaming them didn't help, but they had a hand in their fate. It was just sort of a fact or reality that happened. They would learn helplessness, give up their power, and blame the government for all their problems. Getting stuck became a self-perpetuating cycle. Regardless of whether someone was malingering, service members were influenced by financial and other incentives to remain in a sick role. Incentivizing the sick role resulted in financial handcuffs that contributed to the trap they were in.

Research that Never Changes the Trajectory

On a late Friday afternoon at Naval Medical Center Portsmouth, I sat through a four-hour lecture about military suicide, one of many across my career. The lecturer was a professor from a university and had received a multimillion-dollar grant for studying the problem of military suicide. The lecturer discussed assessment and management of military suicide and proposed common terminology and obstacles for providing high-quality care, such as biases of mental health providers.

Every five years or so, I observed and participated in several similar initiatives. There always seemed to be a new fresh look and set of terminology to describe problems. There were always new screening forms to administer patients and verbiage to document risk indicators and treatment planning into the clinical notes we wrote. Despite all this, the same big problems persisted. The military suicide graph, trajectory, and outcomes remained the same. The annual DoD report on suicide in the military from 2022 illustrates this. It shows that the military suicide rate has remained around 20 per 100,000 since 2011, just above the US population average, with minor variances (DoD Under Secretary of Defense of Personnel and Readiness 2022).

There was a downside to the military's reliance on outside consultants for research. The military invested a lot in the recruitment and retention of highly skilled mental health providers. "Deck-plate" is a colloquial term used to describe the deck of a ship where sailors work. This is the ground or front-line level where work occurs. As military mental health providers, we worked at the deck-plate level. We experienced everything firsthand and were ideally situated to have insight into problems, conduct medical research, and make recommendations. I witnessed situations where our recommendations were disregarded, and it impacted morale. Why doesn't the organization value the input of its own people more? Why weren't we allocated time, resources, and leadership support to participate in research?

Research seemed impractical and never addressed the underlying problems or where the rubber met the road. There never seemed to be a way to effectively address the issues of service members having difficulty accessing care, the high churn rate, and attrition of military mental health providers and stigma. From the perspective of the mental health provider, it was frustrating. There were unanswered questions about the value of the research. There was a feeling that the money would have been better spent toward improving access to care.

CHAPTER 10

The Doctor, Patient, and Military Relationship Triangle

EARLY ON IN my Navy career, I was taught that the rank device was worn on the right collar and the Medical Corps oak leaf device went above the heart on the left collar. Most of the time, those devices were aligned, but serving as a Navy psychiatrist was a struggle to balance those different priorities. It was a challenge to balance my own personal wellness, my family's wellness, my ability to get the mission done, and my career progression.

Military mental health providers had a dual role relationship. We worked for the patient and the government simultaneously. Patients were frustrated when there was disagreement with the doctor about their diagnosis or military disposition, especially when it was seen as negatively impacting their career, personal goals, or disability claim. Understandably, patients wanted to take care of themselves, their families, and their needs. When the doctor was perceived as disappointing the patient, it set them up for frustration. The patient wanted to change providers or drop out of treatment.

Veterans Affairs successfully implemented a separate lane for disposition and disability, called compensation and pension ("C&P"). Under this system, the mental health provider works with the patient to provide care, and the C&P section addresses the disability issues. This frees up mental health providers and patients to focus on their relationship and the patient's medical needs. Implementing this at the Naval Medical Center Portsmouth would have been a game changer. Having a team of professionals to independently author disability evaluations and manage medical boards would have improved workflow, reduced stress, and protected against provider burnout. I was told that something similar was being done at Walter Reed Army National Medical Center, and it worked well.

Mental Health Duty Screenings

One of the jobs I had as a military mental health provider was to conduct various duty screenings. Clearing a service member for a specific duty was well intentioned. Disqualifying someone was intended to protect the service member and ensure mission success. I spoke to a junior naval officer who was flown off a ship after she was found to be struggling with an eating disorder and was forcing herself to vomit to lose weight, sometimes several times per day. We felt it wasn't safe for her to return to a ship until her behavior was under control. She wasn't happy about the decision, but it was for her protection. The ship was not equipped to assist someone with this condition. Sending a service member where they had a low chance of success was not fair to the member. If a service member was at high risk for decompensation, we thought the chances are they would continue to struggle, especially in an austere environment, and have a significant risk of being sent home. The process of sending them home would be expensive and burdensome to the military. There were low-hanging fruit situations where a service member who had a history of multiple inpatient psychiatric hospitalizations and recurrent suicidal behaviors was likely to continue to struggle with the same issues and needed to be disqualified.

In practice, my experience was that disqualification was overly conservative. There was a low threshold to disqualify someone for even the slightest "risk of decompensation." For all the energy that was invested in screening processes, there remained unanswered questions about the screening effectiveness. The *USS George Washington* investigation report suggested that one of the sailors who died by suicide had done so with a firearm despite receiving a screening from the ship's psychologist. Screenings were frustrating, and we felt we were spinning our wheels, doing something that had questionable value. Our time, energy, and professional skill set would have been better utilized helping people rather than chasing paper tigers.

Most frequently, I encountered the consequences of the screening process going wrong. Disqualifying someone unnecessarily felt harsh and discriminating from the service member's perspective. It contributed to increased stigma and mistrust of the Navy's mental health system.

I spoke with service members who had minimal mental health issues that were adequately controlled but were deemed unfit during a duty screening evaluation. They were directed to be placed back on limited duty or to undergo a medical board. The personnel actions were unwanted, there was no disability or functional impairment to drive such actions, and they generated a lot of work. The providers were caught in the middle of these situations, required to perform unnecessary work, and were easy targets for the patient's frustration and complaints.

Sometimes it felt as if the military did not want to deal with individuals with mental health issues and had a propensity to disqualify or discharge them. That type of mentality was short-sighted. It wasn't using resources wisely to invest hundreds of thousands of dollars into a service member and then not permit them to do their job based on a small technicality without clear and sufficient justification. A family member's disqualification during the overseas screening could result in a geographic family separation. The service member would travel overseas unaccompanied, and their spouse would remain behind in the continental United States.

There was a news article that described a scenario where two children received mental health treatment inside the DoD health system while their parents were deployed. Years later, when they became adults, they tried to enlist. Their childhood electronic records were scrubbed. They were disqualified from military service based on those records (Jowers 2018). The article said that despite receiving multiple clean bills of health from civilian and DoD behavioral health providers, they were denied waivers to enter the military.

My professional colleagues and I tried to advocate for our patients as best we could to counter and negate the consequences. Sometimes we were successful, and sometimes the service member got disqualified despite our best efforts. It was a disappointment dealing with these situations.

The Struggle to Determine Duty Status

In many career fields—law enforcement, firefighting, aviation, and military service—there is a fitness-for-duty concept. The idea is that individuals are required to be mentally and physically fit to serve. Fitness for duty is common sense. It is not desirable to have a police officer with violent tendencies, such as a history of recurrent assaults. We would not want a firefighter with uncontrolled alcoholism and recurrent DUIs operating a fire truck.

Military medical and mental health providers were tasked with making determinations and judgment calls regarding service members' fitness for duty and military disposition. Some situations were obvious and easy to solve, while others were much more challenging. If a service member had a broken leg, cancer, recent surgery, or some other visible or easily measurable condition, such as abnormal lab values or radiology studies, it was a simple call to determine whether a service member was fit for duty.

Placing a service member on limited duty had significant implications. A service member would be put into a protected status, likely removed from an operational environment, and classified as nondeployable. Limited duty could result in an unplanned personnel loss for the unit, creating a situation where the remaining service members would have to work harder to make up for manpower loss. Limited duty could also place sailors in a difficult situation where their command and shipmates unfairly blamed them for wanting to quit.

For mental health, a typical scenario was that a service member at an operational command was identified as hitting a breaking point. In the best-case scenario, the service member had an opportunity to receive several mental health treatment sessions prior to being placed on limited duty. Other times, the service member presented to the emergency department asking for help or received a medical evacuation from deployment. The evaluating mental health provider observed that the service member struggling with suicidal thoughts was not able to function in an operational setting and was initiated a period of limited duty. The service member was removed from the command or reassigned to a less stressful job for a time, often six months, for further evaluation, treatment, and recuperation. At the end of the first period of limited duty, the service member was reassessed for return to duty, medical board, or a second limited-duty period, or they were recommended for administrative personnel action.

Physical health and mental health issues were viewed differently at times. There were outlying situations where these issues intersected and there was disagreement between medical specialists. There was a female service member in her early twenties who started out on limited duty for mental health issues. She was found to have a pelvic mass, had surgery, then complained of chronic pelvic pain. She was later diagnosed with endometriosis. The psychiatrist wrote that the patient was fit for full duty and recommended she be returned to duty, although it clearly wasn't the case. Maybe her mental health issues had improved, but overall, she was not fit for duty. The patient was encouraged to follow up with her surgeon to be placed on limited duty for her physical health issues. I became familiar with the case a year or two later after she developed an opioid addiction to painkillers. I was surprised to see that she was never recommended for further limited duty or a medical board. Another patient suffered from ulcerative colitis and developed anxiety and panic attacks. He started out on limited duty for physical health issues but developed debilitating mental health issues. There were situations where a service member had numerous small medical conditions. None of the conditions by themselves were impairing, but when aggregated together, the overall result was significant impairment. These situations were challenging because, rarely, a medical provider would initiate limited duty or a medical board for someone like this. Making the correct judgment call required a medical provider to take a step back and evaluate the overall whole person.

There was another twist to fitness for duty. Service members could be deemed fit for duty but not suitable for continued military service. If a service member had a short time in service and immediately fell apart after arriving at their first duty station, they could be considered to have failed to adapt to military life. If a service member had a difficult personality, they could be deemed incompatible with military life. Mental health providers, service members, and commands often found themselves in challenging situations regarding these issues. Service members hit a breaking point and had difficulty functioning. Commands were frustrated that their service member couldn't do their job or needed a replacement, and the medical provider was tasked with deciding whether it was a fixable condition, a defect of character, or a medical disability. Commands and mental health providers were pressured to prevent unplanned personnel losses. If a service member experienced a mental health crisis in response to a toxic environment, such as the *USS George Washington*, one way to look at the situation was that they suffered a psychological injury and needed a period of limited duty for treatment. Another way to look at the situation was that the service member failed to adapt, was flawed, and was incompatible with military life. These determinations frequently fell to a medical provider's judgment call. If a medical provider found a service member fit but unsuitable, service members faced administrative personnel actions that resulted in discharge from military service. Separating service members who did not want to leave the Navy sent a viral message to other sailors not to participate in mental health treatment.

In my experience, the Army, Navy, and Air Force all had different procedures, standards, and computer systems for implementing, managing, and tracking limited duty. The Air Force had a lower threshold to put people on limited duty, and the Navy had a higher threshold. If a patient had an inpatient psychiatric hospitalization in the Air Force system, they were placed on limited duty for at least a brief time. The Navy did not do this. Many patients left the hospital, returned to work, and went on deployments, including multiweek ship underways. I can recall a situation early in my career when a Navy ship called the inpatient psychiatry unit asking when their sailor was going to be discharged so they could pick him up and take him on a Middle East deployment. Not surprisingly, a short time after leaving for deployment, the sailor received an aeromedical evacuation back to the inpatient psychiatry unit after he decompensated again.

In the Naval Medical Center Portsmouth Tri-Service Market, there were Navy bases, an Army base, and an Air Force base. There was a Navy installation located in Yorktown, Virginia. The closest military treatment facilities were Army and Air Force clinics located at Joint Base Langley-Eustis. Receiving the right help included treatment from a medical provider, being provided the right referrals and medications, and receiving the appropriate administrative and personnel actions. If a sailor received care at an Army or Air Force clinic, they did not receive Navy-specific personnel actions due to service-specific differences and lack of integration. If a sailor was evaluated in an Air Force mental health clinic, ideally the provider could log into a unified DHA information system and initiate a limited-duty period using DoD standards, but that wasn't possible. A sailor would receive the appropriate mental health intervention and be referred to a Navy mental health clinic for the appropriate personnel actions. Sometimes a sailor would be told they needed to be on limited duty, but a Navy medical provider would later make a conflicting judgment call that it was not warranted.

I spoke with a Navy psychiatrist who served at a large joint military hospital. She frequently provided mental health treatment for airmen but could not access the ASIMS limited-duty system to complete the necessary limited-duty paperwork. She complained that the Air Force also utilized a different set of terminology for their limited-duty paperwork as well.

There were screenings to serve at overseas duty stations, to maintain flight status, to serve on a submarine, and to be a recruiter or a boot camp drill instructor. Each of their services had different guidelines and nuances for how these situations were handled. I served on a joint Army and Air Force base. Soldiers went to the Army mental health clinic on one side of the base, and airmen went to the behavioral health flight on the other side of the base. One day an airman and soldier were both considered for overseas PCS to South Korea with the same mental health condition, PTSD. The determination from the Army was that the soldier could PCS overseas, but the airman going to the same geographic location was disqualified, placed on limited duty, and not permitted to PCS. Each military service had some form of aviation medicine. The Navy and Air Force had different standards for evaluating pilots.

Other situations I encountered during my career were patients who successfully completed mental health treatment or had mild mental health issues yet were directed to be placed on limited duty or receive a medical board. Service members found themselves in limbo situations. They were doing very well and had no disability, but on paper they were being directed to undergo limited duty or a medical board.

The services viewed and managed substance use disorders differently from a duty status perspective. The Air Force and Army placed service members on limited duty when they struggled with significant substance use disorders. The limited-duty status designation was important. The Air Force considered an airman nondeployable when they were participating in substance use treatment. The Navy did not. Contemporary thought was that substance abuse disorders were medical conditions and a disease model was recommended, but from a limited duty perspective, substance use disorders weren't handled like medical disorders in the Navy.

Time elapsed since a previous mental health incident was an issue that came up regarding military disposition and clearance determination. What was the time cutoff to disqualify someone based on a prior suicide attempt, previous inpatient psychiatric hospitalization, domestic violence incident, or alcohol incident? Clearly, if a service member had such a behavior in the past month, they were at increased risk of having another. Some felt the time cutoff should be six months, twelve months, two years, or even longer. I witnessed situations where personnel actions were initiated against service members because of something that happened five years ago or more.

From a DoD perspective, it is logical that the same standards should be used across all services. How mental health issues, substance use disorders, and other issues are managed should be the same. From the healthcare provider perspective, there were too many policies to look at, and it was confusing. It would make sense to clearly spell out when and under what circumstances a patient should be placed on limited duty. From the service member standpoint, there was conflicting guidance and increased stigma, and this resulted in fear about receiving mental health assistance.

Fit for Duty but Disqualified

A young service member in the office where I worked told me her story, which illustrated challenges with fitness for duty and the medical boards process. In March 2019 she noticed a golf ball-sized lump in her neck. She went to her ship's medical department and was given reassurance. About a month later, she began having a cough and went back to medical. Soon after this, she was diagnosed with Hodgkin's lymphoma, a form of cancer, and was placed on limited duty and removed from the operational environment. By the late fall of 2019 she completed six courses of chemotherapy and achieved remission of her cancer. In early 2021 her doctor determined that she was fit for duty but recommended assignment limitations. She needed frequent follow-up and imaging studies for cancer surveillance and was disqualified from working in an operational setting. She communicated with the detailer and was directed to undergo the medical boards process. She found herself in a Catch-22 situation. She felt her doctor and the Navy had conflicting views or standards for the medical boards process. She felt caught in the crossfire and forced to have a medical board. She was told she was medically fine but operationally not fine. She explained that she worked in nuclear power but could no longer work in radiation due to her history of cancer. She complained of anxiety about relapse and suffered complications from the chemotherapy, including joint pain. The medical boards process was delayed by the COVID-19 pandemic, and it took eighteen months to complete. She felt negatively impacted by the process. She lost eligibility to get promoted and lost competency in her career field. In August 2021 her medical board results came back. She was awarded 60 percent disability by Veterans Affairs but 0 percent from the Navy. She did not feel the decision was fair. She complained that she was found fit for full duty despite the fact that she couldn't do her job and was nondeployable. She had a formal board in October 2021. She felt the panel decided before the hearing that she was fit for duty, didn't listen, and found her fit for duty again. She was frustrated by the experience. She felt the medical board's process was worse than cancer and the paperwork was more important than the person. Instead of undergoing a medical board, she felt she should have been allowed to receive a PCS to a different command.

Overseas Clearance for Family Members

An Army spouse wrote an op-ed about a negative experience she and her husband, an active-duty soldier, had with the overseas screening process while serving in El Paso, Texas (Flory 2022). The couple received orders for their dream assignment in Germany. They put their house under contract for sale, sold their vehicles, and prepared their family. She was receiving nonmedical counseling for anxiety and had minimal mental health needs. She was disqualified from the PCS, and the orders were changed to make the assignment an unaccompanied tour for her husband. She and her husband felt harmed by an overly conservative personnel decision. It caused anxiety, relationship distress, and financial loss. She wrote in her op-ed that a lesson learned was to check *no* on any mental health screening questions. She wrote that the military was driving those in need underground with situations like hers. She was enrolled in the EFMP program. She wrote about feeling ashamed and concerned that her anxiety and EFMP status would negatively impact her husband's future career assignments. There is a good chance serving in an overseas tour was a career milestone, and not being able to access such an assignment impacted his promotion opportunities and career progression. She recommended an overhaul to the EFMP program in her article.

The exact details of the situation were unknown. She did not discuss any recurrent suicidal behaviors, inpatient psychiatric hospitalizations, or repeated substance abuse incidents that would have been clear grounds for disqualification, but we can read between the lines. I witnessed these situations repeatedly across my career. The medical provider conducting the review used conservative screening standards, and the gaining command didn't want to take any risk of having to deal with a difficult case. Screening guidelines were murky, and there were no protections in policy. There wasn't a clear way for her to file a complaint or seek redress regarding the situation, and there was no accountability for those making the decisions.

A colleague who served with the Air Force told me the story of a situation that occurred with a career LtCol/O5 and his medical group commander. The Air Force officer needed an overseas assignment for career progression, but his spouse had severe depression, and he was recommended for disqualification for overseas assignment in accordance with policy. The commander intervened and asked for the request to be approved, but the colleague declined. Ultimately, my colleague was overruled. The overseas clearance request was granted. The officer and his wife received an overseas transfer, and there was a positive outcome. How situations were handled were inconsistent at times. Sometimes the military had a very low threshold to disqualify someone. Other times the military could turn a blind eye if the situation was seen as in the military's best interests.

Substance Abuse Evaluation, Management, and Treatment

Each military service has its own substance abuse treatment programs. The Navy had the SARP and command DAPAs. The Coast Guard had the Substance Abuse Prevention Program and Command Drug and Alcohol Representatives (CDARs). The command DAPA and CDAR were collateral duty, peer volunteer positions that performed administrative functions, service coordination, and education. The Army had the Substance Use Disorder Clinical

Care (SUDCC), and the Air Force had the Alcohol and Drug Abuse Prevention and Treatment Program (ADAPT). The Army and Air Force did not utilize peer volunteer positions for their substance abuse programs. Administrative and case management functions were performed from within the SUDCC and ADAPT programs.

I worked at a residential treatment program for the Navy. We performed substance abuse evaluations and delivered all types of treatment, including level 0.5, 1, 2, and 3 treatments. The level 0.5 and 1 treatments were brief several-day treatments. The level 2 and 3 programs were thirty-day programs. The difference between level 2 and 3 was that the latter was a residential treatment program, and patients slept at the facility. We even had a virtual level 2.1 program where patients participated by video for six weeks. We had a medical screening form that documented a physical exam, labs, and a service member's physical health needs. We had a continuing-care program where patients participated in aftercare following level 3 residential treatment. Our program conducted drug testing to ensure sobriety. Our facility had a first right of refusal. If we didn't have any bed space, we could defer a patient to a residential treatment facility in the area.

There were interesting nuances between the services. The access to care and referral timelines differed. When I worked for the Air Force, service members were placed on limited duty when they were receiving substance abuse treatment. The Navy did not do this. The issue was a problem because there were sailors who had a DUI incident immediately prior to a shipboard deployment. They could be assigned to a shore detachment to undergo treatment, but sometimes their treatment was delayed, they were deployed, or they later suffered another alcohol incident at a foreign port or second DUI after they came home. A similar situation occurred when a service member was identified as having an alcohol problem immediately prior to PCS. They were told they were fit for duty and to enroll in substance abuse treatment after arriving at their new duty station. When service members changed duty stations, they frequently slipped through the cracks, only to turn up a year later after another alcohol incident. The *USS George Washington* investigation report described a situation where a sailor was referred for help with alcohol issues but was noncompliant with follow-up with the command DAPA and slipped through the cracks.

Among all the services, there was debate about when and under what circumstances a patient could be deferred to the network. Our department head was under pressure not to defer patients to the network due to cost savings. There was variation between the services in how readily able they were to send patients to the TRICARE network. Many network substance abuse treatment facilities performed in-house detoxification where patients could be treated for alcohol withdrawal and then immediately begin residential treatment. At our facility, patients were hospitalized on the internal medicine or psychiatry inpatient units first. It felt like a roll of the dice for them to receive a bed-to-bed transfer to our facility to begin care after their withdrawal was treated.

How substance use disorder patients were tracked for referral and compliance was an issue. There was no centralized information technology system for this. Sometimes patients referred to substance use treatment and were lost without being seen. Other times they would complete their referral, be recommended for a high level of treatment, and then disappear. It was not uncommon for patients to be diagnosed with a substance use disorder immediately prior to deployment, PCS, get lost, and never complete treatment, only to turn up months or years later after another incident. Another scenario that occurred was when the command DAPA left with no replacement or turnover and service members were lost to follow-up.

The DoD IG published a report on active-duty service member alcohol misuse screening and treatment that highlighted many of these problems (DoD Inspector General 2022). The report found that service members were not assessed and treated in a timely manner because guidance was unclear and inconsistent. Thirty-nine percent (104/270) service members did not have an intake assessment to diagnose an alcohol use disorder within DHA or service-established time frames, 36 percent (98/270) did not receive the recommended treatment in a timely manner, and three service members were diagnosed but did not receive their recommended treatment. The report recommended that the DHA establish a maximum number of days between a substance abuse referral and an intake assessment and establish the maximum number of days to provide treatment following a diagnosis.

The military was making a transition to adopting a medical disease model for substance abuse and to improve care and recognition of co-occurring disorders. One of my predecessors, a Navy psychiatrist, was notorious for being dismissive about co-occurring disorders, removing diagnoses, and abruptly discontinuing medications. She would tell patients with both PTSD and alcoholism that their main problem was alcohol and to stop all their PTSD medications. The Navy went through a difficult time period in the early 2010s and was known for overdiagnosing sailors with severe alcoholism. The diagnosis was based on local leadership, personalities, and twisted thought processes. I think there were some good intentions behind the practice. I suspect they wanted to definitively help sailors and stop alcohol issues before they got worse. Overdiagnosing sailors with a substance use disorder could result in a black mark on a member's record and discharge if they declined care, and it stacked the deck against them by setting them up for discharge in the case of relapse. There was also this twisted dynamic that the individuals involved acted as if they were the Navy mental health police and were motivated to remove sailors with these issues to improve operational readiness. Thankfully, in recent years, there has been a shift to using more objective criteria and adherence to treatment guidelines.

The policies and procedures concerning substance abuse were broad and lacked specifics. It wasn't clearly defined when and under what circumstances a patient would be admitted to the hospital. An active-duty service member presented to the emergency room requesting detoxification from alcohol. He reported drinking fifteen beers and eight shots of liquor per day. In the triage area, he was counseled in front of his chief/E7 that he could not be admitted because he was not a harm to himself or others. The patient had worked up the courage to go to the emergency room and ask for help from his chain of command. He felt hurt and discouraged. He returned home and resumed drinking. It was true he wasn't suicidal, but the command was furious, and the patient felt hurt. He couldn't control his drinking. In the command's eyes, he was hurting himself due to his drinking, volume, and frequency of alcohol use. The situation had a good outcome. About a week later he was admitted to the hospital, received an alcohol detoxification, and received a bed-to-bed transfer to our residential treatment program. Other times, a patient would make it into the emergency room and would be sent home with a prescription for an outpatient benzodiazepine taper. Someone coined the term "Librium in a box" for this. I don't think I ever saw an "outpatient detox" work. Often, a patient would take the benzodiazepine, relapse alcohol use on top of that, and end up back in the emergency room days later. I was told outpatient treatment had its advantages and was preferred because sailors were protected from career consequences of having certain diagnoses, such as a severe drinking problem, in their record.

When the decision was made to admit a patient to the hospital for detoxification, there was often a Samuel Shem *House of God*-style turf battle between internal medicine and psychiatry regarding who should perform the detoxification. The emergency room and patients were caught in the middle. The psychiatry service would argue that the patient wasn't suicidal or would exaggerate clinical concerns about possible withdrawal complications. I was aware that one of the psychiatrists had created a quick reference guide of medical justifications for declining admission to the inpatient psychiatry unit, backed up by references. Most of the time, the patient would end up on the internal medicine service. The internists did a great job. The hospitalization was effective at getting through withdrawal, but the internal medicine unit didn't have the therapeutic milieu that the psychiatry unit had. Patients would sit and watch TV during their stay. Internal medicine did not have the mental health discharge planning capability that the inpatient psychiatry unit had. Often, a patient with severe alcoholism was discharged home or back to the command without adequate care coordination. Some would immediately relapse and rapidly bounce back to the hospital. Others would slip through the cracks and be lost to follow-up, only to turn up a year later after another incident.

Similar issues occurred with opioid withdrawal. Patients with heroin addiction, suffering from opioid withdrawal in the private sector, were admitted to the psychiatry unit and prescribed medications, including buprenorphine and clonidine to ease their withdrawal. In the Navy system, patients were counseled that they weren't suffering from a life-threatening illness and often would be discharged home. From my perspective, if a service member was struggling from uncontrolled addiction, they were optimally treated in a healthcare setting, where they could receive a medically supervised detox and not access the substances they were using, to break the cycle of addiction. Placing service members in a healthcare setting freed up commands from trying to self-manage substance use disorders so they could focus on getting the mission done.

Service members were reluctant to disclose the use of illicit drugs during residential treatment, even after being confronted about positive urine drug screens. They were terrified to be honest and make further disclosures about illicit drug use out of fear of getting in more trouble and losing their career or military benefits. It was a disappointing situation for both the treating providers and service members. The military was sending them to an expensive substance abuse treatment program, but the service members couldn't get the most out of it due to fears of getting in more trouble.

How situations regarding medical compliance drug testing results and treatment failures were handled and played out was inconsistent and chaotic. There was an unwritten rule that a service member hadn't "failed treatment" until level-three residential treatment was completed. We were told relapses were part of the treatment recovery process, but there wasn't clear guidance on how this should look. It wasn't clear when commands would be notified about positive drug tests. Sometimes patients "popped positive" one to three times, a treatment team meeting was conducted with the command, and then they were deemed a treatment failure. Separation from military service due to treatment failure was selectively enforced. There wasn't clear guidance about time frames between relapses. If a service member went five years between relapses, they should get a second chance compared to someone who went a few months without drinking. There were high-risk patients who suffered numerous substance abuse treatment failures who remained on active duty and others who were treated much more harshly. Sometimes service members with unresolved or unaddressed substance abuse issues were identified during the duty screening process. They got stuck in a limbo-type situation where they weren't qualified for transfer to the gaining command but were not processed out for treatment failure. Service members suffering from substance abuse issues faced multiple lanes of adverse actions. They could face separation due to personnel actions, be placed on limited duty due to medical reasons, or face disciplinary action and discharge due to misconduct.

Early in my training, I recall a memorable case. A soldier joined the Army to get off cocaine. He lasted a very brief amount of time. He had an inpatient psychiatric hospitalization. The Army planned to discharge him. Two years later, I got a call from a lawyer asking about the case. The Army retained him on active duty, and he continued to struggle with cocaine addiction.

The Challenges of Being a Uniformed Healthcare Provider

Many uniformed healthcare providers joined the military through a commissioning program where their medical school or other professional education is paid for. In exchange, they owe a payback of time and service. Graduates of the Health Professions Scholarship Program program owed four years. The military has its own medical school, USUHS. USUHS graduates accumulated a seven-year payback. There were some who felt they made the right career decision, but there were others who were miserable, felt like indentured servants, and were vocal about it.

Active-duty healthcare providers were told they were soldiers, sailors, and airmen first. They were under constant pressure to keep the chain of command happy, achieve career progression, and gain advancement. Sometimes promotion was highly competitive and a do-or-die scenario. If a service member was passed over twice for promotion, they faced potential release from military service. The career path for a medical officer didn't seem to make sense. Getting promoted didn't equate to being the best leader or top healthcare professional. It frequently equated to navigating political processes, qualifying for military special warfare devices, earning military awards, and looking good on paper. There was a feeling that the balance was off, and the career progression system needed to be tweaked more toward healthcare professional core competencies. Time and brain power would have been better spent worrying about how to assist service members, getting them back to the fight rather than having to navigate the career progression system. Promotion and career progression criteria would have been better focused on the education, knowledge, and skill sets needed to improve readiness and a successful health system.

Active-duty medical providers were undervalued except during times of crisis and got a bad rap for being expensive. It was a frustrating situation. The reality was that nonmilitary physicians outside of the military health system had higher compensation than military physicians. One could argue that active-duty providers weren't as productive as their nonmilitary counterparts; however, that comparison was apples to oranges. Nonmilitary providers had better IT systems, weren't concerned with fitness-for-duty issues, and didn't have military collateral duties.

Medical Readiness Mindset

During my time at Naval Medical Center Portsmouth, a senior medical flag officer from the DHA spoke at an all-officers' call about the state of the military medical system. He showed a photo of a small military boat with a dozen crew members. He estimated that, due to medical issues, limited duty, and other issues, three of the twelve crew members were unable to serve on the boat due to a combination of medical and other issues. He asked the audience which three service members were nonessential and should be picked. My colleagues and I were under constant pressure to keep service members in a full-duty status. Another perspective was that it would be a much better situation to be undermanned and have nine healthy service members on the boat. With an additional member with a severe health condition, the remaining nine members would have to invest considerable time and energy supporting the ill one instead of getting the mission done. On a different note, how about fixing the underlying personnel system issues by increasing baseline manning above 100 percent to anticipate predictable unplanned personnel losses?

There were legendary military tales where service members showed up for an overseas deployment asking for medication refills for their kidney transplant or methadone refills for their heroin addiction. Service members were taken on deployment prematurely only for the military to send them back at great expense. Forcing someone to do something they didn't feel ready or able to do rarely ended in success. If there was any question or concern as to whether a service member was medically ready, the best choice was to err on the side of caution and keep them behind.

From the perspective of a healthcare provider, senior leadership had a love-hate relationship with medical. When a service member needed emergent medical help or there was an urgent medical mission to be accomplished, we were rock stars. During the rest of the time, medical received a bad rap for taking members out of the fight and being expensive. Medical professionals were told that our recommendations decreased manning, increased workload of the remaining service members, and decreased the lethality of the military. The reality was that the service member's medical condition and, more frequently, work environment issues were more important factors contributing to attrition. Squeezing medical providers to improve medical readiness increased our stress and burnout levels.

Command Influence

The orders, needs, and desires of the chain of command were a powerful driving force. The command had so much power in the military. The command's input heavily influenced promotion and career progression through performance reviews. The command controlled professional qualifications, place of work, pay, leave requests, awards, and disciplinary actions. Commands had the power to remove a service member from their position, deny them any meaningful work, and essentially ban them from coming to work with little recourse.

One of my colleagues was an Air Force Cpt./O3. He served as a Family Advocacy officer during a Family Advocacy Case Review Committee. The committee unanimously voted to find a domestic violence allegation unsubstantiated. Much to everyone's surprise and horror, the deputy wing commander, a col/O6, unilaterally ordered the finding to be substantiated. He refused to back down even when presented with the relevant Air Force instructions.

He took my colleague to a private room and lectured him for half an hour. Everyone on the committee was put in a compromising position, and no one wanted to cross the deputy wing commander. Fortunately, the medical group commander, another col/O6, convinced him to reverse his position.

I spoke to an Army mental health officer, Maj./O4, who was both a psychiatric nurse practitioner and a licensed clinical social worker. His supervisor was a LTC/O5 doctoral-level psychologist. The psychologist felt threatened by his ability to prescribe medications and refused to provide endorsement for the clinical privileges necessary to do so. The psychiatric nurse practitioner had no recourse and was caught in a compromising situation. The psychologist who refused to grant the clinical privileges was also the person that signed his annual performance review. If the psychiatric nurse practitioner complained over his head, there would have been consequences.

The service member's commander was an employer and prosecutor simultaneously. If a service member was perceived as crossing the command, they quickly found themselves in a compromising position. A senior Navy psychiatrist described this to me as "getting crushed." There was an unwritten annual performance review category for maintaining loyalty to the command. Service members who were perceived as disloyal ran the risk of getting blackballed and having their career derailed. There was a constant threat of retaliation and retribution. Service members who were perceived as not being on the team found their whole career getting stagnated and sandbagged in a cascade of negative personnel actions. I spoke with a psychiatrist who was a USUHS graduate and had a lengthy multiyear payback. She came to work every day with anxiety and lived in fear. She felt terrified of the military and didn't want to make anyone angry. She wanted to be viewed as part of the team, loyal to the command, and not be denied any career opportunity.

The military medical system was sometimes a bullying-type environment where medical providers were frequently pressured and second-guessed. Most of the time, military leaders worked collaboratively with the medical department, but there were many times when there was an adversarial relationship between the two. A unit commander complained to their flag officer about something that happened. For example, the command disagreed with the diagnosis, military disposition recommendation, or wait times in the emergency department or for an appointment. Then the hospital commander or other senior medical official was attacked. The toxicity rolled downhill to the department head and then to the individual provider who was trying to do the right thing. "How does this make us look?" we were told.

At times there was pressure to make or avoid a major diagnosis as well as initiate a medical board or limited-duty period by senior officials. There was pressure to either return or disqualify patients from duty, depending on the situation. In some cases, a high-ranking officer would call and pressure a military mental health provider to remove or facilitate certain personnel actions for so-called "command interest" high-visibility patients.

I encountered several situations where rank was used to cross professional boundaries. There were several situations where a mid-level provider of a higher rank would scrutinize and torment a physician of a lower rank. They could never get away with this behavior in most employment settings except in the military.

When I was a young LT in Okinawa, Japan, I was consulted on a marine who was incarcerated in a military brig for cocaine addiction. I was asked to sign off on him deploying and had a disagreement with his senior marine commanding officer, a col/O6. The marine commander told me what would help the marine with his drug addiction was taking him out of jail and putting him on deployment. I disagreed and expressed concern that it was a risk to the organization, command, and the service member. Ultimately, the marine commander did exactly what he said he would do and overruled my recommendation. The marine was freed from jail and taken on deployment. To my surprise and relief, everything worked out well, and there was no backlash.

Working in the military medical system was trying to achieve balance between the rank and medical corps collar devices. Most of the time, it was aligned, but there were occasions when the chain of command directed and influenced the outcome of situations, and it was frustrating and stressful for the healthcare providers, patients, and other parties who were caught in the middle.

Promotion System Drives Everything

Service members who were effective in career progression were adept at ladder climbing. They were always thinking about and planning for the next assignment and looking for the next ladder rung. I had a mentor once who carefully studied who was promoted to flag officer. He made a list of the jobs that served as stepping stones for promotion and sought after them. Service members were looking at how to make the person above them look good to lock in a performance review or award necessary to reach a career milestone and facilitate promotion. If an important assignment opportunity opened, a service member had to be ready to PCS on short notice to pursue a critical career opportunity.

The annual performance review system required that each sailor be given an overall classification: *Early Promote*, *Must Promote*, *Promotable*, or *Do Not Promote*. Early Promote was the highest ranking, and commands had a limited number of those ratings that can be assigned. There were "murder boards," where commands "racked and stacked" candidates, internally debated, and determined who should receive the most highly sought-after ratings.

Frequently, who needed to be promoted drove decision-making in the military health system. I had a conversation with a colleague who was struggling to gain advancement. He had to apply for a job he didn't want solely to facilitate his promotion. If someone was leaving military service, they would be removed from leadership roles, and a junior service member with career potential would be put into those roles to beef up their résumé. Individuals who were leaving the military were low-hanging fruit. They could be assigned lower rankings on their performance reviews to free up the better rankings for those who needed them for career progression.

I was told by multiple military medical officers across different services that active-duty officers held the plum positions and leadership roles, while everyone else, including federal employees, contractors, and officers from different services, "did the work." There wasn't much choice about it. Active-duty officers had to have leadership positions to be considered for promotion. There was a lot of talent in the workspace, but often the more junior and less experienced service members were put in charge of operations, and they struggled. I never experienced an optimal mix or ratio of active duty, civil service, and contractors.

A psychiatrist who served at a large military hospital talked about a similar phenomenon between services. At this facility, the Army had a heavy presence and held most of the leadership positions. There were a smaller number of sailors. She felt there were aspects of the Army and Navy's cultures and priorities that clashed. She was concerned about career progression issues while serving at a non-Navy facility.

An article about flag officer promotion by Capt. Kevin Eyer, US Navy (retired), captured the pressures naval officers face. He described a secret "watch list" system (Eyer 2016). He wrote this to achieve promotion:

> You must be fully supportive of Navy policies, whatever they may be. Cynical compliance will not be welcome. Actually, cynicism of any sort is unwelcome. You do not want to be identified as one of those poor souls who simply doesn't "get

> it": *More than one promising officer "died" by perversely (if sensibly) opposing the Littoral Combat Ship. . . . You must execute your job with unfailing enthusiasm, even in the face of what may be surprising expectations.*

Capt. Eyer's specific example of the littoral combat ship (LCS) is especially relevant because, in recent years, the LCS program has struggled, and many LCS ships have been decommissioned prior to the end of their anticipated life expectancy (US Government Accountability Office 2022). His words capture the plight of the active-duty service member. In many organizations, there is pressure to be a "yes man," but it's especially true in the military. Service members find themselves in situations where they must bite their lip, put on a pleasant face, and carry out the mission even if it doesn't make sense.

CHAPTER 11

Information Technology Issues

WE WORKED WITH numerous information systems that had different functionality and were independent of each other. The result was fragmented data, closed systems, and inefficiency. The main medical records system was called AHLTA. This was where the clinical progress notes were stored. We had another system called CHCS that was a legacy command line system where appointment scheduling was done. It was necessary to access both the AHLTA and CHCS systems because CHCS contained information AHLTA did not. For example, we conducted urine drug testing. AHLTA would not display labs that were pending or requisition numbers, so we had to log into CHCS to see if the drug screens had been drawn by the lab. Also, only CHCS could display future appointment dates.

There was a system called the Behavioral Health Data Portal (BHDP) that was a measurement-based care initiative. Patients would sit at a kiosk in our clinic prior to their appointments and complete scientifically validated mental health rating scales. Frequently, this would delay appointment start times. The system was opened to the internet in early 2022 so patients could complete their information from home or work prior to their appointment.

There were delays in implementing remote access for years due to various roadblocks, including security concerns. There were two other systems we used. One was called HAIMS that was intended to contain scanned records from network providers to coordinate care, but the records rarely made it there. Another system was called the Joint Legacy Viewer (JLV). JLV was used to access records from the Veterans Affairs Medical System. Each of the services had different systems to track limited duty. The Navy used LIMDU Smart, the Air Force used ASIMS, and the Army used eProfile in MODS to track limited duty.

For inpatient records, Naval Medical Center Portsmouth used a system called Essentris where hospital discharge summaries were stored. There was a separate system used by the emergency department called T-System. Emergency department notes were not input into AHLTA or Essentris. One day I was asked to consult on a service member in the emergency department. I was surprised to see that my T-System account had been deactivated. I was told the system was overloaded with too many users. It took some wrangling, but I was able to get my account restored and access the necessary information.

I attended a presentation at Naval Medical Center Portsmouth given by one of the senior DoD officials managing one of the above systems. He complained that the services were reluctant to adopt the system, although it had been congressionally mandated. He described internal issues his team was facing. He complained that the system's contract went up for renewal and the outgoing contractor was outbid, although they were doing a great job at a critical point in the development process. The outgoing contractor left on a Friday, and the new contractor came on a Monday. He indicated that the government might have saved short-term money on the contract, but there was disruption, delay, and long-term cost increases. He discussed efforts to integrate the system into other associated DoD systems. He said, technologically, it was an easy fix, but a contract amendment was required, and the vendor requested a multimillion-dollar payout to make the change. This made improved integration impossible.

The state of Virginia had a sophisticated prescription monitoring system for tracking controlled substance use, but it wasn't integrated with the above electronic systems. Medicines ordered through the military system did not make it into the state database. Toward the end of my time at Naval Medical Center Portsmouth, forward progress had been made achieving this.

There was another system called the Protected Health Information Management Tool (PHIMT). Healthcare providers were asked to record protected health information disclosures anytime they disclosed medical information to the command. Another electronic system received electronic DoD Suicide Event Reports (DoDSER) to improve suicide surveillance efforts. From my experience, the DoDSER and PHIMT systems were rarely used.

To conduct an outpatient visit, medical providers had to coordinate and integrate information across all these systems simultaneously. For a really complex patient, I reviewed notes in AHLTA, reviewed labs in CHCS, used CHCS to check for possible future scheduled appointments, reviewed self-reported rating scales in BHDP, reviewed inpatient records in Essentris, checked scanned records in HAIMS, queried the state prescription monitoring program for possible controlled substance misuse, and accessed the limited duty system to see if the patient was on limited duty or if a medical board had been initiated. On top of all that, I had to read and respond to emails about the patient.

Acquiring, Deploying, and Maintaining Information Technology Systems

Across my career, I experienced the rollout of different military information systems. The DoD struggled with AHLTA and again with the MHS Genesis rollout. When I worked for the Coast Guard, it acquired the Epic medical records system, but the project was ultimately canceled. The Epic system was purchased by the Coast Guard in 2010. There were roadblocks and delays, and the project was canceled in 2016 (Sullivan 2017). The military faced a different set of challenges and obstacles regarding the procurement and maintenance of technology compared with the private sector.

I was involved in situations where various information technology system bugs, glitches, and feature requests were identified and submitted. I attended meetings, participated in telephone conferences, and sent emails to developers, but it was always an uphill battle to get things fixed. On the other hand, I had a part-time job working for a large private health system that implemented a successful rollout of Epic in a short period of time.

The DoD and military services were at a significant disadvantage due to the procurement process. Unlike the private sector, the government couldn't go after a specific system or company when it wanted to procure a system. The government had to generate a list of requirements and then have a highly regulated open competitive bidding process. In the private sector, a company had more flexibility and could purchase the best piece of equipment no matter what the cost, but government procurement didn't work that way. The government faced pricing and other limitations. Contracts were highly sought after by vendors, could be worth billions of dollars, and were locked in for years. Frequently, vendors who missed out on contracts filed challenges and lawsuits against the government, which resulted in excessive delays.

Often, after a contract was executed, the government discovered it needed more functionality. The government can go back to the vendor to request a contract modification to increase functionality, but that was an uphill battle. In that situation, the vendor had leverage and could request an exorbitant amount of money for the modification or a new module to add the desired functionality. Often, it was cheaper and faster for the government to procure a second system with the new desired functionality rather than modifying the first system. The vendors' mission was to make money, and there was little incentive for the vendors to collaborate with each other. The result was closed systems with fragmented data. I discussed how I interacted with ten different information systems while serving as a Navy psychiatrist. I suspect a lot of that had to do with the issues I just described.

Email Misuse, Online Training, and Information Fatigue

All personnel were issued an email account that was secured by the DoD Common Access Card (CAC). Users would physically insert their CAC card into a reader, and the email software would prompt the user for a pin to access encryption certificates. The system was glitchy. Frequently, the system would hang, and there was excessive lag and latency. Email helped sometimes, but frequently, it sapped productivity. Leadership used email in place of regular meetings to send out information and discuss work issues. With email, there was no opportunity to have meaningful dialogue or ask questions. Overreliance on email created misunderstandings and tension. There were excessive amounts of email, sometimes 50-100 per day. When email responses were sent out, the writers tended to widen the audience by adding more and more people to the carbon copy line. Email threads got larger and snowballed. As the number of people on an email chain increased, the effectiveness and productivity value decreased exponentially. Personnel would get distracted by the volume of incoming emails and important emails, and critical issues would get buried in the pile.

There was a legendary email event that captured the scope of the problem. A Navy two-star admiral sent out an email to a global distribution list entitled, "The Ongoing Power of Navy Medicine." I suspect the permissions on the email distribution list were set incorrectly because someone replied to the email. The response went to everyone: "I've moved to a different duty station. Please remove me from this list."

Following this, the email thread went viral. For days, there were hundreds of similar replies. There were replies that said not to reply, but even those got replies.

Email was weaponized, abused, and used defensively. Leadership would purposely give vague guidance via email. A number of my colleagues told me they avoided electronically writing about or documenting certain issues. Emails were also frequently sent as *cover your ass* maneuvers in case situations went south. A senior doctor I worked with told me she emailed as many people as possible to associate them with situations to protect herself.

Emails and taskers asking for a complicated issue to be addressed ASAP were frequently sent immediately prior to a suspense date or after a deadline had passed. Receiving an email like this was stressful. It was clear the overdue tasker was sent because someone didn't do their job, and it left you with a feeling that your professional and interpersonal boundaries were violated. When leadership would task you with something important that was due three days ago, it was like getting punched in the gut.

There were numerous online click-through trainings to accomplish across different systems, including Joint Knowledge Online, Relias Health, and service-specific websites. Selected topics included the information security cyber awareness challenge, counterintelligence, and insider threat awareness training. There was also the run, hide, fight, and active shooter training and a lengthy fall prevention training. At one point, there was comprehensive training on chemical and biological weapons. From a healthcare provider perspective, the organization had too many training requirements. Once a month, the command would send out a delinquency training list. If your name was on the list, it had to be addressed.

Once, we were beginning a mandatory online training at my duty station. One of the senior doctors forgot to turn off her webcam. As soon as the training started, she got a big smile on her face, grabbed her jacket from the back of her chair, and walked out of her office. It was obvious she ditched the training and was headed for lunch. Shortly afterward, she ran back into the room with a bright-red face. She sat down, pretended to watch the training, and then turned off her webcam.

Challenges Implementing Technological Solutions

I worked in a Navy substance abuse treatment program. Our facility conducted diagnostic assessments of service members for possible substance use disorders, made treatment recommendations, and provided in-house treatment. Referrals came in from commands, including from the command DAPAs or through a medical pathway. A mental health provider in the outpatient clinic could directly refer a patient to our facility. To admit a patient to the SARP program, we needed a solid diagnosis most often completed by a military mental health provider, a physical exam, and lab work. We had a fixed number of beds and a census and would determine the next available bed date for patients. If there were lengthy delays, we would submit a network deferral so the patient could receive treatment through the TRICARE network.

Our referral process consisted of encrypted emails, scanned documents, and spreadsheets. When emails came in, spreadsheets on the network share drive were manually updated to track referrals. Frequently, we would get emails from commands and healthcare providers asking to check the status of the referral. If there was a problem with the referral, we would troubleshoot by querying the spreadsheets and sending emails. Frequently, emails would get lost or buried in the pile, resulting in scheduling delays. We hoped for a web-based system where referrals could be submitted electronically with status update emails and a dashboard for tracking key numbers and metrics. The process was begging for modernization and a technological solution. There were so many touch points where human error could and did occur. So much time and energy was invested in maintaining the email and spreadsheet system.

We were aware that many private sector organizations were utilizing SharePoint or similar systems to generate and store online forms. We had access to the DoD 365 office enterprise cloud. We developed innovative ideas and approaches using SharePoint, Microsoft Teams, and DoD 365 to overhaul our processes, but with each attempt, we were told the functionality was locked down due to security concerns and were not authorized for storing personally identifiable information or protected health information (PHI). Despite our best efforts, we could not find any viable solution to address the issue.

During one email thread where our modernization project was being discussed, our hospital's chief medical informatics officer wrote, "I wish it were better news. . . . It rarely is. The Military Health System is where good ideas go to die!"

Air Combat Command Master Control

It was disappointing that software issues could be fixed, but no one was able or wanted to put the time and energy in to do it. Often, mental health providers in the field were left to develop innovative solutions to solve problems. One of the best examples of a homegrown information technology hack I had seen was a Microsoft Access database developed by an Air Force psychologist, Capt./O3 Rabecca Stahl, around 2013. Prior to becoming a psychologist, she worked for a technology company, creating and maintaining databases. She was the director of psychological health at Offutt Air Force Base in Nebraska. The database she created was called Air Combat Command Master Control, or "ACC-MC" for short. The database assisted in the operation and management of her mental health clinic.

Her system tracked patients, prevented them from slipping through the cracks, and provided metrics and sophisticated statistics about service utilization. The Air Force supported innovation and embraced the project. It was designated as best practice by the Air Combat Command and was rolled out to multiple bases. Anytime an airman was checked into the clinic, the psychiatric technicians logged them into the database. I'm sure the psychiatric technicians felt like it was double work because they also had to be logged into DHA systems. The success of the database relied on Capt. Stahl to help maintain it. The system eventually faded away. I don't know exactly what its fate was. I think its demise had to do with her getting promoted and changing duty stations.

Creating a Mental Health Intelligence Database

The military struggled to alter the course of military suicide, substance abuse, assault, and mental health issues despite significant amounts of manpower, time, money, and attention being invested. Prevention and Force Health Protection were part of a comprehensive system, including prevention, postvention, treatment, and recovery.

Early on in my career while serving in the Navy, I discovered a book written by Dr. Douglas Bey, an Army psychiatrist who served in Vietnam from 1969 to 1970, called *Wizard 6: A Combat Psychiatrist in Vietnam* (Bey 2006). The book was written years before I was born and decades before I would go to medical school or serve as a military psychiatrist. It was amazing; the lessons learned from the book were directly applicable to my work as an operational psychiatrist in the Marine Corps during the early 2000s. Dr. Bey discussed a public health approach to operational mental health, including keeping detailed records of the soldiers he treated and evaluating the records to search for trends to prevent psychiatric casualties. His team would identify units with clusters of referrals and would then travel to the unit to try to determine what was causing the stress that led to the referrals and conduct interventions. When stress indicators for a unit increased, his team would contact command, interview service members, and assign an enlisted psychiatric technician to live in the unit and work with the unit's enlisted men to gather information about the unit stresses. Dr. Bey wrote that they would report back to the unit, and the process was effective in assisting the unit focus on the emotional aspects of the organization and solving problems.

Dr. Bey wrote, "We began charting stress indicators for every unit in the division. We monitored the number of chaplain visits, accident rates, sick-call rates, mental health visits, inspector general complaints, Article 15s, courts-martial, and malaria rates (this was a command indicator because it reflected unit discipline—if men didn't take their pills as ordered, they got malaria)." He and his team graphed the stress indicators for each unit, identified organization stress periods and factors, and were successful in impacting positive change via command intervention.

When I served as a Navy psychiatrist with the Marine Corps in the early 2000s, there were population health initiatives to track key mental health indicators, high-risk behaviors, to create a database dashboard and provide mental health intelligence data to military leaders so they could provide intervention. The Marine Corps Expeditionary Force I served in created a hodgepodge methodology for doing this. Each month we contacted law enforcement, safety, family services, and the Navy hospital to ask how many suicide attempts and deaths by suicide occurred. We tabulated other mental health indicators, such as alcohol incidents, domestic violence incidents, and the number of inpatient psychiatric hospitalizations and mental health-related emergency room visits. We keyed the numbers into a spreadsheet and presented them during monthly briefings. The numbers were forwarded to a Marine Corps headquarters element at Quantico. The process was like what Dr. Bey and his team did during Vietnam, but we used Microsoft Office to track and graph data.

The process was frustrating and time-consuming, and there

were many roadblocks. Everyone felt understaffed, and no one wanted to take ownership of the initiative. We encountered turf wars, and individuals and organizations were reluctant to record and share data. Everyone suggested it was someone else's responsibility to provide numbers. For example, some felt the command, not the substance abuse treatment program or law enforcement, should provide numbers for alcohol incidents. When we asked for participation, we were met with resistance and asked to show policy that directed disclosure of the numbers. It is important to note that the Marine Corps mental health program managers had not succeeded in providing such a policy or methodology. At the Marine Corps division, there were three mental health personnel, including myself, another psychiatrist, and a psychiatric technician. At one point, we tried to create a Marine Corps expeditionary force or division instruction to establish the methodology in writing, but it was over our heads. It was a noble effort, but we couldn't get it done. We felt what was needed was a Marine Corps order.

Later in my career, I completed a tour of duty with the Coast Guard, but this time I was at the managerial level. The Coast Guard had a similar initiative to try to set up a database dashboard. Coast Guard leaders wanted to use the dashboard to study and conduct workplace and environmental interventions. There was no effective method to collect data passively from the field. For most data pulls, we contacted personnel in the field and asked them for numbers. We experienced the same resistance and pushback I encountered during my time in the Navy and Marine Corps. The numbers provided were by self-report, varied depending on who was reporting the data, and were exaggerated. The personnel in the field felt they were underutilized, were fearful their employment could be impacted, and tended to exaggerate numbers. Coast Guard policy said primary care personnel were responsible for collecting numbers pertaining to suicide, but the medical personnel didn't do it and felt the work-life personnel should be doing it.

Everyone agreed the military would benefit from having a sophisticated health intelligence database to track high-risk behaviors across military units and report the results in a dashboard. No one could agree who should be tracking what or the methodology for doing so. The other problem was that there were numerous closed information systems with poor cross talk. Ideally, a health intelligence database would passively pull and aggregate data across multiple systems and organizations. We encountered information technology policy restrictions. For example, we were told it was a great idea, but we couldn't put it on SharePoint.

Across my career, lots of money and time were invested trying to develop and implement solutions for health intelligence databases, dashboards, and systems for tracking and intervening on treatment participation and compliance. There were promising initiatives, but there was never a finished project or fully effective solution. My colleagues and I felt the best solution was to have a policy explaining what indicators were to be tracked, where the data sources would come from, who would be responsible for the work, and the precise methodology for doing so. We felt there needed to be checks and balances, including inspections, to ensure the tracking was being done and corrective actions when there was noncompliance.

CHAPTER 12

Obstacles the Military Faces Addressing Mental Health Issues

THE DOD IS a war-fighting agency. The mission of the military has been described as putting "warheads on foreheads." "Medical" was important, but it was lower down on the priority list. A moment in my career I will never forget was hearing the chief of naval operations speak during an all-officer call. He said he would rather buy bombs and bullets than pay for health care. Feeling supported by leadership is a critical protective factor for burnout and hearing the most senior leadership make critical remarks about medical and the work I was doing was demoralizing. The admiral's remarks were a common theme that would be repeated over the course of my career. We were told, "Why do you cost so much? Why are you chewing up my budget?" When medical and military hardware were in competition, bombs and guns almost always won out. I read reports about a politician and Army veteran who spoke about deficiencies with the marines' barracks. He said he wanted marines focused on bullets on bad guys, not on maintaining heating, ventilation, and air-conditioning systems. That mentality was pervasive. Health care and living conditions were important, especially during times of crisis, but almost always there was a more important mission.

The military medical system is focused on the medical readiness of individual service members, operational readiness, and supporting combat units, not health care. When I worked for the Navy, the Navy surgeon general sent out regular emails. He said the purpose of Navy medicine was to contribute to lethality by improving the survival of our warfighters. He wrote that Navy medicine provided medical experts, capable of operating in austere conditions on expeditionary platforms, operating as high-performance cohesive teams to project medical power in support of naval superiority.

The military is agile in some ways. It can launch a kinetic response, sending anyone or anything anywhere in a short period of time. On the other hand, it is a massive slow bureaucratic organization, and its primary mission was not to run a high-reliability healthcare organization.

Challenges of Running a High-Reliability Military Healthcare Organization

A marine col/O6 whom I very much respected and worked with said creating a military COSC program was like trying to paint a train while it was moving. It was more difficult than that. It was like trying to paint a moving train while 30 percent of personnel rotated out of the command every year, including the conductor. At the end of three-to-four years, everyone had rotated out, negatively impacting continuity of care and operations. By the time a service member had mastered their job, it was time to rotate to the next assignment. At the same time, while all this was occurring, the funding source kept changing or drying up.

In between my time in the Navy and the PHS, I worked at a Community Service Board in Virginia. This was a state and local mental health agency. The medical director, many doctors, and nurses had been there for years. Operations were mature, efficient, smooth, and cost-effective. In addition to being seasoned, experienced, and mature, the personnel knew every patient in the area, especially those who received long-term care at the state hospital. The team knew exactly what worked and what didn't work for each patient when they struggled. The team developed many effective long-term initiatives. One initiative they were known for was cutting the agency's pharmacy budget in half. This was accomplished by factoring medication cost into treatment plans and utilizing generic drugs whenever possible.

The military's health system didn't have the luxury of stability. Just when we got to know a patient and their needs, it was time to move on. Either the patient or healthcare professional deployed or received a military move, and it disrupted the relationship. It was challenging for service members and their families to receive help with chronic and complex problems.

A successful healthcare organization strives for a solid framework, policies, stable staffing, communication, quality control, and long-term planning. In an ideal situation, an organization is mature, and there are skilled, experienced, long-term, and stable personnel solely focused on health care and providing measured excellence. The military was great at winning wars and fighting battles. The Navy has done a fantastic job throughout history fighting historic battles with bravery, improvisation, and quick decisions. Consider that a small group of warships, a Navy squadron, is deployed and one of the ships was sunk by the enemy. The remaining ships rapidly adjust and change tactics. The Navy accomplishes the mission no matter what and finds a way to win. That mentality works for battle but isn't as effective for health care.

The military health system excelled at straightforward health issues. If a patient suffered from strep throat, it was easy to go for an acute care appointment, get tested, and receive treatment with antibiotics. High blood pressure or low-grade chronic depression were conditions readily responsive to treatment and were easily treated.

It was a different story for chronic, more complicated problems that took months and years to solve. The problems of military suicide, mental health, and substance abuse are complex. To tackle those issues effectively, a system-based integrated team approach is needed, with stable personnel. There needs to be prevention and training, early identification, early intervention, and tracking of high-risk patients, with rescue interventions for those who drop out. The healthcare providers involved in the care need to possess the appropriate skill sets and have reduced distraction to free them to focus on their work. There needs to be communication and care integration with commands and across helping services.

I was at a briefing where a cardiologist at Naval Medical Center Portsmouth was discussing the challenges of trying to maintain accreditation for a sophisticated chest pain program. She said the hospital started the year off with ten cardiologists but lost six of them due to contracting issues. She said the DoD's medical information systems wouldn't interface with the accreditation organization's system, so a nurse was "hand-jamming" case data into a web interface. She discussed how she was deployed on a short-notice six-month mission and how this resulted in the project being set back.

There were competing priorities between hospital and operational requirements. Anytime something happened in the world, staff and resources were pulled, clinical operations were disrupted, and the result was chaos and confusion. Even the hospital cafeteria would close or reduce services. A lot of times, operational events felt like a wild goose chase. Often, there was a lot of last-minute planning and scrambling, but in the end, it was all for nothing, as deployment plans were canceled.

In the military system, active duty were tasked with things that competed with the healthcare mission. It contributed to a feeling of organization chaos, inattention, and a fly-by-the-seat-of-your-pants feeling. In an optimal situation, it was desired for patients to have a surgical procedure done by a healthcare team who had done the procedure a hundred or more times and had a solid system for assisting them in the immediate post-operative recovery process. I doubt this was ever fully achieved in the military system due to the issues described above.

Stigma and Consequences of Getting Help

Much to my surprise, during a briefing with a battalion of 1,000 marines, the division general told the marines not to get help, and if they did, make sure it didn't go in their record. At the time, I was taken aback by his comments. Years later, there was truth and wisdom in his comments. He knew service members and their families needed and benefited from help, but he knew about the stigma and the consequences of getting help. Despite all the interest and attention military mental health has received, a decade after his speech, the same issues persist. Service members face consequences for getting help, including negative career impact, job disqualification, and loss of security clearance. Career service members just like the general distrust the system. They have witnessed the consequences of getting help from their brothers and sisters in arms, and many have vowed not to talk to anyone unless they are outside of the system or until they have left military service.

Service members have a warrior mentality. It is said that marines and soldiers will march until the soles of their boots are worn off and then on bare feet until they can march no more. A similar saying is "Soldiers always march forward." They are strong people who are determined to get the mission done and take care of their families. With that mentality where strength and independence are valued, it isn't easy to raise a hand and ask for help.

Service members face stigma and consequences for asking for help. Often, their peers and chain of command have a negative view of mental health. They view leaving the unit as quitting and see mental health as something that takes service members away from the fight and causes unplanned personnel losses. A service member asking for help violates the ship, shipmate, and self code. They are perceived as selfish, putting themselves in front of the unit, making a choice, and they face scorn and contempt from others. Service members who need help are blamed and labeled as having a character defect or lack of willpower, including by helping professionals. Patients complained to me that their mental health providers were laser-focused on duty status instead of helping them and accused them of trying to get out of work or the military. I've had patients complain that after starting treatment and being recommended for limited duty, they were pulled into an office, confronted by their chain of command, accused of screwing everyone else over, and asked why they couldn't suck it up and deal with it. I worked with a sailor who told me the command refused her requests for help, she hit a breaking point, she went to the emergency room, and she was then accused of circumventing the chain of command. It was another Catch-22 situation. She couldn't get help from her chain of command, so she had no choice but to go elsewhere, but then she was accused of violating the chain of command. She complained that she was verbally abused and retaliated against by being given increased workload, adding to her distress levels. Once, there was a junior marine who worked up the courage to get help. He spoke to a psychologist, engaged in therapy, and got started on medication. The next thing that happened was one of the most senior enlisted marines, a sergeant major/E9, confronted the junior marine. He made him stand at attention and dressed him down. He told him he was disappointed in him; all he needed was "the Marine Corps" and not mental health treatment.

There were social consequences to mental health issues too. A friend of mine served as a marine GySgt as an artillery operations chief. The military occupational specialty was a small community. When word spread that he was medically retired due to mental health issues, he lost a lot of friends and was blackballed professionally. His son joined the Marine Corps about six years later and served in the same specialty. His son faced stigma too because of the situation regarding his father. The marines who remained his friend looked after his son, while those that had changed their opinion of him gave his son a hard time. His son was told, "Your dad was the GySgt who got out due to mental health issues? You aren't going to enjoy it here." The situation led to his son defending his father from his superiors, and he got into trouble for being disrespectful. His son ended up leaving the Marine Corps after four years and joined the Navy.

Commands had the difficult task of balancing the needs of a service member against getting the mission done. Losing a service member was challenging because it made it harder to get the mission done since the remaining workload was divided among fewer people. The underlying issue here is the personnel system. If units aren't adequately staffed or able to get a replacement for an injured or ill service member, it would be better to address the personnel system problems rather than placing blame on the service member for issues that are out of their control.

Labeling a service member who is lost from a military unit with defection or betrayal is short-sighted. The service member is recovering, getting stronger, and preparing for the next fight. Blaming the service member hampers the recovery process. It would be better to look at it like lines of infantry swapping places during the firearm reloading process of the eighteenth century, where the infantry line in front was shooting and the line in back was reloading with a ball, powder, and ramrod.

Service members faced judgment and humiliation in front of their peers when their issues went public at the command. I witnessed situations where emails between medical and senior leaders were forwarded down the chain of command, and service members felt hurt. No one wanted to break uniformity and stand out in a negative way.

Stigma was also self-imposed. No one wanted to be that person to ring the bell and quit. They don't want to go home and say they experienced a personal failure and failed to provide for their loved ones. No one wanted to be the person who made work harder for everyone else and let everyone down.

There were real, immediate, and significant career repercussions for asking for help. Once, I worked with a sailor who had the courage to open up, stop drinking, and complete alcohol treatment. The gaining command completed an orders screening and disqualified him from the assignment. The sailor felt harmed by the adverse personnel action. I had a conversation with the medical officer who conducted the review. He said it didn't matter if the member completed alcohol treatment successfully and had a good prognosis. The command had a member who was recently involved in a DUI fatality, and the command had zero tolerance for any alcohol issues. The gaining command didn't want to deal with even the slightest suggestion or risk of alcohol issues.

One of my patients had a suicide attempt and was reassigned from his command via the limited-duty process. His security clearance was pulled on the way out. His ability to work was compromised by this. He lost access to the information technology system. The patient felt that the security clearance action was punishment for leaving the command. The patient was provided feedback from the security clearance manager, there was a backlog of mental health security clearance evaluations, and it would take months to have the clearance restored. Service members with mental health issues were commonly screened out for overseas duty. Patients felt the process was stigmatizing and overly conservative. Mental health issues impacted special status and military duty. Consider a pilot, for example. If significant mental health problems were identified, they would be grounded immediately. While serving at Veterans Affairs, I worked with a former pilot. He seemed to be withholding information or minimizing the extent of his suffering. I asked him about it, and he told me, "That's the aviator in me, Doc." He explained that he learned "don't tell the flight surgeon everything." He explained how he learned to conceal his health issues to protect his career and duty status.

Street drug use was infrequent but not uncommon. Service members were young and at the age where experimentation with alcohol, drugs, and other related behaviors was prevalent. It was understood that there was a zero-tolerance policy, and frequently, service members who were found to have used drugs were given the boot. If a patient tested positive for an illicit drug, frequently, this would be followed by a phone call to the patient's command, informing them of the results. Sometimes patients who wanted to leave the military took advantage of this by intentionally ingesting illicit substances to achieve a positive drug test and facilitate discharge. The military invested a lot of money, sometimes hundreds of thousands of dollars, into training an individual service member. If they had the courage to ask for help, face their demons, and successfully kick a drug problem, zero tolerance didn't seem right, especially when they were motivated for continued service. The service member used illicit drugs but learned their lesson and would never do it again. After going through a self-improvement process and completing treatment, they would be expected to be a more productive service member. Instead, the service member becomes a public service announcement for reasons to avoid getting help.

Leaders Are Fearful Situations Make Them Look Bad

When I worked with the infantry, when something bad happened like a suicide, there was a tendency for military leaders to become fearful. The gut reaction was "Did the service member receive their required post-deployment health assessment?" and "What happened wasn't my fault." Leaders would lock up and get defensive.

I remember a situation many years ago where a service member who was intoxicated died in a fall. There was discussion about if it could have been a completed suicide, and I was approached for an opinion. There was concern how the situation, if it was deemed a suicide, could reflect poorly on the unit. I don't remember how it turned out. I think it was ultimately impossible to determine exactly what happened.

I was asked to provide an opinion about how to improve Healthcare Effectiveness Data and Information Set metrics for mental health. I provided a well-researched and well-thought-out briefing backed by factual information. The responsible management official said they wanted everything spun in a positive light. They said, "I don't want to have to deal with the DHA. I don't want them calling me. Do whatever it takes to satisfy the requirement." They said they didn't want to hear anything negative. They didn't want to hear "We don't have the staff to do this."

Service members, especially military leaders, are under tremendous pressure. They are under pressure not to make the command look bad and to perform at a high level to achieve career progression. When an incident happened, acting out of fear and blaming the parties involved did not go well. The best outcomes happened when leadership addressed the situation in a nonpunitive manner.

Organizational Stovepiping

There were many military helping programs at different levels with variable funding sources. Programs were at the DoD, service, and local levels and had different implementations across the uniformed services. Help also came from Veterans Affairs, nongovernmental and nonprofit organizations.

Military programs typically had a program management component at the DoD level and service levels and were operated at local levels. Helping programs such as Military OneSource and Military and Family Life Counseling were at the DoD level and were run by contractors.

Each of the military branches had community service and family readiness programs. Programs run under the community services umbrella were typically considered "nonmedical" and "nonclinical" and had a different funding source, oversight, and management chain of command. Such programs included new parent support, domestic and child abuse prevention/support, financial management, transition, and relocation assistance. Hospital-based and operational-embedded mental health providers and programs were considered "clinical" and received oversight from medical commands and military treatment facilities.

The terminology was confusing because a licensed clinical social worker could provide service members in both realms. A social worker could provide both nonmedical counseling and clinical individual therapy. The main difference was under what roof the service was being provided, including under what program and who the payer was. If individual therapy was offered at a military medical treatment facility or paid for by TRICARE, the service was clinical individual therapy. If Military OneSource was funding the service or it was provided at a community service center, it was nonmedical and nonclinical.

At larger hospitals, inpatient and partial hospitalization services were offered. Services at smaller facilities were often outpatient-based. Mental health providers conducted individual therapy, group therapy, prescribed psychotropic medication, and other treatments to assist patients. Some commands had operational-embedded mental health providers or chaplains embedded in the units whose duty was to help service members and coordinate with the command.

There was great diversity in mental health providers in terms of training, education, background, clinical approach, and specific services offered. Mental health providers were medical doctors, doctorate and master's level psychologists, master's level social workers, master's level counselors, and licensed substance abuse counselors.

Programs such as sexual assault, family advocacy, and substance abuse had volunteer, peer, or collateral duty advocates. These volunteers received specialized training and achieved qualifications to assist service members in distress, navigate the programs, and coordinate care between the commands and the services.

At the deck-plate level or in the field, the mental health system and available resources were confusing and contradictory. A retired Navy captain, John Cordle, wrote an essay about this phenomenon (Cordle 2023):

> *The Navy already has a wide range of mental health and suicide prevention programs in place. Unfortunately, these programs are often in competition with each other, fighting for the same promotions and funding. This need not be the case. The following programs are already in place across the fleet but could be more impactful if properly applied and resourced.*

Captain Cordle's remarks were consistent with my experiences and feedback I had received from senior military leaders throughout my career. The programs were confusing and fragmented, and there were questions about their effectiveness.

The military helping system struggled with "stovepiping." Often, the programs were developed and executed in isolation from each other. With all the different programs and personnel, there was suboptimal cross talk and integration between programs. The mental health providers at the hospital could not review the notes written by the counselor at the family services program who provided individual counseling and vice versa. The mental health department at the naval hospital could not access the family advocacy or sexual assault program electronic records, although ideally there would be coordination, integration, and cross talk to ensure the best outcomes.

The 2007 DoD Task Force on Mental Health documented similar findings: "The multiplicity of programs, policies, and funding streams ... may also lead to confusion about benefits and services, fragmented delivery of care, and gaps in service provision" (Department of Defense Task Force on Mental Health 2007). The report also documented that no single mental health program existed across the DoD and pointed out the considerable variation in mental health service delivery among the military services and TRICARE.

A RAND study in 2011 (Weinick 2011) captured the issues with stovepiping. The study set out to develop a comprehensive catalog of programs sponsored or funded by the DoD to address psychological health or traumatic brain injury. The researchers noted it was a complex task to identify 211 programs. The study documented barriers to maximize program effectiveness: information was decentralized; programs were developed in isolation from the existing care system; there was inadequate funding, resources, staff capacity, and stigma; and issues with program evaluation delivered unclear outcomes. A key finding from the study was that no branch of service maintained a complete list of the programs, tracked the development of new programs, or had appropriate resources in place to direct service members and their families to the full array of programs that best met their needs.

Turf Battles and Interservice Rivalries

The way the services approached and managed problems varied widely, sometimes drastically so. There were various initiatives over the years to achieve Tri-service consensus, but achieving this was on a rare occasion.

The Army had the reputation of being the biggest service, and there was a perception that the Army got everything it wanted. Given the size of the Army, it had the most political clout and lobbying power. When the Army needed someone for deployment, it had the ability to pull from other services. Whether or not this was entirely true, I observed resentment toward the Army. I discussed the issue with a senior Navy psychiatrist. He said the Army had done some really good work, but other services were reluctant to adopt it due to interservice rivalry and tension. I contributed to the development of the Marine Corps' combat and operational stress control program when I served as a Navy psychiatrist with the Marine Corps. Throughout the initiative, leaders criticized the Army's work and vowed to go in a different direction. The truth was that the Army did great work, and we all might have been better off playing nice in the sandbox and developing a unified approach.

An example of this was the Army's BHDP program, a measurement-based care initiative. The system administered scientifically validated mental health rating scales and tracked the results over time. Research has shown that measurement-base care improves outcomes when utilized in mental health. A senior military psychiatrist told me the Navy did not agree with the system and was dragging its feet on the implementation. Despite being directed to adopt the system, the Navy consistently had low rates of adoption. The Air Force used BHDP religiously in the outpatient clinic, and it was helpful in assisting service members. By the time I left the Navy hospital, BHDP compliance was still an issue, and there was a new initiative being discussed to provide the Navy a monetary reward if BHDP compliance hit a certain completion target. In hindsight, the Navy had a reputation for underdiagnosing sailors and overutilizing administrative separations. If a sailor consistently scored in the severe range on the rating scales, that would suggest a more severe diagnosis. The BHDP system created some accountability for diagnosing, and that might have had something to do with the low implementation rates.

There were turf battles and disagreement within services as well. The Navy SARP building where I worked was an example of this. The building needed renovation. Historically, from what I understand, there had been a series of disagreements about who owned and was responsible for facility maintenance. The base owned the building, but it was being utilized by Navy medicine. Everyone agreed the building needed renovation, but no one agreed who should pay for it. The base said the hospital should pay for it. I suspect the hospital said the Navy Bureau of Medicine and Surgery should pay, and they likely suggested the DHA should be financially responsible.

Turf battles impacted everyone at every level. Inside the hospital, there were turf battles between clinical services. I wrote about how there was tension and disagreement between psychiatry, internal medicine, and the emergency room regarding management of alcohol withdrawal treatment. The psychiatry service argued that internal medicine should conduct alcohol detoxification, and vice versa.

Around 2019, the DHA began a takeover of the administration and management of health care at all military medical treatment facilities. A common sentiment among my professional Navy peers was that the DHA was impeding on their turf, and everything should be turned back over to the individual services. A colleague relayed to me a story about how there were frequent disagreements between a senior psychiatrist at BUMED and the DHA. I had a part-time job working for a large healthcare organization and experienced the benefits of standardization across hospitals. I covered two inpatient psychiatry units at different hospitals in the same hospital system, and they were run in a similar way. The documentation templates were identical, the order sets were the same, and it was easy to jump between hospitals. We would have benefited from a DHA mental health division and clinical practice manager to actively manage mental health and substance abuse treatment facilities to include setting policies, establishing documentation templates, monitoring productivity, managing personnel, addressing facilities issues, and troubleshooting situations.

Identifying, Tracking, and Intervening on High-Risk Individuals and Groups

Historically, military mental health was focused on face-to-face interactions between individuals and mental health providers.

Responses to situations were reactive. One problem with reactionary response was that by the time individuals in need of help were identified, the problems had reached a breaking point, and they were past a point of no return. Another problem was that individuals dropped out of treatment, slipped through the cracks, and suffered in silence until their problems reached a critical mass, bringing them back into the system. Often, individuals would drop out of treatment after a PCS. High-risk individuals who experienced access-to-care issues had a second incident while waiting for initial service from the first incident. In the Navy's substance abuse treatment program, I came across sailors who had a second alcohol-related incident while waiting months to get into treatment for the first one. Individuals who suffered from domestic abuse issues were transferred overseas despite an open Family Advocacy case, arrived at their new duty station, and suffered repeat domestic violence incidents.

The problem of military suicide was complex and vexed many highly intelligent and capable people. I participated in numerous meetings and internal debates where ideas were discussed on how to address the problem of military suicide. At the DoD level, a form was created called the DoDSER. The idea was to complete a DoDSER report for any suicide death, suicide attempt resulting in hospitalization, and suicide attempt resulting in evacuation from theater. The intention was to study the results to assist in suicide prevention efforts. At Naval Medical Center Portsmouth, I never saw a single DoDSER report being filed or discussed, although there were patients identified with these issues frequently. A critical issue regarding this initiative was that buy-in for the DoDSER program was lacking. The initiative didn't positively impact a patient's care or have any visible benefit to the local organization, and the annual reports were delayed or nonexistent. There also was no additional time allocated during clinical visits to complete the form.

When I started my career in psychiatry, suicide terminology

included "attention seeking," "suicidal gesture," and "contracting for safety." Toward the end of my career, military mental health was moving toward a system of using common terminology and risk factors to describe suicidal thoughts and behaviors and stratify risk levels, track patients, and target interventions based on risk level. Consider a patient who had recurrent inpatient psychiatric hospitalizations and recurrent suicide attempts, who was going through major life stresses, including a relationship breakup and military legal problems. The service member was assigned an aggregated high-risk level and flagged. There were efforts to track progress and treatment participation on a weekly basis by a case manager and a multidisciplinary team. Instead of discharging patients from the clinic for noncompliance, there were efforts to contact the service member in question, check on them, and communicate with the command to discuss ways to assist the member in re-engaging in care. There was an additional benefit to tracking indicators across military units. If a unit was identified as being an outlier with a high number of high-risk cases, then it became a potential target for intervention.

Health, Wellness Checks, and Securing Firearms

I encountered situations where a chain of command went to the home of a service member who was struggling with significant mental health issues, suicidal thoughts, and substance abuse issues and conducted "a health and wellness check."

A command was concerned about a service member's behavior, went to the service member's house, found drug paraphernalia everywhere, and discovered the service member was huffing. There was no lab test for huffing, so observing the aerosol containers and balloons was critical. The command assisted the member in removing all the drug paraphernalia from the residence and facilitated enrollment in alcohol and drug treatment.

Throughout my career, I experienced situations where a chain of command went to a member's home to bring them in for help. There was a situation at Naval Medical Center Portsmouth where a service member had been absent without leave at their residence for several weeks, was missing appointments, and was complaining of feeling depressed and making suicidal statements via phone and email. I asked the command to conduct a health and wellness check. The command didn't feel comfortable going to the service member's home due to safety concerns, and they called local law enforcement. Local law enforcement felt that the Navy should be responsible for conducting the check. The service member remained at home until a mental health provider decided to take matters into his own hands, picked up the service member, and brought him to the hospital.

When service members were considered high-risk, a best practice was to inquire about access to firearms and other weapons. If weapons were identified, we would work with service members and commands to secure them. Sometimes firearms were secured by family members, inside a base armory, or by another service member. Frequently, this was a win-win situation for all parties involved.

The practices of in-home health and wellness checks and securing firearms were best practices that assisted service members and command. I never saw a clear DoD policy or service level policies defining these practices, and they varied from base to base.

Lengthy Medical Board Processing Times

Issues with the medical boards and limited-duty processes were identified as impacting the sailors in the MARMC suicide cluster. The medical boards process was a multistep process that included actions by the Veterans Affairs medical system. A lot of the process was congressionally mandated. I served at Naval Medical Center Portsmouth during the height of the pandemic, and there were lengthy delays getting patients through the medical boards process. A rule of thumb was that it could take nine to twelve months to get to the end. At one point, there were an estimated 1,000 service members on limited duty, and a subset of those were undergoing the medical boards process.

The medical boards process started with identifying when a service member needed one. It wasn't easy; sometimes patients were stuck on perpetual limited duty. When patients suffered from more than one condition and were receiving care from multiple specialists, it wasn't clear which specialist would initiate the board and when the appropriate medical board initiation point was. The medical boards process included writing a narrative summary and associated paperwork and for the service member to complete Veterans Affairs evaluations. That process took several months. Then it took several months to process everything and send the final board package off. It took an additional three months to await findings. If the service member appealed the decision, the process would take longer.

There were pros and cons to the medical boards process. It might have been a necessary evil, but at times it put patients in a bad situation. Most boards had a high probability of medical discharge, and the patients were away from their support systems. Most suffered from chronic mental health conditions that were not going to be solved on active duty. For these service members, the process delayed getting back home, starting fresh with their new lives, and establishing care at Veterans Affairs. Occasionally, there were outlying situations, especially in the Navy when a service member suffered from severe issues but was unexpectedly returned to duty.

Of all the medical board cases, there was a small subset of high-risk mental health cases that would have benefited from expedited processing, but there was no way to do this. These were patients suffering from severe mental illness, including schizophrenia, schizoaffective disorder, bipolar I disorder, and recurrent suicidal behaviors. These individuals had difficulty functioning, even wearing a uniform, and required daily assistance and frequent redirection. Another patient population that struggled were those undergoing the medical boards process with co-occurring substance use disorders. There were patients undergoing the medical boards process who would suffer from repeated alcohol incidents despite participating in substance abuse treatment. My colleagues and I felt it would have been more therapeutic, better for all parties involved, especially the patients, to expedite these service members out of the military so they could return home and begin long-term treatment through the TRICARE and Veterans Affairs medical systems.

Measuring Workload and Productivity

Our department head facilitated a meeting inside the conference room of a building that was in desperate need of renovation. He was standing in front of a big-screen TV that was damaged, with one side of the screen suffering from green discoloration and distortion. On the screen was a spreadsheet showing the workload of every provider. He said our department was being looked at due to concerns that we weren't using resources efficiently. He talked about his experiences working in military mental health where providers spent more time looking productive than being productive. He talked about how the system was gamed to inflate productivity numbers. He suggested if we could document and code better, we would be considered for more resources and the higher-ups would leave us alone. He discussed the Defense Medical Human Resources System-Internet (DMHRSi). He said it was used as a "moderating variable" that, together with our relative value unit calculations, made it harder for us to get the people we needed. I heard something along these lines at every DoD facility I had ever worked at.

DMHRSi was a biweekly electronic time card that was utilized to measure productivity. When I left the naval hospital, there was a 38-page list of 529 work task codes that were utilized to document what work was done during the workday. Healthcare providers submitted a snapshot of their daily workload, for example six hours face-to-face time with patients and two hours administrative time, into the system. Many submitted "crazy eights," showing eight hours of daily productivity that didn't accurately capture the work being done.

We were told staffing numbers could improve if commands and personnel did a better job of recording their time. If this was the case, I never saw it at any DoD facility. From the command and healthcare provider perspective, the system added little or no value to operations or clinical care. The time cards were stamped, and there was never any meaningful feedback about the codes that were used.

When requests for staffing and resources came in, senior officials referred to a summation of DMHRSi numbers. While serving with the Air Force, my department head, hospital commander, and a more senior official met to discuss staffing issues. The staffing request was immediately declined with the feedback that the DMHRSi numbers did not support the request. It was a frustrating and all too familiar situation. We were told a reasonable and valid staffing request couldn't be addressed due to a superficial number or technicality.

An email from Naval Medical Center Portsmouth's mental health directorate business manager captured the pressure medical providers faced surrounding DMHRSi:

> *Good Morning All:*
>
> *If you have completed your DHMRSi entries and submissions—Thank you.*
>
> *If you have not completed your DMHRSi for this time frame please take a few moments to do so. I cannot overemphasize the importance of doing so in terms of our funding. Please ensure that you are recording your time accurately and using the task codes for the work being performed. This is especially important for providers to show what time they have been available to the clinic to see patients, and equally important, when you are not available due to training, tad, etc. The amount of time available is used*

to gauge productivity. So if you're saying you are available 8 hours a day to see patients but you were not in reality—Then you look like you are under producing.

Hope this helps. Remember the Command Executive Board and leadership outside of our Command scrutinize these reports closely. Compliance and accuracy are key to our future success.

My professional colleagues and I spent a lot of time and energy wrangling over DMHRSi and billing codes, although there was no visible exchange of money. The private sector had annual bonuses for clinical productivity, but the military health system had nothing like this. The highest producer got paid the same amount as the lowest producer. Workload standards and billing codes waxed and waned over time, and there was conflicting guidance.

Serving Reserve and Guard Members

Reservists and National Guard members were different from full-time active military, and working with them was always like being thrown a curveball. There were Guard and Reserve members who drilled on weekends and completed two weeks a year of annual training. There were others who were called to full-time active duty. Sometimes Guard and Reserve members would develop medical conditions while on active duty. There were differences in policies, procedures, and service eligibility regarding these individuals. For example, when activated, service members and their families were eligible for TRICARE Prime, and when inactivated, they were eligible for TRICARE Reserve Select.

Guard and Reserve members who were injured while on active duty faced unique challenges. They were kept on active duty away from their homes and support systems. I worked with a reservist from California who was injured on deployment overseas, and he was sent to Naval Medical Center Portsmouth for care. He found himself in a prolonged limbo status and struggled with living on the East Coast, far from home. There were also Guard and Reserve members who were perceived as intentionally delaying their demobilization and wanting to remain on active duty for as long as possible.

Defining Who Qualifies for Help

Those who could receive care in the military system included the service member and immediate family members. From the service member's perspective, "family" could include those outside of the policy eligibility definition, including a longtime partner, a child's parent, the service member's sibling, parent, grandparent, or even a godparent.

I spoke to a junior service member who was struggling to find help for her ten-year-old sister who was struggling with child abuse and neglect issues back home. Another service member had a parent who had a stroke in Central America and had poorly controlled diabetes. Her parent was not an American citizen and non-English speaking. The service member hoped to bring her mother to the United States, but it was unclear how her mother could receive health care. These were critical members of the service members' lives that comprised the family unit, but they had limited eligibility for care.

Service members were prioritized for service access, and services were frequently closed or restricted to family members and retirees. There were many times across my career where the issue went back and forth. Early in my career, family members and military retirees were told they had to receive care at the military hospital, the hospital had a first right of refusal, and there were many complaints. Later, they were told the hospital was closed to them. Service availability to family members and retirees flipped in a predictable sin wave pattern every five or ten years in my experience. Every time the flip occurred, there was chaos and confusion. Care was disrupted when providers changed, and the system scrambled to accommodate an influx of patients. The messaging surrounding the changes impacted people too. Family members and retirees didn't feel valued when they were told to seek care elsewhere.

Inspections, Oversight, and Accountability

Programs looked and sounded good on the surface, but the challenge was to objectively study and measure them. Once, I was involved in program management and oversight. One program had no way to measure workload or that the work being done achieved positive results. The program managers sent out solicitations to the field, asking for feel-good stories and photos about the program. It was a tactic to avoid discussion of objective outcome and cost-effectiveness measures. During flag officer briefings, the program managers would give presentations with pictures and descriptions of the people who were helped. Management was frustrated that objective data was lacking. How many were helped? Were the programs achieving what they were supposed to be doing? Were they cost-effective?

In the private sector, money drove the system. If the service rendered wasn't medically necessary or professionals didn't document properly, the organization didn't get paid. There was scrutiny by insurance companies and government payers such as Medicare. This wasn't the case in the military system. Personnel were paid no matter what happened.

Oversight and accountability in the military health system was a significant challenge. I participated in numerous discussions and meetings where personnel shrugged and said, "It is a manning issue. We just don't have the bodies." There was always some truth about manning issues, but it was also an excuse for mismanagement.

A few times across my career, I was involved in inspections. During a FAP inspection, one of the clinicians explained that she kept no records whatsoever. She worked at a remote site and had little day-to-day oversight. Her clinical supervisor worked at a different geographic location, and electronic means and self-reports were relied on for day-to-day supervision. The issues she was having went on for months undetected.

Site inspections were most helpful when a solid policy existed that documented procedures, workflows, and measurable criteria. When we were asked to conduct inspections without a solid policy, it didn't go well. How do you conduct an inspection when there aren't clear metrics or standards? I participated in site inspections and "assist visits" where there were no consequences. Our feedback was received and appreciated. At the same time, the site being inspected had little or no motivation to change or comply with our recommendations. In the worst case, the personnel being inspected didn't prepare or take it seriously. We felt time and resources weren't effectively utilized when there was no solid policy or consequences that defined what was to be inspected.

DoD Instruction 5010.40 required internal controls to assure programs were operating as intended and to evaluate the effectiveness of controls, but oversight and accountability in the mental health programs I experienced was lacking. For most programs, key benchmarks and inspectable criteria were not defined in policy. How can an inspection be conducted if the program standards and measurable criteria aren't written? What if access-to-care standards were busted? Who checked to see if the DoDSER forms were being generated? Where were the accountability and corrective actions?

CHAPTER 13

Challenges in Assisting Service Members

Mental Health Issues Spin Around Multiple Axes

MILITARY SUICIDE AND associated conditions such as alcoholism are easy to understand but difficult to get a handle on and alter the trajectory. Mental health issues, heart disease, and cancer are common universal health conditions. It is estimated that as many as one in five individuals suffer from a mental health condition during their lifetime. Everyone has been touched by a family member, friend, or coworker who has suffered from a mental health disorder. The population rates of cancer and heart disease are relatively constant over time. So are the rates of mental health conditions, suicide, and drug and alcohol incidents.

Just like cancer and heart disease, there are a fixed number of cases that occur. The good news is that many are modifiable and preventable. The challenge is to figure out which ones are good candidates for intervention and how to enact the change. Military leaders are under pressure to eradicate behaviors like suicide, alcoholism, and sexual assault. There was nothing like the experience of having a congressman or senator question a military leader, demanding to know why sexual assaults occur and why more wasn't done about it. The challenge is to find the sweet spot between what can and cannot be fixed.

There are numerous factors that influence mental health, substance misuse, maltreatment, domestic violence, and sexual assault. They are multilayered and intertwined in a complex way. Designing and delivering interventions for these issues is a challenge. Giving a group of service members a motivational presentation was helpful, but the presentation was not going to solve or even change the trajectory of problems. To effectively address these problems, other simultaneous, meaningful interventions are required.

Conceptually, there are similarities between military suicide and fevers. There are many causes of fevers and contributing factors. Military suicide has often been described as a confluence of factors. Sometimes military suicide was impulsive, brought on by acute external stresses, and fueled by alcohol intoxication. Other times it built up over time across numerous concurrent processes and was the final step in a pathway where the factors converged in a perfect storm.

Consider a service member who had a challenging childhood and academic difficulty in school and joined the military. They suffered from mental health and suicidal behaviors prior to service, received mental health treatment, but made it through the military screening process. The operational tempo at their first duty station was high. The leaders in the chain of command were irritable, mean, with behaviors bordering on workplace abuse. The service member sought camaraderie in peers who were turning to alcohol to cope with problems. They learned poor coping mechanisms and began to drink as well. The service member was terrified to seek help from the operational mental health provider because they witnessed peers who asked for help being deemed not compatible with military life and recommended for discharge. Maybe they tried to get help one time, had a bad experience, and never returned. Finally, one night after a terrible day at work, the service member's alcohol use escalates, and the service member dies by suicide. The situation captured the complexity of the problem of military suicide. One psychologist described military suicide as resulting from "death by a thousand paper cuts" (Marshall-Chambers 2023). There were predisposing factors, risk factors, a stepwise progression, stigma, difficulty accessing care, and peer pressure.

Inexact Science

The *Diagnostic and Statistical Manual of Mental Disorders Fifth Edition* (DSM-5), published by the American Psychiatric Association, provides standardized criteria for the diagnosis of mental health disorders but is far from perfect. Despite diagnoses being clearly defined, there was overlap between conditions, and often the diagnosis and prognosis fell on the individual healthcare provider's judgment call. Frequently, different healthcare providers saw things from different perspectives and arrived at different diagnostic conclusions. Post-traumatic stress disorder was almost always associated with severe anxiety. Severe anxiety was frequently associated with depression. Individuals suffering from post-traumatic stress disorder could hear voices, suffer from paranoia, and have hallucinatory-like experiences. For example, they might hear the voice of a buddy in combat calling out for help after they were wounded. There was no "psychotic traits" diagnosis for the condition. Individuals suffering from childhood trauma frequently suffered from borderline personality traits. Inattention and impaired concentration were common in patients suffering from high stress levels, anxiety, and trauma issues and were not always symptoms of ADHD.

Physical health issues overlapped with mental health disorders. Sleep apnea, chronic pain, and obesity impacted mood, energy levels, motivation, concentration, and an individual's overall feeling of health and wellness.

In the military mental health clinic, frequently, a service member complained of various stresses and was diagnosed with adjustment disorder. This is a condition where mental health symptoms are transient and in response to acute life stresses or transitions, such as getting divorced, moving to a new command, getting deployed, or coming back from deployment.

I reviewed a case where a service member was underdiagnosed with adjustment disorder. The military mental health provider documented, "There is less evidence for a mood disorder such as major depressive disorder as his depressive symptoms are acutely tied to his current interpersonal issues, inflexibility with current beliefs, world views and general paranoia/suspicious of others."

The narrative illustrates issues with mental health diagnoses. There is much overlap between conditions, and the diagnosis is left up to the individual provider's judgment call.

Similar issues applied to personality disorder diagnoses. Patients frequently presented in acute crisis with poor coping mechanisms and exhibited primitive behaviors while under duress. Some mental health providers associated these behaviors with "character pathology." Service members tended to be young, and the behaviors were consistent with a normal development pattern of someone in their early twenties making a transition to adulthood. For example, young adults experimented with brief unstable relationships.

There was an unwritten playbook for diagnosing service members with personality disorders in the military. Service members could be diagnosed with narcissistic personality characteristics if they were seen as self-centered, entitled, and requesting special treatment. Did a service member disagree with the chain of command? Were they demanding to be removed from an operational environment such as a ship? Did the service member have an unreasonable expectation that they needed to be reassigned to a different duty station?

Was the service member young, female, and immature? Did the service member have recurrent suicidal thoughts? Did they make a string of bad relationship choices? Was the service member frequently upset and struggling with mood swings? Those symptoms could be documented as unstable self-image, recurrent suicidal thoughts—signs and symptoms of borderline personality.

Did the service member fail to conform to social norms? Were they irritable, impulsive, irresponsible? Did they show a lack of remorse? Those could be interpreted as signs and symptoms of antisocial personality.

Was the service member odd or aloof? Did they make weird posts and videos on social media? Once, our clinic was asked to consult on a service member who dressed in goth during off-duty hours and made concerning posts on social media, including one that was perceived as a bomb threat. He was worked up for schizotypal personality.

It took an extended period to get the right diagnosis right, sometimes through trial and error. It took weeks and even months for stress levels to subside and for patients to develop a relationship with their provider, to open up and discuss their issues. Even with the correct diagnosis, it could take a substantial amount of time to get the treatment right. Different patients responded to different treatments differently, even if the diagnosis was clear.

A young female patient suffering from musculoskeletal pain came to the emergency room. She said she was tired of the pain and suffered from suicidal thoughts. She complained that she had a disagreement with her surgeon at the Naval Medical Center Portsmouth and wanted to have a medical procedure from a TRICARE network provider. The military surgeon disagreed and recommended the patient not be granted a network deferral. The patient ended up in the inpatient psychiatry unit, where she expressed her frustration and was diagnosed with histrionic and borderline personality disorder. After the hospitalization, she was referred to a nonmilitary mental health provider in the TRICARE network who diagnosed post-traumatic stress disorder, depression, and anxiety. The diagnoses between the nonmilitary and Navy mental health providers conflicted with each other. The patient coped with the situation by dropping out of treatment at the military treatment facility. Her medical record clearly indicated when the disagreements started because all the future visits from that point on were replaced with no-show telephone notes and efforts to reconnect with care.

Screening Service Members Who Underreport Symptoms

The idea of a periodic health assessment was logical and appealing. Once a year, service members' mental health issues were assessed. The results were reviewed, and referrals were generated for those identified with issues to facilitate the help they needed. In practice, it didn't work quite so well. Logistically, it was difficult to identify service members who were due for a periodic health assessment, get them in a room, and administer the assessment. There were issues finding building space and computers, and personnel needed to conduct the assessments.

The biggest barrier to screening implementation was service members' reluctance to answer the questions due to stigma and the consequences of getting help. A retired Air Force M.Sgt./E7 told me he was always afraid to answer "yes" due to concerns about his career. He explained that documenting concerns made problems worse, and the military had a bad track record addressing issues. I spoke to another senior enlisted service member in the Air Force who identified as having possible PTSD on a mental health screening. After it became apparent that his upcoming overseas transfer was threatened due to the concerns, he quickly recanted everything. Another issue with the screenings was access to care. It was one thing to identify an issue, but it was something else to ensure the service member had access to care within a reasonable time frame. A colleague told me that a service member expressed an opinion that he received "a million-dollar screening and two-dollar care afterward" due to difficulty accessing care and quality-of-care issues.

There is a legend about recruiters telling military recruits to answer negatively to medical screening questions. Recruits were told "YES means Your Enlistment Stops" and "NO means New Opportunity." For a career service member, mental health assessments were an intelligence test. Answering yes on a screening form was like pressing a self-disqualification button. A service member had little or no incentive to admit they had a substance abuse problem or were struggling with suicidal thoughts.

On a rare occasion, there was some question whether screenings were even being accurately reviewed before being off. Once, I reviewed a case where a service member died by suicide. A couple days later, a Periodic Health Assessment (PHA) review of the deceased was signed off "good to go" by the reviewer. The review indicated that the patient had no mental health issues days after dying by suicide.

The concept and intention behind screenings was good. If a service member in the early stages of a disease process was detected, intervention could be conducted to address the problem and prevent it from escalating. The military invested a lot of time, energy, and resources into screenings. While they weren't perfect, they helped some receive needed help and intervention.

Placing Injured and Ailing Service members

A pivotal moment for both service members and commands occurred when a service member reached the point of not being able to function in the unit. I worked with a service member who worked in an aviation career field. He developed anxiety being around aircraft and an intense fear of flying after being involved in a near airplane crash. He was reassigned from aviation duties as part of his recovery plan. There were also female sexual assault victims who felt uncomfortable serving on ships due to the preponderance of males. They suffered from anxiety from being around males and were reassigned from serving on a ship.

The issue of where disabled or impaired service members were sent was a perennial problem. There was an unwritten code across military commands not to send perceived problem service members to other units, and commands were reluctant to do so. The Marine Corps had Wounded Warrior Battalions. The Army had Soldier Recovery Units. The Navy had limited-duty commands like MARMC and a section for limited-duty sailors at the military treatment facility. Frequently, the Air Force kept service members at their current commands until the medical boards process was complete.

In my experience with the Navy, service members complained that there were too many in the limited-duty pool, the limited-duty section was understaffed, and service members got lost. Service members complained that they lost their job when they were reassigned from operational units, lost purpose, felt underutilized, and lost competency in their career field. A significant number of individuals in the limited-duty pool had poor mental health and were disgruntled, and there was a rotten-apple-in-a-barrel effect where the service members negatively impacted each other.

There was one exception, and that was culinary specialists. The cooks told me they worked harder on limited duty. I worked with a cook who appealed his medical board finding that he was unfit for duty. In his appeal, he wrote that he demonstrated he could perform the duties of his rate because he worked harder in a galley on limited duty than he did at his previous assignment.

Assisting Members Who Aren't Ready to Receive Help

The military had policies and procedures to involuntarily hospitalize service members and compel mental health evaluations via the CDE process, but there was no methodology for compelling someone to participate in treatment. The closest thing I saw to this was the Air Force's high interest list, which had similarities to outpatient involuntary commitment.

I worked in a military program that took care of patients with severe mental illness, such as bipolar disorder and schizophrenia. The patients tended to be junior service members who experienced their first psychotic break. All of them were undergoing the medical boards process, and our program was trying to help alleviate their symptoms and assist them in transitioning out of the military. Frequently, the patients would stop their medication, and they struggled with poorly controlled symptoms. The patients with the most severe conditions tended to lack insight, argue about their diagnoses, and refuse medication. The command designated our program the place of duty for the members but couldn't require them to participate in treatment or take medication.

Our inpatient psychiatry unit would treat patients with severe mental illness for weeks and months on end, even though patients refused their medication. In the private sector, at a civilian hospital in the state of Virginia, there was a judge who conducted hearings for involuntary hospitalization and for medications given over objection. The administration of medications over objection was routinely done, went much more smoothly at a nonmilitary hospital, cut down hospitalization days, and alleviated patient suffering. We could have significantly cut down hospitalization days and alleviated suffering if there would have been a solution for giving medications over objection in the military setting.

A similar issue was patients refusing substance abuse treatment. My experience was often that patients would refuse, but when they discovered they were in a positive helping environment, they would open up and start participating. Perhaps there should be a similar mechanism to order a service member into treatment while they are in uniform, at least to try for a few days before designating them a treatment failure or refusal.

I spoke with a psychiatrist who participated in a meeting at a large joint military hospital where potential use of long-acting injections through a medication-over-objection process was discussed. She complained that leadership dragged their feet, made excuses, was risk-averse, and didn't want to do it, even though it was a best practice. She told me a solution was to send a service member to a nonmilitary hospital where they could receive the medication.

Safeguarding PHI and Protecting from Unauthorized Disclosures

An important issue was safeguarding PHI. At various points in my career, legal entities, like a military criminal investigative service, would send formal requests to the mental health clinic, asking for information regarding service members:

Ref: (a) 45 CFR 165.512(f)

1. *The military investigative service is conducting a criminal investigation into [redacted]. As part of the ongoing investigation, we are requesting all medical and psychiatric records for [redacted] received at unspecified medical facilities. In order to conduct a thorough and comprehensive criminal investigation into this incident, we must accomplish a thorough and complete review of his medical records for the period set forth below.*

2. *There, we request disclosure of all medical records regarding [redacted] for the time period of [redacted], inclusive. Pursuant to reference (a) and in accordance with Health Insurance Portability and Accountability Act (HIPAA) of 1996, the medical records in question are believed to contain information that is relevant and material to a legitimate law enforcement inquiry; this request is specific and limited in scope to information pertinent to the investigation; and de-identified information could not reasonably be used.*

3. *In accordance with HIPAA and reference (a), I request that you temporarily suspend the above named individual's right*

> to receive an accounting of any disclosures of protected health information to us. Informing [redacted] that his medical records were disclosed to us would impede our investigative activities. This temporary suspension is effective until [redacted].
>
> 4. I certify that the examination of these medical records is required as part of an official investigation. Should you have any questions regarding this request, please contact the case agent.

We would forward such requests to the hospital attorney and the release-of-information officer. We were told these were "fishing expeditions." How the requests were handled depended on the interpretation of the attorney and the specific circumstances of the situation. As a rule, we followed legal guidance and provided the minimal amount of information necessary. As mental health providers, we did not want to take any action that would create stigma or further discourage people from getting help.

One of the main DoD instructions for military mental health was 6490.08, command notification requirements to dispel stigma in providing mental health care to service members. This instruction established protections for disclosure of participation in mental health services. Once, I read an email thread between a military mental health provider and a military hospital attorney that explained how to exploit a loophole in the policy. There was language in the instruction that impact to the mission was a justification to disclose information to the command. Almost any situation could result in negative impact to the mission and provide justification for a mental health provider to communicate with command. Any situation has the potential to result in unplanned personnel loss, which could negatively impact the mission. An example of this was positive drug tests. It was understood that medical lab tests could not be used for administrative or legal action. If a service member had a positive drug test for an illicit drug in the emergency room or as part of outpatient treatment, a mental health provider could contact the command on the basis that illicit drug use interfered with the service member's fitness for duty and operational readiness. After receiving notification, the command could order a legal drug test and prosecute the service member.

The issue of malingering might have been similar. I witnessed a number of cases where a mental health provider contacted a command and expressed concern that a service member was feigning illness, and this resulted in legal investigations or charges. The HIPAA statute had a military exception or loophole that allowed for disclosure regarding military readiness issues.

It was understood that military mental health providers had a duty to report crimes. There was a military regulation that stated persons shall report as soon as possible to superior authority all offenses under the Uniform Code of Military that come under observation. Earlier in my career, there were situations where service members were reported for homosexual behaviors, having affairs, or experimenting with cannabis. The helping professionals told the service members they were there to help them, but they had to report their alleged misconduct, and the situation didn't go well.

CHAPTER 14

How the Military Environment Impacts Personnel

WHILE SERVING WITH the Coast Guard, I participated in a meeting where difficult issues were discussed. One of the senior leaders, the deputy commander of Health, Safety and Work-Life, discussed his experiences. He said, "This organization, the Coast Guard, does things to people. The organization challenges personal sanity." His remarks were very insightful and applied not only to the Coast Guard but to all branches of the military. These organizations impact their people. The *USS George Washington* and MARMC reports captured how the Navy impacted its people. To understand how the military impacts its people further, it's helpful to drill down into organizational demographics, nuances, culture, and contextual factors.

The US military is a massive organization, roughly 200 years old, with approximately 1.4 million personnel on active duty and an annual budget of 700 billion dollars. If the US military was a company, it may very well be the biggest and most successful company in the world. It has bases all over the world. The logistics that power the military are impressive. It has massive personnel, payroll, information technology, supply chain, medical, travel, and other systems that drive its operations.

According to the 2019 Demographics Profile of the Military

Community Report (DoD Office of the Deputy Assistant Secretary of Defense for Military Community and Family Policy 2019), there were over 3.5 million military personnel. The largest branch of the military was the Army, followed by Navy, Air Force, Marine Corps, then Coast Guard: 39 percent of personnel were active duty, 29.6 percent were ready reserve, and 25.5 percent were civilians.

Here are a few more stats: 82.4 percent of the military were enlisted and 17.6 percent percent were officers; 83.1 percent were male and 16.9 percent were female; 45.7 percent of enlisted personnel were twenty-five years of age or younger; and 24.3 percent of enlisted were pay grades E1-E3 while 48.3 percent were E4-E6.

Much of the military consists of young, healthy individuals in their early twenties. From a developmental perspective, this age group is going through a dynamic time, making a transition from childhood to adulthood, and maturing emotionally. At times, older adults enlist, including those with a college degree. Such nontraditional service members face challenges fitting in because their peers are younger, with a maturity gap. Another challenge of enlisting as a second career is money. Frequently, older adults who enlist take a significant pay cut to change careers.

The typical career path of an enlisted service member is to join the military after graduating from high school. A large percentage of service members leave after their first tour of duty, and a smaller percentage go on to serve a full twenty years. Those who serve twenty years retire in their late thirties, early forties, and go on to work in the private or public sector.

Historically, the military has tended to be male dominated, although that may be changing. Having an 80 percent preponderance of males creates situations that are ripe for challenges in gender dynamics.

Each military service has its own history, traditions, look, feel, and way of doing things. Each has its own organizational goals, uniforms, culture, and congressional budgets. Each service has a unique motto and cultural and contextual factors that impact its operations and personnel.

A book entitled *The Culture of Military Organizations* (Mansoor and Murray 2019) explored differences between services in depth. The Army is infantry, tanks, and conducts field operations. The Army is famous for massive land campaigns and is the largest branch of the military. Army culture was described as focused on designing and executing major combat operations and struggling with the aftermath. A senior mentor described the Army to me as a 900-pound gorilla or massive bulldozer that rolled over the enemy and itself in the process.

The Navy drives ships and submarines, conducts beach landings with marines, and operates aircraft. Sailors are known for struggling with austere environments and lonely separateness associated with sea service. The Navy is known for "OpNav Culture," a culture focused on sea service and technological solutions to achieve operational challenges. The Marine Corps is part of the Navy and is famous for combined-arms tactics—using land, sea, and air simultaneously to fight battles on a shoestring budget. The culture of the Marine Corps is family, tribal values, and loyalty and has been described as an "armed priesthood with unmatched commitment." The Air Force operates aircraft and airports. The Air Force has a reputation for technological supremacy, precision, careful planning, good organization, uncertainty avoidance, and taking care of its people. The Air Force's approach to addressing the problem of suicide, including the high interest list, exemplifies these characteristics.

The Coast Guard is considered military but is not part of the DoD. The Coast Guard is the smallest military branch, with a very diverse mission set. During peacetime, the Coast Guard operates under the Department of Homeland Security but can become part of the DoD and operate under the Navy during times of war. It has operational heavy icebreakers, and the Navy does not. The

Coast Guard is known for flexibility and being able to do anything, anywhere, with minimal resources. It is unique for the Coast Guard Auxiliary, a civilian volunteer organization that assists and supports the Coast Guard in various missions and activities. It is also known for taking care of its people.

One of the most famous battles in US military history was the D-Day Normandy Beach invasion. I am proud to say my grandfather Melvin "Sam" Marietta was there and survived. He served as a sergeant/E5 in the Army. Estimates were 155,000 Allied troops successfully stormed and held the beaches. The battle captured the toughness of the American warfighter. They drove on to achieve the mission no matter what the cost. The military is a culture and organization that struggles with a "suck it up," "soldier up," and "drive on" mentality that gets the mission done but results in barriers for seeking help.

The military is a massive bureaucracy with overlapping lines of control. On the ground, a service member ultimately reports to a senior operational commander through various levels of the organization. Simultaneously, the service member reports to a service-specific headquarters. A colleague described the DoD as a 100-foot-tall man, with service members being likened to the toes on this colossal entity's feet. Service members find themselves at the bottom, disconnected from senior leaders at the top, with numerous levels in between. A Navy psychologist described the military to me as an unkind and uncaring machine, with service members like cogs in the machine sometimes being unintentionally chewed up.

A critical concept behind the military is the notion of public service and "freedom is not free." Serving in the military is a civic duty, giving back to the country, a form of public service. Service comes with sacrifice, benefits, and opportunities, including personal growth. Service members learn, grow, receive educational opportunities, and make money, but that is not the primary purpose. I encountered individuals focused on rigid personal goals that did not share this mindset. Some had specific educational goals, geographic goals, and were focused on maintaining family businesses and pursuing financial objectives. Such individuals tended to become frustrated with military service after a short time and leave.

Regardless of the specific uniformed service and its nuances, the individual service member is both the common thread and lowest common denominator of the military. Ultimately, the Army, Navy, Marine Corps, and Air Force are hundreds of thousands of individuals. These individuals form a superstructure or backbone of the nation's military.

Uniform wear is not a requirement to serve in the military. Military spouses, children, family members, contractors, federal employees, and volunteers serve and make sacrifices too. They may not have a rank or receive a paycheck but are part of the military too.

The Impact of Political Winds and Congressional Budgets

After every election cycle, regardless of who comes to power, new administrations bring new initiatives and priorities. Change is also driven by world events. When this happens, directives are canceled, budgets are realigned, and people and materials shift rapidly. Regardless of which administration takes control, there is a whole new series of priorities, social directives, and online training to match.

Service members find themselves fighting a war. Soon after a new administration comes into power, the political priorities change drastically. Now, instead of fighting, the mission is changed to retreat. We are pulling out, cutting losses, and redefining victory. The pros and cons of political change can be debated, but the impact it has on the military and its personnel is irrefutable.

Periodically, if not annually, Congress determines the military budget. The politicians engage in power struggles and conflicts with each other. The services, service members, and families are caught in between. If Congress doesn't agree on a budget, the result is a dramatic government shutdown. Paychecks are missed, and services such as tuition assistance and travel are cut.

The Military Is the Gun Club of the United States

A Marine Corps colonel I served with affectionately referred to the military as the "Gun Club" of the United States. He described it as "the real 1 percent." Only a small percentage of the US population raises their right hand and volunteers to serve in this elite group. There are no conscripts in the US military. Serving in the Gun Club is a privilege, an honor, and an opportunity subject to certain rules. With the privilege comes a combination of duty and opportunities described above.

Gun Club rules include the following:

- Swearing an oath of allegiance
- Following orders
- Wearing proper uniform
- Adhering to grooming standards
- Maintaining physical fitness and body fat standards
- Maintaining personal conduct standards
- Maintaining medical readiness
- Using alcohol responsibility
- Zero tolerance for illicit substances
- Being ready to deploy at all times

Service members are held to the highest standards and are under pressure to follow these rules. They wear a uniform and are required to be neat and clean in appearance. Across my career, I encountered individuals who ate uncontrollably, weighed 300 pounds, and used alcohol and street drugs excessively. Some were extremely good at their jobs, but the military was not the right place for them.

Perpetual Manpower Issues

A typical military assignment or set of orders is one to five years, with the average military assignment being three years. At any given command, an estimated 30 percent of personnel rotated each year. If a military unit was staffed with 100 people and each year thirty people rotated out after three-to-four years, a 100 percent turnover rate was achieved.

Military manning numbers ebb and flow in a cyclical manner, swinging back and forth like a pendulum. One year, the determination was made that a particular career field was overmanned. Promotion rates plummeted, and service members were offered incentives to get out or were forced out through reduction in force initiatives. Soon after, the determination was made that too many personnel left, the same career field was critically undermanned, and service members were offered retention bonuses and increased promotion opportunities.

Service members are subject to the crunch and pressure from ever-changing manning numbers and unpredictable environments. The manning at military units turned over rapidly, and career field manning periodically oscillated back and forth. In addition to planned personnel losses, there were unplanned losses. Manpower issues and the feeling of being undermanned is frequently a top stress cited by service members suffering from mental health issues.

The Clash Between Individuality and Uniformity

The Borg Empire from the *Star Trek* science fiction universe is a part humanoid and android species that evolved over many centuries to forcefully assimilate other species. The Borg kidnap people, take over their bodies, and steal their knowledge and resources to increase their numbers and advance their society. Borgs communicate and share their minds through a collective consciousness. There are similarities between the Borg and active-duty service members. Much like the Borg, active duty looks the same and acts the same. They work together and follow orders from above to work collectively to accomplish the mission.

Camaraderie was great but at times counterproductive. A patient told me everyone at his command was stressed, depressed, and drinking alcohol. Another discussed learning how to drink in an unhealthy way from his military peers. There was a collective feeling that "going through the suck" was a shared responsibility. He felt pressure to conform to negative behaviors. He knew he was at his breaking point but told me he didn't want to sit on the sideline and let his team down by being positive and moving in a healthy direction.

Service members in distress complain that the message they receive is to "work, work, work" and feel treated like a number. They feel under tremendous pressure, and the message they receive is to get the mission done no matter what the obstacle. Sailors complain that they don't feel treated like human beings, and there is a mentality that as long as the ship is moving, no one cares. Service members feel pushed to the side. They receive a message that their problems don't matter, and they need to handle them on their own. If they leave work due to hitting a breaking point, for a medical appointment, or to take care of family members, the message they receive is production is lost and they let the team down. Service members complained to me of verbal abuse, including being told they were useless since they couldn't contribute to the mission. It was explained to me by one of my patients that verbal abuse was a bad leadership strategy because it made his issues worse and further sapped his productivity.

In the private sector, one can have a meteoric career rise by rapidly moving up the food chain based on the success of their ideas and work. The military was not like this. Service members start their careers at a low rank and progress slowly up the food chain. There were early promotions in the military but more barriers to career progression compared with the private sector. Each step of the way, career progression was closely scrutinized by the chain of command, individuals of a higher rank, and the promotion system.

Individuals who value freedom and individuality above all else quickly tired and hit a frustration point in the military system. Individuals who overperformed, underperformed, or didn't conform stuck out like a green thumb and drew negative attention or scrutiny from their peers and those above. I received accounts of being punished for both being a high performer and a low performer from the service members I worked with.

When a mortgage, car loan, or employment agreement is finalized, there is a lengthy multipage legal agreement. The military didn't operate like that. There is little in writing, no guarantees. An Army veteran discussed his experiences with me. He told me he had witnessed "too many guarantees thrown in the trash" and did not trust the military. The choice the service member has is whether to put on the uniform, to sacrifice some degree of individuality, and to serve. The recruiter made promises, and even if they were kept, things frequently changed. The famous financial book *The Simple Path to Wealth* by J. L. Collins recommended readers stockpile a stash of "F-You money" so they had the freedom to walk off a job. The military doesn't operate like that. Service members can't leave easily. Once they put on a uniform, it becomes difficult to leave military service.

Military Power and Family Dynamics

The military is significant for a strict rank structure and hierarchy. Service members are at the mercy of their superiors and bureaucrats and must obey orders. The plight of the service member is to do whatever the government asks them to do. This includes "other duties as assigned," for example working in the file room, and there is little recourse. The Stanford Prison Experiment was conducted in 1971 and examined interactions between guards and prisoners. As the experiment progressed, the guards abused their authority and power imbalance to exercise arbitrary control. The guards verbally and physically abused the prisoners and disrupted their sleep. They dehumanized them and used isolation as punishment. The prisoners rebelled and exhibited signs of psychological distress. The signs and symptoms included psychological breakdown, depression, mood swings, anxiety, emotional numbness, and social isolation. The experiment was canceled after a week.

There are parallels between military life and the Stanford Prison Experiment. In the military, those senior exhibit power and control over those junior. Service members aren't incarcerated, but the environment is controlled, and they must obey. Service members are limited in what they can and cannot do and are confined at times, for example on a ship or small base. There are similarities between the impact military life has on its people and the psychological distress the prisoners in the experiment experienced. One key difference between the Stanford Prison Experiment and the military is that the power leaders wield is not unchecked. Service members have protections through the Uniformed Code of Military Justice (UCMJ).

A news article describing toxic work environment issues onboard the *USS Scranton* illustrated Stanford Prison Experiment-like dynamics (Ziezulewicz 2022). The commanding officer was documented as being frustrated that sailors were not at work or in the hospital and ordered a sailor back to the ship who was later found to have a torn rotator cuff shoulder injury. The command was abusive; the sailors suffered and felt helpless.

In the military, I observed and was subject to twisted power dynamics, where people had power over others due to rank, went on power trips, and used authority to inflict psychological distress on others. In the *Highlander* series, immortals battle each other to the death, and the victor gains the deceased's magic in a dramatic display of lightning bolts to gain strength. Across my career in uniformed service, I observed and received firsthand accounts of similar phenomena. There are service members who achieved a promotion and abruptly changed the way they interacted with others, including detaching, exhibiting power and control, and becoming malignant. There was a cycle of mistreatment, stemming from a tradition of negativity being transmitted through generations. In this scenario, a victim transforms into the perpetrator, imparting the same negative influences they suffered onto others. There have been many news articles about commanding officers and senior enlisted leaders who were fired for toxicity. I suspect, if interviewed, they would report having been subject to similar toxic behaviors. The line-crossing ceremony, or blood-pinning ceremony, where service members were physically assaulted due to tradition, were good examples of this. The abuse was perpetrated under the guise of cultural tradition and improving resilience, but the reality was that a cycle of abuse was perpetuated that had negative effects. These traditions of hazing continued until the perpetrators were ordered to stop.

Most active-duty service members are in their early twenties. The typical junior enlisted sailor performs scut work—cleaning, sweeping, waxing, painting, and paperwork. There is a lot of forced downtime. Leadership chases young junior sailors around all day to ensure tasks are accomplished. There is an age gap between junior and senior enlisted. There is a parent-child dynamic. Service members complain that they are treated like children and struggle with independence issues. Expectations are high, and service members complain that leadership has a high propensity for disciplinary action. Service members are ostracized for leaving work an hour early. On an Army deployment where soldiers were working twelve-hour shifts, soldiers complained to me that they were pressured and discouraged to go to medical appointments. Soldiers complained and were told that their morale didn't matter. They were asked if they were trying to screw over their buddies and were encouraged to reschedule appointments so they occurred during their one day off. Soldiers perceived that their leadership was trying to drive them extra hard to get their numbers up for their annual performance review.

A Navy surface warfare officer told me they were forced to get out of bed early for no reason at all except to be malignant and malicious. I had little experience with male-on-male sexual assault until I served with the infantry in a Marine Corps unit. I was told by my patients, male-on-male sexual assault, "tea bagging," was an initiation ceremony into the unit.

Service members have been compared to indentured servants. The military tells them where they can live, what to wear, and how to groom. The military tells them what to do and sets their work hours. Service members can't quit without passing over extensive hurdles and obstacles. In the best case, the command is a strong family unit where senior leaders take care of the junior service members. In the worst case, the military is a dysfunctional family. Military family dynamics can mirror the situation that occurs when parents are in an abusive marriage and the children suffer. If the parents are struggling with severe marital problems, the children feel the pain and are unhappy and struggling too. If the command is struggling, the pain is passed on to service members.

Trauma and pain roll downhill far too often in the military. The commander, deputy commander, and senior enlisted leadership experience pain and kick the can. If they are hurting, everyone will feel it too. I encountered an example of this during a Joint Commission medical inspection. The inspector identified issues with the paper clinical charts. The hospital commander ordered our clinic to provide twenty-four-hour in-house coverage to review thousands of charts by hand, find all clinical chart deficiencies, and correct them. Another example of this was the *USS Gerald R. Ford*, a large multibillion-dollar Navy ship, the first of its class. It was over budget, had extensive delays, and was under intense scrutiny. My patients told me the command was under extreme pressure from Big Navy and Congress. Sailors complained that the misery and pain were passed down on to them. Everything rolled downhill, and everyone felt miserable.

Maltreatment was a cancerous thing that spread and negatively impacted individuals, units, the organization, and the overall mission. Abuse and toxicity hurt people, caused them to shut down, impeded communication, and sapped productivity. Service members who are bullied are more likely to suffer mental health issues (Kime 2023). Maltreatment creates a situation where service members act out, become oppositional-defiant, and engage in passive-aggressive behaviors. From the perspective of a perpetrator, malignant behavior was career enhancing because it allowed them to achieve more at someone else's expense, but it was short-sighted and had an overall negative impact on the organization. I had an interesting conversation with a refugee from Afghanistan. He said he had a childhood friend who was smart, handsome, and athletic but joined the Taliban. He explained that it was "nurture." He felt that the environment was so toxic, many joined the Taliban to survive. There were similarities in military culture. One strategy to survive in a toxic environment is to become toxic.

The Milgram Shock experiment, conducted in 1963, showed that participants would repeatedly shock subjects due to obedience of authority even to the point of death. People tend to obey orders from others if they recognize their authority as morally right and/or legally based. I experienced this phenomenon while serving in the military. Service members do what they are told to do. In every discussion of improving military mental health, the need to achieve cultural and institutional change is raised. To achieve this requires somehow breaking the cycle and improving these dynamics.

Healthy Boundaries, Privacy, and Constant Chaos

A healthy personal or business relationship occurs when there is mutual respect between parties. The parties can agree to anything, but effective communication and informed consent are required. If one party says no, the other party respects this.

Military service is a challenging environment for service members, their families, and those who are employed by the DoD. Military life is significant for frequent transitions, moves, and unplanned and unwanted changes. There is little or no control when political and policy decisions are made ten levels above where the individual sits in an organization.

An individual could say no to abusive spouses, parents, or business partners, but it's very difficult to say no to the military. I was told that, technically speaking, a service member can refuse an unlawful order, but that is shouldering a big risk. Refusing a lawful order is insubordination and can result in UCMJ legal charges and retaliation. I experienced the Navy to be mafia-like at times. I was once told that a three-star Marine Corps general had so much power, they could have someone killed. How is one to cope with someone who has so much power?

Military life is significant for issues surrounding lack of privacy. When service members are on flight status to pilot billion-dollar aircraft or have clearance to handle nuclear materials, everything they do is known and scrutinized. There were pros and cons to lack of privacy. If the military knew a service member suffered from alcohol problems, additional monitoring and accountability was provided to assist the service member in achieving sobriety. A lot of times, when Uncle Sam got into someone's personal business, there were positive outcomes, but there were times when it backfired.

Service Members Are Perceived as Gaming the System

A toxic belief I encountered while serving with the Navy was that leaving the ship was a choice, a form of quitting and letting down the team. The belief system included that service members were trying to get out of work. Often, service members in distress presented to the command, medical, or another helping agency with the complaint, "I can't go back." They were labeled and tagged with negative stereotypes and biases such as "malingerer." The negative biases applied to family members too. Family members were referred to as "dependapotamus," "dependa," or other negative terms. Gaming the system did happen, but my experience was that it was overblown.

Service members, especially junior ones, were at the bottom of the food chain. Given their age and life experience, they were at increased risk for poor coping mechanisms. If they were in a toxic, hostile environment, couldn't access care, or found themselves at a breaking point, one power they had was to try to get out of that environment. Recognizing one was at a breaking point and trying to get out was being street smart.

Often, it was difficult and humiliating for a service member to approach the chain of command or a peer and say they were at a breaking point, wave the white flag of surrender, and ask for help. They didn't want to be the one breaking the Ship, Shipmate, and Self code and looking bad. It was hard for them to ask for help from someone who was signing their annual performance review. It's unfortunate because, chances were, a system problem or some other issue fueling their distress could have been addressed by command, the first line of defense to address issues.

Too often, when a service member presented to medical or the command asking for help, there was a presumption that the service member was at fault or had ulterior motives. It was the easy way to turn it around and blame the service member for issues they were experiencing. Dealing with a complaint and vetting an interpersonal conflict was a headache. The outcome of an interpersonal dispute or conflict could be positive and had the potential to positively impact other service members and strengthen the organization.

When service members were at a crisis point, they were overloaded with emotion and frustration, and it was difficult for them to communicate about issues effectively. Too often, there was a knee-jerk reaction from the command and helping system that lacked empathy and compassion. Everyone else chooses to go to work, sucks it up, and pushes on in the face of numerous problems, so why can't others do this? I served along with mental health providers who assumed service members were disability-seeking and trying to increase their disability percentages. I witnessed mental health providers pressure service members to go back to the ship when they didn't feel ready, and it was a gamble. Consider the scenario of forcing a service member who can't swim into a training pool. Sometimes "sink or swim" is effective, but a lot of times it isn't and has ended in death.

I spoke with a sixty-five-year-old Army E7 retiree who experienced a bad outcome from that exact scenario. His unit was involved in water-based training of soldiers. He went to the 2nd lieutenant, who was new, and told him he had concerns about the safety plan for the pool exercise. The commanding officer overruled him, and later he was called to the pool after a soldier was found dead at the bottom. He was from the islands, a good swimmer, jumped in, pulled him out, and administered CPR, but it was too late. The command tried to turn it around on him, but when it was discovered that the first sergeant was lying, Article 15 was dismissed, and the commanding officer was fired. My patient suffered psychological and moral injuries and developed PTSD and substance abuse issues, and it took him years to recover. For many reasons, especially risk management, it doesn't make sense to send service members who are not medically and mentally ready into an operational environment.

If a service member hits a breaking point, it is best for all parties involved to examine the situation and either fix the underlying issues or remove the member from the environment. If an issue is critical enough to negatively impact one service member, there is a high probability it was impacting others. If a service member is truly engaging in dysfunctional behavior, that pattern becomes apparent with time, and the member can be dealt with appropriately.

Family members served too. If a child couldn't access the pediatrics clinic or their medications from the pharmacy or receive a timely sports physical, it was a legitimate issue. Not having these issues addressed increased stress at home, impacted the service member's performance, and contributed to mental health issues. Families sacrificed a lot to serve in the military. They gave up career and educational opportunities to serve. Writing off family members as "dependapotamus" was simplistic and counterproductive.

There were outliers, but for most, "gaming the system" worked like taxes. Most optimize their tax return to minimize tax liability. Military beneficiaries try to optimize the benefits and perks of service. Negative biases against service members and toxic cultural beliefs didn't help military readiness and made things worse.

Benefits of Service

This chapter contained a lot of discussion about how the military environment negatively impacted people, but there were positive impacts too. Serving in the military is a great opportunity and has many positive benefits.

Military service is a civic duty, an honorable tradition. It is rewarding. It benefits other people, the community, and the country. There is an intangible benefit of doing something for the mission to achieve something higher. After getting out of the Navy, I worked in the private/public sector for a brief stint. I made more money and was treated better, but it felt like *Groundhog Day* and as if something were missing.

Service members are called to work in dynamic, challenging, austere environments. They learn practical skills such as leadership, organizational structure, teamwork, discipline, and communication. The military wrote the book on these topics. Service members learn how to cope with loss of control, frequent moves, and changes. Military service is a personal challenge that results in growth, increased flexibility, and mental and physical toughness. Service members develop resilience and skills to cope with any stress or situation.

Time spent in uniform is frequently a stepping stone to a larger career. Many companies, organizations, and governments value and seek out military veterans.

Serving in the military brought once-in-a-lifetime opportunities. When I served in the Navy and PHS, I did things I will remember for the rest of my life, like living in the community in Okinawa, Japan, experiencing a different culture, and learning to appreciate new foods that I continue to enjoy to this day. I'll never forget deploying to Puerto Rico for earthquake relief, staying in the oldest hotel on the island, and experiencing an earthquake. I was fearful that the building would collapse. I'll never forget deploying to Liberia and working at an Ebola treatment facility. I remember our team getting a phone call from the secretary of health during the Christmas holiday, being told we were in her thoughts and prayers, we were on a no-fail mission, and no expense would be spared.

The perks of military service were tremendous. The housing allowance was nontaxable and lowered my tax bracket. The post-9/11 GI bill covered college expenses, providing around $20,000 per year. It included a monthly housing allowance and book stipend. The benefit was transferable to family members, and I utilized it to help pay for my children's college education. Serving with Veterans Affairs taught me about the extensive benefits veterans have available to them. Veterans can receive medical care, disability payments, and assistance with education, training, and housing.

CHAPTER 15

Mental Health and Support Resources

THE NEXT PART of the book is focused on resources for getting help, common issues service members face, and recommendations for coping mechanisms.

The scale and magnitude of the assistance and resources the DoD offers its people is impressive. It offers direct patient care through medical providers at military treatment facilities and pays for care through the TRICARE network. The military provides operational mental health providers and chaplains that are embedded in military units. For substance use disorders, the military has its own substance abuse treatment programs, and TRICARE covers the cost of a thirty-day residential treatment program. It provides the Family Advocacy and Sexual Assault Prevention and Response programs. In addition to the services offered by the DoD, the Department of Veterans Affairs provides resources that go above and beyond.

In preparing for this book, it was difficult to find specific itemized budget numbers for all these programs. An estimated billion dollars annually, likely even more, was spent by the DoD to fund these initiatives. Across 1.4 million active-duty service members, a rough estimate was between $1,000 to 2,000 was spent per service member annually.

Many organizations and companies can't afford or access the services the military offers.

What other organization invests as much time and energy in people as the DoD does? Unfortunately, there is no comparative data. How much possible similar programs, like the militaries in China, India, and Russia, have invested is unknown.

Besides specific programs offered, numbers and dollar amounts, the people in the military community form a family. The service members and their dependents are part of that family. In a healthy unit, the chain of command, fellow service members, and coworkers are part of that family too. The military family works together to support each other, achieve a shared mission, and celebrate camaraderie.

Family and Friends

The first stop in getting help is often a spouse, close family, or friends. The immediate support system includes a battle buddy, wingman, or best friend. There is an understanding that no one takes care of an individual like blood. The people who have close, healthy, positive relationships with a service member know them best, are in the best position to identify a problem, are trusted to handle issues with sensitivity and kindness, and have their best interests at heart. Research has shown that having a good support system, to include family and friends, is a positive prognostic factor for mental health issues.

The Command

A lesson I learned early in my career as a military psychiatrist is that the chain of command is an unidentified family. Active duty lived, worked, and breathed together, especially on deployment, just like family. The service member's relationship with command was key. In an ideal situation, the relationship between the service member and command was healthy, and commands were invested in their success. Just like real family, commands have internal problems and relationship dynamics. The command has a tremendous amount of power and ability to impact many situations. All requests, leave chits, workplace qualifications, and performance reviews require endorsement from the command. A lot of times, service members were reluctant to ask for help, but for many situations, asking for help from the command was critical. Commands had the power to address work environment issues. Including the command in a service member's care and treatment plan ensured the best outcomes.

Navy chiefs and Air Force first sergeants, in my experience, were often a first line of defense for service members struggling with issues. They had been around a long time, knew how to work situations, and were familiar with helping resources and could connect service members to them.

I spoke with a forty-four-year-old female veteran who retired after a twenty-year career in the Navy. When I asked her about the *USS George Washington* and MARMC suicide clusters, she said anytime there are problems, her reaction is "What is going on in the chain of command?" She said operational tempo and other factors impact sailors, but in her experience, issues with the chain of command determine how sailors fare. She explained that sailors do best in a healthy chain of command where people are put first.

Mentors

Finding an older, more experienced service member to sit down and talk with on a regular basis is strongly recommended and a best practice. I spoke to a service member in the Navy who received mentorship from a retired Navy chief at her church. Her mentor explained the nuts and bolts of her career field and how to navigate the Navy. This was a turning point for the sailor and the issues she was experiencing. Mentors are farther along in the career path, have been through what junior service members are going through, and offer wisdom and a broader perspective. Mentors experienced many things and have seen people come and go. A mentor offers insights, guidance, and suggestions for coping with career issues, including discussing unwritten standards and practices. A mentor is also a valuable resource in times of crisis.

It was documented in the *USS George Washington* reports that "multiple sailors interviewed stated they did not have a mentor." Not having a mentor was identified as a factor that contributed to the deaths.

Community Services

Each military service has "community services" programs that are configured differently. The Army has Army Community Services. The Navy has Fleet and Family Services, and the Marine Corps features Marine Corps Community Services. The Air Force has Community Service Centers. The Coast Guard has resource-sharing agreements with the military services, and coasties utilize the above programs depending on geographic base proximity. Community service programs include transition and relocation assistance, family employment, financial services, and counseling. The community services programs also offer gaming and computer hubs, recreation, and instructional classes.

Military OneSource

The Military OneSource program is a twenty-four seven call center, referral hotline, and website for service and family members run by a DoD-funded contractor. It is managed by the Office of the Deputy Assistant Secretary of Defense for Military Community and Family policy. Military OneSource screens callers and makes referrals. Military OneSource maintains a referral network of thousands of counselors where individuals can receive counseling outside of the military system. Sometimes, if a problem is too complex or too severe, callers are referred back to the military service and the military health system. The Coast Guard has a similar program called CG SUPRT. Military OneSource's areas of focus include confidential and nonmedical counseling, family and relationships, financial and legal, health and wellness, education and employment, on and off base living, and deployment and transition.

Military Treatment Facilities

The military medical system maintains medical facilities and medical providers to provide direct care. Healthcare professionals in the military medical system include doctors, dentists, nurses, pharmacists, physical therapists, laboratory experts, optometrists, and more. There are surgical subspecialists such as cardiothoracic surgeons and neurosurgeons. It has operational medics or corpsmen, medical providers, and medical personnel embedded in military units.

When I started my career in the Navy, the military hospitals were open to family members and retirees, but the primary focus was always on active-duty service members and medical readiness. Service availability to family members and retirees has shifted over the years. Overseas military hospitals and clinics provide care to family members because there is no off-base option. When I served in Okinawa, Japan, there was no TRICARE network to fall back on. Service members and families had to receive care from the naval hospital, out-in-town from the Japanese health system, or be flown home for care.

TRICARE Network

The DoD operates its own healthcare insurance system called TRICARE. When there are no local resources or there is nonavailability, service members and their families are deferred to the TRICARE network for care. A network deferral allows beneficiaries to receive care from a nonmilitary provider. Military retirees utilize TRICARE for health care.

I encountered service and family members who requested to receive care outside of military facilities. The reasons varied.

Sometimes they had difficulty getting care in a timely manner, a negative experience, or simply a preference to receive care from a nonuniformed medical provider. They found themselves in a difficult situation because the military facilities had a right of first refusal and were reluctant to send them to the network.

Substance Abuse Treatment Programs

Each military service has its own substance abuse treatment program. The Army has the SUDCC program. The Navy has SARP, and the Air Force has ADAPT. There were several ways a service member could be referred for assistance with substance issues. The preferred pathway was self-referral. It was always better for service members to self-refer for treatment because policy conveyed legal protection. If a service member came forward, asked for help, and disclosed driving while intoxicated, without getting in trouble, they had protection from prosecution. Other referral pathways included referrals from the command after an incident or from a medical provider. If a healthcare provider had a strong clinical suspicion of a substance abuse disorder, they referred a service member directly to the substance abuse treatment program. If there was public knowledge of a situation or if a service member was arrested after a DUI, the situation was considered a command referral. I spoke to service members who presented to medical asking for help the day after being arrested for a DUI, requesting self-referral, but it wasn't the case. There were also incidents where a service member had a public episode of intoxication, including on social media, and were referred by others.

Unit Family Readiness Programs

Unit family support programs are staffed with volunteer spouses who, in some cases, receive compensation. They perform a vital role, acting as a liaison or coordinator between families and the military unit. Functions include distributing information from the command to families, acting as a support and communication bridge, advocating for community resources, and assisting families with maintaining readiness, resilience, and a connection to the unit. Each service has different names for the program. In the Army, the program is referred to as the Soldier and Family Readiness Group. The Navy calls it Ombudsman while the Marine Corps calls it the Family Readiness Program. It is referred to as the Key Spouse program in the Air Force.

Exceptional Family Member Program

The EFMP provides resources for families with special needs. Spouses, children, and dependent adults who require special medical services for chronic conditions were enrolled in the program. Medical and military personnel departments assist service members and families to coordinate assignments to ensure they are stationed at a location where special medical and educational needs are met. The EFMP program also helps connect families with resources and support, including providing nonclinical case management.

A nurse coworker told me about a situation she encountered while serving overseas. A single mother of two was stationed overseas on a small island. One of her daughters began having severe mental health problems, including psychotic episodes six months into her three-year tour. The island didn't have the resources to provide care for the child. She enrolled in the EFMP program and was recommended for tour curtailment, and the military assisted in relocating the whole family near a large military treatment facility so she could receive care.

Chaplains and Spirituality

Chaplains were an underappreciated, underutilized, and misunderstood resource. I observed a chaplain delivering a pre-deployment briefing to a group of marines. He said the mission was a righteous, just cause, and a higher power had our backs. I'd been to many mental health pre-deployment briefings, but that approach was powerful and offered something that was missing. A lesson I learned in life and working with patients is that some problems are so big and complex that they are in God's hands. Across my career, I've observed patients struggling with catastrophic problems, such as a woman who was pregnant with triplets who lost two of her babies. Medications and talk therapy helped, but religion offered peace and hope. I've observed, personally and professionally, that spirituality exercises a part of the brain that medications, therapy, exercise, and other activities do not.

Military chaplains have the highest level of confidentiality. They can keep anything a secret, unless it involves child abuse or neglect. A Marine Corps chaplain took me aside and explained that he had a loophole to work around confidentiality issues. He said he would never disclose private information, such as suicidal thoughts, but would never leave a service member's side to prevent something bad from happening if needed.

Chaplains embedded in a military unit provide another resource for getting help. At times, service members don't want to talk to a mental health provider but are willing to speak to the chaplain. My colleagues and I observed that the chaplain had what we referred to as "the privilege of the cross." The chaplains could connect with people in ways and do things we, as embedded mental health providers, could not. Many marines had a distrust for Navy medicine and healthcare professionals, and the chaplain was not part of the medical system. He could address issues coming from a different angle. The chaplain I served with in the 3d Marine Division had a seat at the general's table. He had a direct line of communication with leadership. He could make things happen that we could not.

For some, religion is a top priority in life, a strong foundation that drives all thought processes. Others have a different sense of spirituality. When service members are in a dark place and have nothing going for them, spirituality is a source of hope. The practice of religion and prayer is a healthy way of coping. Places of worship can provide a sense of community and belonging that are critical for healing, mental health, and wellness.

Sexual Assault Prevention and Response Program

The SAPR program (pronounced "saa per") varied between services but overall offered services for sexual assault victims through a network of Sexual Assault Response Coordinators and Sexual Assault Prevention and Response Victim Advocates (SAPR VAs). The sexual assault program featured a twenty-four seven crisis intervention support hotline called the DoD Safe Helpline. Service members filed unrestricted or restricted assault reports concerning sexual assault incidents. The benefit of the restricted report was that they were kept private while facilitating help for service members. Unrestricted reports resulted in formal legal investigation. Victims filed confidential information about their assailants into the Catch a Serial Offender (CATCH) system that was pooled and analyzed. If a pattern of assault allegations against a specific perpetrator was discovered, the victims were connected and could work together to pursue prosecution. SAPR offered something the other programs didn't, and that was the expedited transfer program. Service members could request an assignment change to create geographic separation with their assailant and to facilitate their recovery. In my experience, the expedited transfer program was a trump card that topped everything. A victim would present to medical to report a sexual assault, and then shortly thereafter, they would be eligible for transfer to a different military unit. The expedited transfer program didn't always work out. Some victims felt it was unfair they had to relocate instead of their perpetrator. Victims could also receive legal representation from Special Victims' Counsel and Victims' Legal Counsel.

One afternoon in the mental health clinic, someone realized a sexual assault victim and her alleged offender were scheduled for outpatient appointments simultaneously with different providers. Both suffered from mental health issues, including suicidal thoughts. The victim struggled with obvious issues, and the alleged offender felt falsely accused and struggled with career-ending legal actions. I think the situation was solved by one of them going through the clinic's back door. We had to be vigilant about these sorts of situations. In case they had to be hospitalized, we had to ensure the victim and alleged offender were not both hospitalized in the same inpatient psychiatry unit.

Family Advocacy Program

Family Advocacy provides intervention and tracking for domestic violence and maltreatment issues. Maltreatment is broken up into different categories, including intimate partner and child abuse.

Family Advocacy is charged with prevention and intervention but was focused on allegations and police blotter-type incidents. When a formal allegation is received, Family Advocacy interviews the parties involved. A committee meets, vets the allegations, and votes to determine whether an allegation was substantiated. Family Advocacy provides recommendations and treatment and coordinates services with commands. There was overlap and similarity between the sexual assault and the Family Advocacy Programs. If a sexual assault occurred within the confines of an "intimate partner" relationship, such as a married couple, FAP offered services and intervention.

Family Advocacy was framed as a helping program, but service members could face legal or disciplinary actions for assault. It was explained to me like this: "Family Advocacy doesn't push punishment, but the command provides allegation information and can do what they want to do." Service members were reluctant to disclose anything that could get them in trouble or jeopardize their career. Many service members complained to me that participating in FAP made their situations worse.

Military Family Life Counselors

Pronounced "M flack," these mental health counselors serve on bases around the DoD. Like Military OneSource, the program is managed by a services contract through the Office of the Deputy Assistant Secretary of Defense for Military Community and Family Policy. One of the biggest advantages of these counselors is that the services provided were undocumented. They do not take notes or keep counseling records. They offer nonmedical counseling to service members and their families, including children. They provide support for a range of issues, including deployment stress, reintegration, relocation adjustment, separation, anger management, conflict resolution, parenting, parent-child communication, relationship and family issues, coping skills, homesickness, and grief and loss. They are also unable to receive restricted reports for sexual assault or domestic abuse.

Education Assistance

The military services offer tuition assistance and reimbursement for educational expenses. Eligibility requirements include having three years' time in service. The tuition assistance program was a way for service members to pay for school while preserving their post-9/11 GI bill benefits. The payback is that service members must remain on active duty for the number of years it took to get the degree. The Department of Veterans Affairs offers the post-9/11 GI bill, which includes tuition, room and board, and a book allowance for thirty-six months. The bill equates to a full scholarship at a four-year undergraduate degree program. The VA also offers Veteran Readiness and Employment services, which include help with job training, education, employment accommodations, résumé development, and job seeking skills.

The Air Force has a program called the Community College of the Air Force. Airmen frequently referred to achieving their "CCAF" degree. It is a federally chartered degree-granting institution that assists airmen in earning an associate's degree in applied science. It is described as a flexible degree program that utilizes technical training, professional military training, credit by examination, and college classes.

Military Welfare and Morale

The Military Welfare and Morale (MWR) program is a great resource for service members and their family. While serving overseas, the MWR program where I served in Okinawa, Japan, had a scuba shop, which offered lessons, gear rentals, and oxygen tank refills. Scuba diving on a regular basis helped me cope with the military stress I faced. There were MWR trips, campsites, cabins, and gear rentals, including bounce house rentals for children. "If all else fails, go outside and camp" is great advice. Research has shown that exposure to natural environments assists with recovery from physiological stress and mental fatigue.

The MWR programs are a great way to get out and meet people with similar interests. Many joined the military to travel and have adventures they would've never experienced in their hometown. MWR provides a service member stationed at a new, unfamiliar place with a guide to adventures that are waiting for them and helps build great friendships and relationships.

Legal

Most military bases have a legal clinic where service members can walk in and talk to an attorney. The military legal clinics assist with wills and power of attorney documents. There are times when service members must use the Servicemembers Civil Relief Act to break an apartment lease due to a military move. When these situations occur, the military legal clinics assist service members in breaking their leases.

Equal Opportunity Program

The military family unit wasn't always rosy. Just like in any family, there was friction, tension, and politics. Service members and civilian employees suffer from discriminatory acts, sexual harassment, and hostile workplace issues. Affected personnel can file formal grievances with the equal opportunity program. There is a forty-five-day time limit from the date of the alleged act to file. A complaint can result in an investigation and legal consequences. Alternative dispute resolution is a collaborative, nonpunitive process to resolve workplace disputes.

IG Hotline Program

The IG program is where service members can file complaints about waste, fraud, and abuse. The IG program is an alternative method to the chain of command when a complainant believes the chain of command is unresponsive or they reasonably fear or have suffered from reprisal. The IG is charged with utilizing an unbiased, impartial approach to ensure issues are properly evaluated, investigated, and, when necessary, corrected by responsible authorities.

Military Relief Societies

Each of the services has relief societies, which are nonprofit organizations. The Army has Army Emergency Relief. The Navy has the Navy and Marine Corps Relief Society, and the Air Force has the Air Force Aid Society. The Coast Guard has Coast Guard Mutual Assistance. These organizations aid with budgeting, financial planning, and offering low interest loans for service members who find themselves in a financial pinch. During government shutdowns, the military relief societies step up and provide aid to service members.

Operational Stress Control and Crisis Response Teams

Each of the military services have operational stress control and crisis response teams. The terminology utilized to describe these teams varies between the services, but they are multidisciplinary teams of mental health professionals who would travel to a command and conduct interventions. The Navy once referred to such a team as a Special Psychiatric Rapid Intervention Team, or "SPRINT." Once, I collaborated with an Army Combat Stress Control team while on deployment with the PHS, and we worked together to provide intervention. Operational stress control teams are used successfully to assist service members and military units coping in the aftermath of natural disasters, workplace accidents, workplace violence, or deaths.

PHA, Screenings, and Questionnaires

There are numerous DoD and service-specific health screening programs that include periodic mental health and substance abuse screenings. There are screenings concerning post-traumatic stress, suicide, anxiety, and alcoholism. If a service member reached a threshold of affirmative responses, assistance and referrals for help were offered.

The ICE Complaint

Service members and their families can utilize the Interactive Customer Evaluation (ICE) system at the DoD level to file a service comment. Technically, comments could be positive or negative, but the system was known for complaints. Sometimes it is true, the squeaky wheel gets the grease, and the ICE system facilitates this process. If an ICE complaint was submitted, it would make its way down to the department level. If a service member complained, they couldn't get an appointment, or their medical provider was rude, the ICE complaint received attention, and positive things could result. Sometimes nothing could be done, but if nothing else, the complaint helped someone air a grievance or get an appointment.

CHAPTER 16

Common Issues Service Members Face

I SPOKE TO tens of thousands of service members and their families across my career. I also worked with service members after they left the military, including retirees. After reflecting on their issues, I pieced together common issues and obstacles that are a frequent focus of attention. Some of the issues are unique to military life, and others impact everyone everywhere. I reflected on the success stories of my patients and jotted down their words of wisdom.

Boot Camp and Basic Training

A pivotal moment in boot camp is when the bus of recruits pulls up, the drill instructors get on the bus, and they start yelling at the recruits.

Having worked at a basic training facility and delivered mental health services to recruits, I observed a dirty little secret of basic training: A lot of it is for show. Why do recruits need to march around, get yelled at about their hygiene, have their rooms inspected, and walk around with a mattress above their heads? Is it all a ruse designed to stress the recruits and filter out the ones that can't handle it? The practice of hazing has been going on for centuries. A lot of it is a rite of passage, a centuries-old tradition. From my perspective, a big part of challenging recruits is to prepare and test them for the stresses and bureaucracy they will experience during a military career. Boot camp was indoctrination into military culture. Recruits face the heat of boot camp because everyone before them did, and it's meant to make them stronger.

Recruits who find themselves in this situation should not panic or get discouraged. Boot camp is like a modern video game, where there is only one direction that can be traveled. Boot camp is designed to get people through, and staff are pressured to maintain a graduation rate. Recruits are wise to go with the flow and do what they are told. Practical advice is for recruits to trust the system and instructors to get them where they need to be no matter how cranky or abusive they may seem. Drill instructors have limits, and there have been serious consequences for those convicted of abuse.

Many service members enlist in the military immediately after graduating from high school. For many, it is their first time away from home and a difficult adjustment. Service members struggle with being away from a sweetheart. Recruits should not be afraid to be away from home or to be geographically separated from a relationship. If a relationship is meant to last, it will survive and strengthen being apart. Recruits would benefit from getting out of their comfort zone and experiencing new things.

Another observation about basic training and military training in general is that breaking people with unnecessary and harsh training contributes to mental health problems. There have been service members who died by suicide while participating in basic training. Sometimes the focus on basic training programs is not having enough mental health providers, but a larger issue is that the training methods and tactics utilized could be adjusted to make them more palatable for the recruits.

Realistic Expectations

Across my career as a military psychiatrist, I talked to patients who experienced crisis levels of distress because their expectations weren't being met. A classic example of this was a sailor who said, "I didn't sign up for this" because they wanted to be in the Navy but not serve on a ship. Other service members told me they wanted to serve in the armed forces but not carry a weapon. They must have never heard the saying "every marine is a rifleman." Another common complaint was that service members were upset because they desired some type of special treatment, accommodation, or duty status. A service member told me they were stressed to the point of suicide because they had very specific educational goals, the recruiter promised tuition assistance, and they couldn't access that. Another service member complained of psychological distress because the command wouldn't modify their work schedule so they could attend college classes.

Expectations must be realistic, or service members are set up to become frustrated and dissatisfied. For those struggling with expectation issues, it is critical to temper expectations and recognize the point of military service as "service." The perks of service come with time, patience, and as circumstances and funding allows. Service members are wise to avoid unreasonable expectations and entitled thinking, as such leads to disappointment and frustration.

Loss of Privacy and Independence

The military is composed of small, tight-knit communities. Everyone knows everything about everyone. Service members are under the microscope and constantly scrutinized. There is a close relationship between the service member and command. It is helpful for service members to acknowledge and accept some degree of loss of privacy and confidentiality and respect and appreciate command involvement.

Service members are told what to wear. Hygiene and body fat standards are enforced. The military has a way of intruding into every aspect of an individual's life. This includes facing hard expectations about what to do, where, and when to do it. There is also a tendency for leadership to be brash, overbearing, and micromanaging. There is a loss of autonomy and independence in military life. It doesn't stop there. At other points in a service member's military career, especially when the service member functioned in sensitive and special duties, the government was even more intimately involved and intertwined in a person's life. The military scrutinizes everything a service member does: who flies aircraft, works with nuclear materials, or possesses a high-level security clearance.

Functioning in an environment like this can be a bitter pill to swallow, especially for someone new to the military. Sometimes service members don't react well, are passive aggressive, or act out and rebel, but this makes things worse. The chain of command responds to such behaviors by increasing efforts to control. Service members who struggle with loss of independence benefit from demonstrating to leadership that they are independent and responsible and can be trusted to get things done rather than fight them. Demonstrating independence assists in helping an overly involved command to back off. It is critical for service members to accept and have expectations about some loss of independence as a condition of military service.

Adapting to Military Life

A good rule of thumb is it takes one to two years for someone to really feel settled after they move to a new location and start a new job. It takes time to form relationships with others, learn a new geographic area, receive on-the-job training, and learn the ins and outs of a new job. Joining the military is a massive adjustment. The military is always changing and is an unpredictable environment. For many, it is their first job and first time away from home. Other service members leave good-paying jobs, take a pay cut to serve, and struggle to adapt. A lot of the perks and financial benefits of military service are hard to see or come long term, and it is easy to focus on day-to-day pain instead of seeing the long-term outlook. Military life ebbs and flows. There are times when it is strenuous and other times when the workload is light. It is hard for service members to see the light when they feel they are drowning in the moment.

Service members adapting to military life are best to maintain a long-term perspective. Those new to the military should find a mentor and set short, intermediate, and long-term goals to formulate a path to success. A helpful skill is to network and communicate with other service members who have been around longer and have had a successful career. Service members should not be afraid to ask for career guidance or help. When talking to a mentor, service members are recommended to learn about the issues their mentor faced and how they coped with them. Another skill is studying other service members, observing those who are doing well and those who are not and the characteristics driving success or failure. Above all, service members benefit from getting into a battle rhythm, finding what works, and having patience.

Dealing with Pay Issues, Paperwork, and Bureaucracy

The military is a massive bureaucracy that is at times suffocating. Policies and procedures are outdated and can conflict with each other. Service members are put into impossible situations. On a rare occasion, I experienced a refreshing unwritten military cultural tradition where leaders bucked policy and took matters into their own hands to get the mission done, including conducting business under the table.

Catch-22 was a famous book by Joseph Heller and is a must-read. It is a satirical book about the military. There is a memorable scene where a service member presents to the personnel section and complains that he isn't getting paid. He is told they can't talk to him because military records document him as being deceased. He tries to argue, but after that point, the personnel specialist completely ignores him. That soldier was caught in a Catch-22. He was serving overseas on a deployment, and there was no way to fix the problem.

Issues with military pay are far from fiction. The military personnel system was slow, dysfunctional, and inefficient, and this contributed to psychological distress. There were stories of service members not being paid for months, suffering unpaid travel claims and disputes over housing allowances. There was a news article published during November 2021, describing military pay delays service members faced (Kime 2011). The article described a service member who resorted to taking a personal loan in the Washington, DC, area because his housing allowance was delayed many months past the deadline.

There is an unwritten rule: The squeaky wheel gets the grease. Sometimes I observed that service members take out their frustration on personnel specialists. The problem is they have a lot of power and can make situations worse. The personnel specialists were struggling with bureaucracy and had their own set of problems. Often, the personnel specialists were doing their job, but the situation was out of their control. Service members struggling with pay issues, where solutions are elusive, are recommended to be courteous and find someone senior at the chain of command to validate the problems and provide advocacy. Sometimes taking on the personnel system one-on-one was effective, but often it backfired. The military had an unwritten tradition of turning things around on service members and blaming them for issues. With a senior advocate, complaints came from the chain of command instead of the individual service member and were taken more seriously. Paperwork tended to collect in a pile on someone's desk, and sometimes it took prodding and leadership intervention to move issues forward.

Red tape and bureaucracy are part of working for the government. Service members coping with bureaucracy are recommended to use humor, pick battles, complain constructively, and find a positive way to cope instead of getting frustrated and destructive.

Balancing Service and Self

On the wall in the ship's cafeteria is a large banner that reads "Ship, Shipmate, and Self." "Self" is the last priority. There are many who served in the military whose blood was the color of their service, including my relatives. They gave up everything to join and serve in the military. They worked to excess at the expense of their family and personal life for the government. They sacrificed themselves for an uncaring, impersonal machine, only to get passed over for promotion or have some outrageous event or thing happen to them that caused their career and relationship with the military to take a dramatic turn. A patient told me his relationship with the Navy was like a domestic violence situation. No matter how hard he tried or worked, he felt that the Navy kept hitting him. He regretted giving so much of himself to the Navy.

A Navy LCDR/O4 I worked with bet his life on the Navy. He served overseas in a high operational tempo environment. On top of that, he deployed. He was passed over for promotion a second time, and it was a psychological injury. To him, it was an injustice. He was crushed, devastated, and experienced a mental health breakdown.

I spoke to a retired Army col/O6 in his fifties. He described how he started off as enlisted, went to Reserve Officers' Training Corps, became an officer, and served for thirty years. He felt institutionalized by the Army, and it was all he knew. He complained that it all came to an end after soldiers complained about him and he was relieved of command. He told me he had a style of being terse and to the point. He said the Army investigation found that he did not violate any specific Army regulation. He felt betrayed by service members he was trying to help and by his chain of command. He felt toxic military politics drove the situation. He concluded that he made the people in power unhappy and was relieved. He felt he couldn't get help on active duty, at one point paid out of pocket to talk to a therapist, and ended up turning to Veterans Affairs for help after he left the Army.

In the middle of a naval battle, "Ship, Shipmate, and Self" was a great ideal to strive for. Working together, service members achieve the mission. At other times, the notion was counterproductive. A doctor at Naval Medical Center Portsmouth told me her mentor gave her some great advice: "The Navy doesn't look out for you or care for you. Get out when you need to and don't feel bad about it."

Service members and families function at an optimal level when there is balance. Service members are more productive when they are happy and healthy and have stable homes. A useful skill for service members is to constantly assess and rebalance priorities between service, family, and self. Service members are recommended to have good boundaries with the military and not let themselves get used up and spit out.

Balancing Personal Problems Against Work

Everyone in life has problems. Common problems are relationships, money, children, health, real estate, legal, and the list goes on. Service members must always maintain readiness, which includes being mentally ready and having personal issues addressed. Those who were bogged down with too many problems, had the problems spill over into the workplace, and were distracted by worry experienced a negative impact in their military performance. Not balancing problems resulted in decreased productivity and an excessive number of workdays missed. Everyone has problems and takes a mental health day every now and then. The challenge is finding a way to keep them in check and optimally balance work and personal problems.

Coping with Problems Back at Home

One of the privileges of working in mental health was hearing the stories of patients. A patient told me they had a rough childhood and suffered from neglect from their parents. They joined the military to escape the situation and to better themselves. They made it through boot camp, then A School. Sadly, what happened next was their parent kept calling them frequently, begging for money, and guilting them about it. This junior enlisted service member was sending money home, which they couldn't afford, they felt distressed, and their work performance suffered. There was a similar scenario where a young service member was trying to adopt their younger brother to save him from neglect. Another junior enlisted service member was housing her mother, sister, and her sister's baby in a small off-base apartment. The service member was trying to save her family from being homeless, suffering on multiple levels, and the situation was dragging her down. The family members weren't pulling their weight. They were unemployed and couldn't or wouldn't get a job. The apartment was too small for all of them, the service member was taking on financial debt, her personal space was violated, and there was sleep deprivation.

Service members who successfully navigated these situations set healthy boundaries. They found balance between their personal life and career. Sometimes a bit of tough love and saying no was required and helpful for everyone. Concerning the latter situation, the service member evicted her family members from her apartment, and this caused them to go back to work. Her work performance improved. Another service member I worked with couldn't make it work. Despite his best efforts, his mind was back at home, and he couldn't fulfill his military duties. He ended up leaving the military and returning home to help with the family business.

I worked with young service members who returned home frequently, suffered from homesickness, and were unable to adapt to the military. The *USS George Washington* investigation report suggested MASR Mitchell-Sandor struggled with the environment of the ship and traveled home frequently, but the extent of the struggle was not evident to leadership. I felt he needed someone to take him under their wing and make him a part of the Navy family.

Promotion and Career Progression Issues

Promotion and career progression are critical parts of military life. Service members compete against their peers to advance in rank. A rule of promotion is the higher the rank, the harder and more competitive it was to gain advancement. Promotion success rates varied from year to year. At junior ranks, promotion approaches 100 percent, but for higher ranks, the promotion rate is as low as just a few percent. There are career milestones, some written and some unwritten. It is important for service members to self-manage their careers, be aware, track milestones, and work toward advancement.

Gaining advancement has been described as ladder climbing and ticket punching. It is personal, and it hurts to get passed over, but it is also a game. It is a paperwork and political game. Service members who encounter roadblocks to career progression are recommended to identify military career milestones that need to be achieved and what actions need to be accomplished to achieve these. A successful strategy for career advancement is to study those who achieved advancement and emulate what they did to accomplish it. Finding an experienced mentor is critical for advancement and career progression. Complete workplace qualifications on time and keep the chain of command happy. Retaliation was very real, but so were rewards for loyalty and being part of the team. Service members have some choice in military assignments, and it's wise for them to pick their next assignment strategically. If a service member is passed over for promotion, it is a learning opportunity to do better, adjust, and focus energy on positive career moves. It is a mistake to get discouraged for any significant length of time. Sometimes there were situations where advancement was impossible. I encountered 5-10 percent advancement rates during my career. In a situation where advancement was impossible, a service member could look at other opportunities, such as furthering education, becoming an officer, or leaving the military. When I served at Naval Medical Center Portsmouth from 2019–2022, the corpsmen complained that the advancement rates were very low, they felt stressed out, and many used the situation to leave the Navy and pursue a college education like nursing school.

Annual Performance Evaluations

Performing at a high level on a day-to-day basis isn't enough to obtain promotion. It is critical for service members to look good on paper for promotion consideration. Each service had traditions and unwritten rules for how performance evaluations were written and handled. Service members are recommended to prepare well in advance for the annual performance review process. It is recommended that service members discuss upcoming reviews with their chain of command and prepare drafts months in advance to ensure optimal success. The promotion process was political. Service members must be perceived as performing at a high level. It is important for service members to advocate for themselves. Last minute scrambles to complete performance evaluations rarely resulted in success.

Awards

Advocating, applying for, and receiving military awards was an important part of military life and necessary to look good on paper and facilitate career progression. A colleague completed an overseas tour. The chain of command told him to submit a write-up for an end-of-tour award, but he didn't do it. A couple years later, he was passed over for promotion and regretted not applying for an award. The scenario for receiving an award was the same over the course of my career. The service member wrote it up, and the supervisor edited and submitted it.

Working Outside of Career Field

An aircraft mechanic in the Navy I worked with completed A School, then was sent to a command, where he worked outside of his career field at a desk job. He did a great job and, over the course of a six-year period, achieved rapid promotion from E3 to E6. The Navy issued him new orders to a large operational unit, where he was expected to function as a fully competent supervisor in a career field he had never worked in. Similar situations occurred on the *USS George Washington* when the ship was in the yards. Service members worked outside of their rate to perform maintenance on the ship and complained of psychological distress.

Service members who find themselves in this situation are wise not to panic, stress out, and beat themselves up. Service members are recommended to have good communication with the chain of command and work with the command to formulate a training and remediation plan. Receiving training remediation was a learning curve situation. Relearning or regaining career field skills might take a while, but it did happen. I knew surgeons who went on a yearlong deployment, were not able to perform surgery, and received training and remediation after they returned home.

Punishment for Being a High Performer

I spoke to a soldier who served in the Army from 1968–1972. He reflected over his time in the Army. He told me a story about how he felt punished for overperforming. He explained that his unit did a really good job, outperformed leadership, and made everyone look bad. He was reassigned from the job and punished. I worked with many service members who reported and experienced the phenomenon of being punished for being a high performer. There is a tendency, especially in a government agency, for individuals to do the minimum and skate by. Individuals who do a good job and are productive tend to become the go-to people when things need to get done, and they get work disproportionately thrown at them. Sometimes it's a path-of-least-resistance thing; other times it can be malicious and a toxic work environment. In a situation where there is a lot of uniformity, high performers and under performers stand out compared with everyone else and are an easy target.

Conflict with Supervisor

The military was a gruff place. The environment was notorious for service members getting yelled at and being told what to do. Early in my career, I was told there was a senior Navy psychiatrist who had a reputation for throwing coffee mugs. I worked with a senior medical officer who sent out rude, confrontational, and condescending emails. People could get away with a lot when they were hiding behind a rank and a uniform. When I was in training, during my psychiatric residency, a fellow resident completed a clinical rotation at a nonmilitary hospital. He communicated with a nonmilitary patient in a manner similar to how he interacted with active-duty service members. It did not go well. My colleague found himself in a situation where his rank and uniform didn't matter. The patient responded by threatening to kill him and eloping from the hospital. The situation was eye-opening. It was a valuable lesson in how the military treats people. We also learned not to take for granted our relationships with patients.

Perhaps in a manner like the Stanford Prison Experiment, the military breeds difficult characters. There is also an unwritten tradition of being happily unhappy. It is my personal belief that difficult and toxic supervisors are a source of morbidity and mortality in the military. There is a quote: "An angry skipper makes an unhappy crew."

Treating people the wrong way is a bad leadership strategy. People get away with abusive, passive-aggressive behaviors and other forms of maltreatment due to rank and other privileges, but from a big organizational perspective, they cause negative impact. How sailors felt they were being treated and valued was a common theme in the *USS George Washington* and MARMC investigation reports.

Finding oneself in a situation like this is challenging because the dynamics of power and control are heavily weighted in the chain of command's favor. Service members find themselves in a compromising situation when they are faced with complaining to the supervisor, who is perpetrating the maltreatment, or complaining over their head. Often, the command is in a situation where it investigates itself. This creates an inherent conflict of interest and makes it difficult to get relief. The risk of retaliation is very real.

A strategy for a service member coping with an abusive supervisor is a face-to-face conversation behind closed doors where common ground, advice for doing better, and improvement is sought. How can the issue be resolved, and a mutual understanding be achieved, without going nuclear? After all, service members are all on the same team and trying to achieve the same goals. Sometimes the strategy doesn't work. If someone was engaging in maltreatment, frequently, they were negatively impacting others in a similar way. It may be a service member's duty to file a formal complaint.

Once, I worked at an Immigrations and Customs Enforcement facility as a PHS officer. A colleague and I witnessed a nurse have negative interactions with an inmate. We were concerned that if she treated inmates in a negative way, it could provoke them to violence. We complained to the nurse's supervisor and were thanked. We were told others had complained about the nurse, but since we complained, they finally had enough to act and address the situation.

Conflicts with Coworkers

Ferris Bueller's Day Off (1986) is a movie about a group of kids who play hooky from school. In *Sgt. Bilko* (1996), Steve Martin plays a well-liked soldier and conman who runs a gambling ring and oversees development of an experimental hover tank. Situations arise where coworkers behave like characters from these movies and have styles that result in personality clashes. Service members who find themselves at odds with a coworker are recommended to try to find common ground. Bringing the chain of command into the middle of a personal dispute is always a gamble. It is said that when someone else is brought in to mediate, the parties surrender decision-making power to that person. This is true for divorce. If soon-to-be-exes can't decide, the judge decides, and neither party may be happy with the outcome. In my experience, the military has this way of punishing both parties in a dispute. The military, especially the Navy, turns situations around on sailors even when the findings were in their favor.

False Guilt

In the mental health world, there is true guilt and false guilt. If one committed a crime, they did something wrong and should feel guilt and a sense of responsibility. False guilt is when someone blamed themselves for something out of their control, something that wasn't their fault. I observed a natural human tendency for individuals, especially service members, to blame themselves when something bad or traumatic happened. I worked with an aircraft mechanic who performed maintenance on a plane prior to the engine breaking down in mid-flight, nearly resulting in tragedy. He was racked with anxiety and false guilt issues even after an investigation cleared him of what happened. When equipment broke, it wasn't necessarily someone's fault. If someone died in combat or from cancer, there was no one to blame except the enemy or the disease.

False guilt applied to organizational problems too. Organizational weaknesses set people up for failure. I observed mental health systems that relied on a single person. The system was only as good as that person, and when that person took time off work or left, the system fell apart. A system where a single person was the point of failure was not a healthy system. Situations like that resulted in one individual constantly trying to save the ship and burnout.

An important lesson I learned was that sometimes things must fail for them to improve. Letting things fail goes against the fiber of a service member and especially a doctor. It is ingrained in our personality to be proactive, prevent problems, and do things the right way. When things failed, there was personal responsibility, but the organization, like the military as a whole and the big Navy, had the lion's share of the responsibility. The situations with the *USS George Washington* and MARMC are examples of this. Long-term organizational weaknesses will be worked out, and the Navy will be better off.

Survivor guilt was similar. If individuals in a unit died in combat or were injured in military operations, the survivors ruminated, wishing they had been hurt in their place. If one missed a flight and all the passengers died in the plane crash, it's not the person's fault who missed the flight. I've asked patients struggling with these issues if the ghost of the deceased was present, what advice would they give them? Usually, the advice is to stop feeling guilt and to live a full life. Guilting oneself or blaming others never helps and only makes things worse.

I talked to a service member who was told by a higher-up in their chain of command that they were a disgrace. This resulted in a psychological injury. In discussing the situation, it appeared the individual might have meant well by trying to challenge the individual, but it was verbal abuse, guilting, and made the situation much worse.

Military Readiness and Fitness

Wearing a uniform is a sacred duty and privilege. Ultimately, the responsibility falls on the service member to maintain readiness, including maintaining the necessary job qualifications and certifications. The military provides training and other resources, but it falls on the shoulders of the service member. It is a requirement to maintain height and weight standards. Similarly, a family care plan is needed that documents who will take care of loved ones during deployment. Service members are recommended to be proactive regarding these issues and ask for help if they are having issues.

Maintaining a healthy diet and exercising are skills that can be learned. Improving health and wellness are great skills to have for everyone at every level and are necessary to maintain military readiness. Service members who struggle with physical fitness issues are recommended to use a smartphone application and smartwatch to track calorie intake and expenditure like a checkbook. A 3,500-calorie deficit results in a pound of weight loss. If the daily calorie intake count is less than the number of calories burned due to metabolism, weight is lost. Service members are recommended to make healthy food choices and eat a stable, healthy diet. Those trying to lose weight are best to do it slowly over time about two pounds per week. Rapid weight loss tends to result in binge eating, and the weight yo-yos back.

Service members who struggle with weight and physical fitness issues are recommended to consult with a nutritionist and personal trainer. Athleticism and exercise are obtainable skills that can be enjoyed even for those who did not play sports growing up.

Security Clearance Evaluations

Service members are required to have a secret or higher level security clearance to perform the duties of their job, such as accessing a computer and protected information. Historically, there have been situations where unstable individuals damaged national security. Controls, such as security clearance evaluations, are intended to ensure the right people are qualified to safeguard information. Service members identified with issues that raise questions about their ability to meet the standards necessary to maintain a security clearance are referred for specialized mental health evaluations.

The Questionnaire for National Security, SF-86, asked, "Do you have a mental health or other health condition that substantially adversely affects your judgment, reliability, or trustworthiness even if you are not experiencing such symptoms today?"

The military is looking for individuals who are trustworthy, stable, and reliable. Many service members suffer from mental health disorders or have had substance use problems. Many had entanglements with the military justice system. What's important is how the problems were dealt with and handled. Were they dealt with in a positive way? Did the service member admit they had a problem? Did they accept or refuse treatment? Past behavioral patterns could be predictive of the future. Were they a repeat offender, or did they learn from their mistakes?

Regarding security clearances, service members were best to disclose when they had issues, seek help, be receptive to feedback, and follow treatment recommendations.

When faced with a security clearance evaluation, service members are best to be honest and open. Often, the investigators had collateral information and knew if a service member was truthful. Dishonesty was a red flag for a security clearance evaluation. If a service member was arrested for DUI, this should be communicated to the investigator who had a copy of all criminal records. Service members are encouraged to pay their bills in a timely manner and apply the same responsible behaviors to financial health as well.

Flight Status and Other Special Duties

Service members who work with billion-dollar aircraft, nuclear materials, and top-secret information are held to a higher standard. Such service members can expect even higher levels of scrutiny and micromanagement necessary for the privilege. An effective strategy for this issue was to reframe thinking to view these things as a necessary part of the privilege instead of an unnecessary hindrance or intrusion.

Information Fatigue, Email Abuse, and Excessive Online Training

Service members have a difficult life. A sailor serving on a ship works grueling hours with a supervisor who is in their face. It isn't uncommon for service members to get called into a half-day PowerPoint training for suicide prevention or some other issue. The worst presentations are when the presenter reads off PowerPoint slides and causes the audience to fall asleep.

A retired Navy captain told me a story about how a suicide prevention presentation made him furious and caused him to take time off work to talk to a mental health professional. He felt the presentation consisted of two slides. The first slide was "we care about you" and the second slide was "don't kill yourself." The presenter read from the slides and had difficulty connecting with the audience. He said someone in the audience asked, "What if I'm thinking about suicide right now?" And the presenter responded, "This is not the forum for that." Such presentations feel like a slap in the face. What the service needs to improve mental health is simple: Stop being abused verbally and physically, shorter work hours, and not burdened with unhelpful training.

If it isn't PowerPoint by death, it is online training. The military is notorious for excessive online training requirements. When I completed online training, it wasn't uncommon for online training to glitch at the 98 percent completion mark, resulting in the training having to be retaken from scratch on a different computer.

Research suggests that email use can be counterproductive (Kadet 2022). In the military, and especially in the military health system, asynchronous communication was overutilized, and we were sent political and passive-aggressive emails that increased psychological distress and required minefield-like navigation.

Successful military members find a way to cope with required training and learn how to use electronic communication and email effectively.

Shift Work and Sleep Hygiene

When I served in Okinawa, Japan, I saw patients at the brig located on Camp Hansen. Several active-duty marines who served as guards at the brig were referred to me for help. They showed signs and symptoms of significant mental health problems and were complaining about their sleep schedule. They described a Panamalike work schedule where they were working three days on, two days off, then two nights, followed by three more days off. I met with the warden and discussed the issues they were having. I explained that the rapid switch between working days and nights disrupted their sleep cycle, and I recommended a circadian-based watch bill. The marines who worked days stayed on the dayshift and those who worked nights stayed on the night shift so they could wake up and go to sleep at the same time. At the end of the month, the marines who worked days and nights swapped shifts. Soon after this was implemented, the guards' mental health and sleep issues quickly resolved.

In many research papers, having difficulty sleeping is frequently cited as a common problem in the military. A GAO report discussed recommendations for a Navy fatigue management program after lack of sleep was cited as contributing to the *USS Fitzgerald* and *USS John S. McCain* ship collisions in 2017 (Government Accountability Office 2021). Sleep deprivation was cited as a factor contributing to the death of one of the *USS George Washington* sailors. Service members have little control over their work environment or work schedule, but they have control over how they cope with it, including setting a healthy sleeping schedule. It is critical for service members to maintain proper sleep hygiene. Service members are recommended to create a sleeping environment free of light, sound, and distractions. It was also a helpful coping skill to find a way to put problems on the back burner to facilitate a good night's sleep. One service member told me, before they went to bed, reviewing a to-do list was a way to put problems down for the night.

I spoke to service members who stayed up long hours playing video games or engaging in other activities. This was poor sleep hygiene and wreaked havoc on their sleep cycle and mental health. This resulted in sleep deprivation, fatigue, and reduced job performance. Excessive alcohol and caffeine use also negatively impacted service members' sleep cycles.

Broken Relationships

Relationship problems are a leading cause of stress and frequently a reason individuals seek help from the mental health clinic. Relationships are extremely personal, intimate, and touch everyone deeply. It wasn't uncommon for individuals in a committed relationship to find out their spouse was unfaithful or be faced with a sudden, unexpected, and unwanted breakup or divorce. Facing this scenario, individuals experience an emotional crisis, devastation, and a feeling that their dream life was shattered. Frequently, a broken heart immediately preceded suicidal thoughts or behaviors and was cited as causing a heart attack in at-risk individuals.

A related issue occurs when relationship problems spill over into the workplace. It was never a good situation when a spouse called the chain of command and complained about their service member's behavior.

Relationship crises are sometimes unavoidable. A relationship crisis or challenge frequently leads to a strengthened and improved relationship, possibly with someone new. There is a balance between fighting for a relationship, cutting losses, and moving on. If faced with a relationship crisis, it's best for service members to stay positive. Service members suffering from severe relationship problems must avoid self-destructive behaviors, verbal abuse, domestic violence, and assault at all costs. Positive communication with other parties and coping in a healthy way are predictive factors for good relationship crisis outcomes.

Aloneness

I was consulted about a service member on a ship. He had a spouse and two kids at home. He worked in a shop with two other people and felt he didn't fit in. He was needy and communicated with his wife constantly. I wondered if she viewed him as a third child. He ended up leaving the ship. He would have benefited from improved coping skills and a support system.

If he had found some way to find buddies and establish common ground and camaraderie with his coworkers, his situation would have had a better outcome. He could have spoken with a chaplain or someone else. There might have been a mental health provider embedded in his unit he could have turned to.

Service members who struggle with loneliness are recommended to find a way to improve independence. Geographic separation is a great opportunity for parties in a relationship to take a break from each other and rekindle passion. Over-relying on a spouse for support creates resentment and more problems.

Substance Abuse

Service members embrace the warrior mentality. They fight hard, work hard, and play hard. Misuse of alcohol is a problem with military cultural roots. Historically, military units had unhealthy customs and traditions of drinking excessively. Unhealthy substance use, particularly alcohol misuse, is a common military problem that negatively impacts service members, their families, commands, and military readiness. My patients told me they took their first drink in the military, were taught to use alcohol in an unhealthy way by other service members, and learned to "drink until drunk." A service member told me part of his recovery was to unlearn that. Another told me he was under significant peer pressure to drink in an unhealthy way, and this was an obstacle he had to overcome.

Service members must use alcohol responsibly and in moderation. Turning to the bottle is not healthy or an effective coping strategy. Drinking to excess is a high-risk behavior and a recipe for disaster. Individuals who use alcohol to self-treat mental health issues learn alcohol is an ineffective medication. Alcohol is expensive, causes weight gain and depression, interferes with sleep, and negatively impacts the liver and other key organ systems.

Street drug use also negatively impacts service members and the organization. Many careers have been lost due to alcohol incidents and the military's zero-tolerance policy for illicit substances. I assisted service members who struggled with addiction to opioids, stimulants, benzodiazepines, and marijuana. Once, I talked to an airman who was ordering controlled substances from overseas and experimenting on himself with them. I'm not exactly sure what he was taking, but it wasn't healthy or legal, and the situation did not have a positive outcome.

Special operations forces were known to use steroids and other performance-enhancing drugs. Once, when I was working on the psychiatry unit, there was a bodybuilder who became psychotic due to steroid use. He paced around what was known as the "milieu," singing Christmas carols. He walked up to a sailor and demanded he stop putting voices in his head. Without warning, he picked up the sailor and threw him. Fortunately, the sailor wasn't injured. That sailor had been exaggerating and embellishing the sick role. A big portion of why he was in the psychiatric unit was because he wanted to get off the ship and saw that as the solution to his problems. After being thrown, he said he was just making it up and asked to be released immediately and returned to the ship. In a comical sort of way, everything all worked out, but steroid use had negative health effects and was no joke.

The best way to receive help is via the self-referral pathway. Service members are better off coming forward with a problem rather than getting into trouble first. If a service member is recommended for adverse personnel action, it is a good thing for them to take ownership of it and address the situation by completing treatment. Having a certificate of treatment completion can help situations.

Stigma

This book has described numerous examples of stigma. This is where service members are viewed in a negative way, treated differently, and made to feel ashamed or worthless due to having mental health issues, which results in them being reluctant to seek help.

One particular patient, an E5 in the Navy, told me he had a history of chronic anxiety and panic attacks. He tried to get help in 2017, saw a mental health provider once or twice, and complained that the session was focused on the possibility of his separation from the Navy rather than the root cause of his symptoms and potential solutions. He said the experience was horrific. He complained that he witnessed other sailors being separated under similar circumstances, and this increased his fear about reaching out for help. He stated a message he and his peers understood: If you can't perform, you are considered "not mentally suited," not in compliance with military standards, and would get the boot. He explained that many sailors chose to suffer in silence. Years later, his situation continued to get worse. His smoking and drinking escalated until his situation hit a crisis point. I met him when he was participating in residential treatment for alcoholism. He stopped drinking and smoking, began treatment with medication that worked, and was able to open up and work through his problems by talking about them.

In my experience, frequently, people in the military are afraid of mental health issues and don't want to deal with them. They are anxious, suffering, and would rather have someone else deal with it. Service members with mental health issues are recommended to identify and work through stigma and not be discouraged. Pushing through stigma is frequently a pivotal moment and a turning point when someone begins to get help and feel relief.

Accessing Care

I participated in a meeting once where mental health provider staffing issues were being discussed. A Marine Corps general made a sarcastic remark: "Ideally, a marine would have a social worker from the womb to the tomb."

In an ideal world, individuals were given time off work, had good access to care, and were given a prompt mental health appointment within a short period of time from a professional who was young, enthusiastic, attentive, caring, and aesthetically appealing, with scheduled openings to allow for consecutive weekly visits.

Unfortunately, that was the exception rather than the rule. Many agencies and organizations had a mentality to keep sending patients and fill schedules months in advance, which impacted appointment availability. They were focused on throughput instead of outcomes. The mental health clinic needed a better system for scheduling and getting the right patient to the right place to the right person at the right time. Mental health providers called in sick or were deployed, and healthcare provider contracts fell through. Facilities were bureaucratic and inefficient, and providers constantly rotated between programs. Facilities shut down due to the weather. There were fire alarms and base incidents that disrupted care. Service members were recommended to be flexible, keep trying, and not give up hope.

Recovering from Life Prior to Military Service

People join the military from all walks of life. Many told me they joined the military to escape situations they were in. Not infrequently, they were recovering from adverse life experiences that occurred prior to military service, such as poverty, sexual assault, child abuse, and dropping out of college.

Childhood abuse includes verbal, physical, and sexual assault. These issues are traumatic, terrible, and gut-wrenching. Poverty is also an issue that service members deal with. The military assisted individuals suffering from these issues with structure, stability, and belonging. The military is a great place, especially for those trying to better themselves and recover from issues. It is a structured environment, with a predictable paycheck and great educational benefits.

Sometimes individuals in a chain of command reminded service members of their assailant or abuser and triggered trauma. That harsh supervisor came across a little too much like that assailant or physically abusive parent. Service members struggling with these issues are recommended to find their power and control. Service members can make positive life choices like asking the chain of command for intervention and getting help.

Coping with Physical and Mental Health Problems

I spoke to a service member in the Air Force Special Forces who developed Crohn's disease, a disease of the gastrointestinal tract. The disease causes inflammation of the digestive tract, which leads to abdominal pain, severe diarrhea, fatigue, weight loss, and malnutrition. He suffered from frequent bouts of bloody diarrhea, pain, and abdominal cramping. He had multiple surgeries to treat the condition, and this resulted in disability. He was a pararescue specialist in the Air Force, enjoyed working in the field and conducting military operations, and had gained rapid advancement over a fifteen-year career of military service. Instead of deploying and working in the field, he found himself flying a desk tied to the close geographic proximity of a bathroom. Instead of achieving his twenty-year career goal, he faced the medical boards process. He was struggling with the loss of his identity, career, and disability. He disliked paperwork and had to learn new skills.

The military is all about transitions. It is constant chaos and change. To thrive, one must overcome and adapt to the challenges.

Medical Board Evaluations

The medical boards process is frustrating and mired with bureaucracy, red tape, and associated delays. Over the course of my career, I authored over 600 medical boards for mental health conditions. The process was frustrating and a source of anxiety for just about every patient I worked with. For most, the process was fair and ended well. A small number of patients appealed their board findings, and a significant number of those felt the outcome was fair.

Recommendations for service members coping with the medical board process are to practice self-advocacy and find a balance. My observation was that members who were demanding, battled the system, and had unrealistic expectations had the most difficulty coping. Recommendations included trusting the medical professionals and the system to get it right. Service members are recommended to have good communication and a positive relationship with their medical board liaison officer.

Filing a Formal Complaint

There comes a time when the behavior of others is so atrocious, a service member has no choice but to file a formal grievance. The military has several programs and pathways where a formal grievance can be filed, depending on the issue at hand. Service members can file Article 1150 and 138 complaints against their commander, according to the UCMJ.

Service members can file grievances for discrimination and harassment through the Equal Opportunity Program.

Formal complaints are also submitted through the sexual assault program. A service member can file an unrestricted complaint, and this triggers a formal investigation.

The IG program vets specific types of waste, fraud, and abuse allegations, such as abuse of authority issues, mismanagement, reprisal, and fraud.

Disciplinary Problems and Military Justice Issues

Everyone makes mistakes. Some rise to the level of a legal offense. There are many individuals who had a lapse in judgment and ran afoul of the UCMJ. Sometimes commands are malignant and try to go after people by creating legal issues for service members. If a service member does something wrong, it is desirable to find a way to take accountability for the mistake and learn from the experience. Military justice is frustrating, unjust, and expensive. Military justice was like a casino: The house always wins. The system seems stacked against the service member. There was also this cultural tradition that the military punishes everyone. So even when you win, you still lose.

What makes it more confusing is that service members face actions from several different lanes simultaneously. Service members faced administrative personnel, legal, and medical actions simultaneously. I had a patient once who was court-martialed for something. Despite being found not guilty in a military court, he was given an adverse annual performance review, and it damaged his career. A service member with a DUI could get off the hook for disciplinary issues but then be medically disqualified from an assignment by a gaining command due to alcohol issues. A service member who was caught using illicit drugs could be considered for both legal charges and administrative separation via a personnel action.

Service members who face legal charges are recommended to consult with an attorney. There are times when service members find themselves in situations where there is no choice but to defend themselves. A recommended starting point is base legal; if they won't help, service members are recommended to consult with a defense attorney. Attorneys are expensive, sometimes hundreds of dollars per hour or more. It is best to look at the overall risk levels. If one was a career military, with eighteen years in the military, and retirement benefits are on the line, or if someone has a senior rank (E7 and could be busted down to E6), spending tens of thousands of dollars on a legal defense could be the most cost-effective course of action.

Board of Correction of Records

Across my career, I saw individuals receive unfair performance reviews or other unfavorable personnel actions. They filed board of correction complaints, and as a result, their performance reviews were pulled from their file. The complaint required specific information, such as the wrong that was committed.

A fellow mental health provider I served with had a dispute with the military about constructive service credit. She had achieved a master's degree prior to joining the military. The military would not award her constructive credit, and she found herself in a situation where she had to apply to the board of correction to receive the credit.

According to military regulations, there were things that could and could not be said in a performance review. If a reviewer cited things that were off limits, that would be grounds to have a record corrected. A board of correction is a situation where assistance from an attorney was helpful. The language and what the board was looking for was very specific.

Changing Jobs

If service members wanted to move, they needed to talk to their chain of command and detailer. A lot of times, there was some type of issue fueling the desire to move, such as a difficult work environment or family issues that could be addressed. A great first step was for service members to talk with their chain of command about issues they were facing. Sometimes a member's work schedule or other issues could be addressed in such a way to improve the situation for all parties involved. Another recommendation was for service members to communicate with community career field managers for advice and long-term assignment planning. Sometimes an arduous tour of duty was followed by a less stressful one.

Getting out of the Military and Retirement

Many years ago, I was in the audience when the commandant of the Marine Corps addressed a thousand marines in an auditorium. He said 60 percent of marines leave the military after their first tour, and he said there was nothing wrong with that. They performed their military duty and returned to civilian life. He said everyone reaches a point of quitting in the military. He explained that the point could be reached during basic training, after completion of the first tour of duty, or even twenty-five years later when a one-star flag officer was turned down for a second star, got disappointed, and turned in their resignation.

Military service was a life cycle. It was completing basic training, serving at different duty stations, overcoming challenges to succeed, and career progression. Leaving the military was also part of the experience. A service member could request a voluntary separation or retire at twenty years or longer. The point was this: Everyone quit, and that was part of the process.

Everyone reaches a point when enough is enough. Military service is voluntary, but there are challenges if a service member desires to break their contract early or voluntarily change jobs. Asking to quit is a last resort and could be premature. Sometimes quitting results in the loss of hard-earned military benefits.

Every service member eventually leaves the military. Service members almost always have some degree of anxiety and apprehension about leaving military service. Leaving the military is a big adjustment for anyone, especially after a twenty-year career. I spoke to an Army veteran. He talked about the change in identity after he left active duty. He told me, in the Army, he felt he was a sergeant and someone important who sent soldiers into combat. He said, as a civilian, he felt he was a nobody and didn't feel respected. Others told me they missed "the brotherhood."

Having served with Veterans Affairs, I'm well acquainted with those who left military service, the challenges, and coping difficulties. Career military lose structure, purpose, camaraderie, and sense of mission. A veteran told me, on active duty, his days were planned out. Every day he was told what to do and he had a purpose. Taking off the uniform was a huge adjustment. He found himself sitting at home without having anything to do, wondering, *What now?* He explained that was a whole different stress on its own.

Some retirees went home for the first time, their spouse couldn't stand them, and they turned to the bottle. They discovered that the military persona didn't work so well outside of the military.

Some service members are reluctant to have a formal retirement ceremony. No matter what the feeling or anxiety level, service members are recommended to have a formal retirement ceremony to help them achieve a sense of closure.

Falling into a Hole

In medical school, I loved physiology. It is the study of the human body's organ systems and how they interact with each other. The heart, lungs, kidney, and bone marrow were in harmony. If one of the systems took a big hit, the other systems tried to compensate. In a critically ill patient hospitalized in the ICU, the result could be the downward spiral of multisystem organ failure and death. Hospitalization was focused on reversing this pathway and restoring organ system function and balance.

I have come to appreciate a similar downward spiral for mental health. There is a lot of discussion about "suicide," but frequently, it's the result of multiple overlapping systems. Active-duty service members and veterans spiral in a characteristic way. They feel depressed and anxious, struggle at work, at home, and in relationships, and start to decline in a negative trajectory. They lose their job or stop working, disconnect from other people, and sit at home. They also turn to unhealthy substance use, including excessive drinking and marijuana use.

In an earlier chapter, I discussed a female veteran who suffered PTSD, depression, and grief after a stillbirth that occurred at Naval Medical Center Portsmouth. She suffered from depression, trauma issues, unresolved grief, and toxic leadership. She fell into a deep depression, and it took her several years to recover. Every year at the anniversary of her baby's death, she experiences a trauma flare-up and has learned to cope. In the Navy, she served as a hospital corpsman and cardiovascular technician. It took her a while for her passion in cardiology to be rekindled. After leaving the military, she went back to school, achieved good grades, and became an echocardiography technician. She explained to me how she climbed out of the hole. She kept moving forward, finding purpose and meaning in her life.

CHAPTER 17

Essential Coping Skills to Thrive in the Military

A RETIRED NAVY CAPTAIN told me he wanted suggestions for things he and his sailors could do to avoid ending up in my office. I observed a common set of traits and coping skills service members who thrived and bounced back from adversity exhibited. These skills helped them survive the military, climb out of "the hole," and turn things around. Frequently, when service members would present in crisis, a turning point in their recovery was identifying coping skill deficits and improving coping mechanisms. Many of the military helping programs in one way or another were geared toward assisting service members and their families with these skills.

Semper Gumby

The military is a dynamic, unpredictable organization. The military is driven by external world events and the political climate and is the output of a massive multilevel bureaucratic organization. The key to surviving and thriving is "Semper Gumby"—being always flexible and embracing change.

Service members change direction rapidly on short notice, sometimes multiple times over a short time frame. There are those who are obsessed about having the perfect career plan. They had their career mapped out on a piece of paper with dates, positions, and geographic locations. Some succeeded, but for many, that type of career plan never happened. It was a source of frustration and disappointment. It almost always ended poorly when service members had unreasonable expectations that the environment would adapt to them. The most successful were those who embraced chaos, and change, looked for opportunities, and adapted to the environment. Flexibility and agility are critical skills for military life.

Just when a service member is doing well in the military and thriving, something happens. Unexpected budget cuts cancel programs service members are working on. I was talking to a colleague, the department head of the traumatic brain injury program at Naval Medical Center Portsmouth. He said the facility was downsizing by hundreds of active-duty providers. He went to a meeting where the possibility of eliminating the traumatic brain injury clinic was discussed. There were acts of God and accidents such as a military installation being destroyed by a hurricane or a Navy ship catching fire and getting mothballed. The military might uproot the service member and their family, forcing them to move across the world. Sometimes the military decides to remove the member's military occupational specialty, forcing them to retrain into a different career field.

Having a positive attitude and changing perspective helps. Civilian life and performing the same tasks day in and day out are boring. Seeing change as positive, embracing it, and looking for new opportunities and adventure is a good way to cope. It is short-sighted for service members to be married to or grow roots in a particular geographic location. Not being able to move results in missed opportunities. When things don't go as planned, expressing an opinion and disagreeing in a constructive, healthy way helps. Fighting the system might have made a difference, but it also backfired and made life a living hell. Change and adaptation is the military way of life. The military doesn't adapt to the member; the member adapts to it.

Being a Positive Team Player

Service members are recommended to approach things from a team perspective. The novel *Ender's Game* was on the Navy's recommended professional reading list. This is a story about how a team utilizes a brilliant strategy to take on an alien race and defeat them in combat. A team can accomplish more than an individual. It is helpful for service members to communicate effectively in a positive manner even when there are differences or tension. Service members are recommended to study their peers and find ways to connect, fit in, and support them. Learning and studying the weaknesses of peers helps find ways to complement, strengthen, and bolster the team. When interacting with others, it is helpful for service members to put themselves in each other's shoes and try to see things from others' perspectives.

The opposite of the positive team effect is the rotten apple effect, where the rotten apple spoils the bunch. The Air Force had a term, Blue Falcon, which referred to an airman who was on the team but not part of the team. A Blue Falcon is someone who threw the team under the bus, someone whose actions harmed his friends but not himself. The optimal situation is a service member with a positive mindset who sparks confidence and enthusiasm. This strengthens the unit and results in a synergistic effect.

Reframing the Perspective

Military life is challenging due to loss of control. Often, service members find themselves in unwanted situations they didn't choose. A senior sailor who successfully recovered from mental health issues told me his life changed for the better when he discovered a simple trick. Instead of thinking, *I HAVE to be on a Navy warship*, he changed his thought process to *I GET to be on a Navy warship*. It's true—serving on a Navy warship is a once-in-a-lifetime opportunity. He got to serve on a fifty-billion-dollar piece of equipment. For those who feel serving on a Navy ship was unbearable, more effective thinking is this: *Serving on a Navy ship was a stepping stone to something greater.* In the grand scheme of things, from the perspective of a young adult, anyone can do anything for a few years. This is especially true when long-term gains are visualized and in grasp.

If a service member is sent to an austere overseas location, it can be viewed as an opportunity, an adventure, and exciting. Instead of fighting the situation, the service member can focus on what can be learned and what new experiences can be had. Service members are recommended to always look for the silver lining. Often, there is limited ability to change situations, but how they are looked at and dealt with can be controlled. There were situations in my life that I would have done anything to stop and prevent, but in retrospect, things worked out much better than I had ever imagined. Looking in the rearview mirror, I regret not embracing change sooner.

I have encountered older service members who complained this was "Not the Navy/Army/Air Force/Coast Guard" they grew up in. That thought process is limiting. The military is a living, breathing organization, constantly evolving and changing based on numerous factors that can't be controlled or predicted. Change brings some good things and some bad. A better strategy is to surf the change and keep moving forward.

Internal Motivation

In the private sector, money was a powerful motivating force. There is a saying: "You reap what you sow." Money made is proportional to the amount of work performed. In the private sector, in healthcare, there are clinical productivity bonuses, such as financial incentives for treating high numbers of patients. The military health system isn't like that. During my first year as a doctor, my internal medicine team was on call every fourth night. On these nights, our patient panel would balloon in size. Overnight, we would admit a dozen patients and spend the next four days working them up and treating them. Many of the patients suffered from heart failure, had an excess of fluid in their system, and suffered painful leg swelling. The treatment involved using medications to improve heart function and increase "diuresis," which was a fancy way of saying their urine production was increased to remove the excess fluid. The saying was that our team would "diurese" by the next call night. There were down days when we had few patients. One such day, one of our Navy attendings, Dr. Monahan, gave a lecture on finding internal motivation in the military health system. He said there was a lot of downtime. He told us that sometimes we didn't have many patients, but we always needed to be able to swing into action, ramp up, embrace the work, and not complain.

Maintaining Resilience, Independence, Self-Soothing, and Self-Care

I worked at a private hospital. There was a medical staff office that managed and filled out most, if not all, my paperwork. There was also a medical provider lounge where lunch and snacks were provided. Doctors were able to quickly grab lunch, eat, socialize in a private area, and get back to seeing patients. The military was not like that. I was expected to complete my own paperwork. There was no lounge or free lunch. Service members are expected to function with little or no support.

Service members had to take care of themselves. If alcohol, an unhealthy relationship, handholding, or some other unhealthy behavior is needed to cope with difficult situations, military service presents a challenge. Service members are encouraged to ask for help and rely on the chain of command and others for assistance, but they must have a self-service mindset and be responsible for their own problems to survive. If things don't go as planned or desired, it is optimal to find work-arounds. Thriving in the military equates to being self-sufficient and resilient.

The military is an invalidating environment. I provided many examples in this book of toxic, abusive leadership. Sadly, this seems to be part of military culture. It is imperative for service members to have a strong sense of self-worth to survive in such a toxic environment. A twenty-year Navy veteran communicated to me that a coping mechanism she learned was to "grin and bear it."

Military life is like an escape room. No matter what the issue is, service members are challenged with figuring it out, solving the puzzles, and navigating bureaucracy. Service members work as a team with others to solve problems, but ultimately, it falls on their shoulders to ask for help and figure a way out.

Patiently Navigating Bureaucracy

The military is a multilevel bureaucracy, mired in politics and red tape. It is notorious for "hurry up and wait," where service members were directed to hurry to a specific location at a certain time, only to wait hours for the event to occur. When I flew from Okinawa, Japan, to the Philippines, I waited hours at the Futenma Air Base due to delays. Too often, the same occurred for pay and travel reimbursements (Ziezulewicz 2023). We were told pay paperwork needed to be submitted by hard deadlines. We submitted our pay paperwork promptly in advance, but there were lengthy delays. Sometimes the paperwork would sit on someone's desk at the local level. Other times the delays resulted from higher levels of bureaucracy.

Service members are wise to be patient, temper expectations, and not expect things to happen immediately. Striving for and achieving a greater understanding of how the organization and bureaucratic processes work is helpful. It is important for service members to try to work within the framework of the system and its limitations. It is also critical to understand the process of enacting change that occurs at a glacial pace.

Finding a Mentor

This best practice has been discussed throughout the book. I had many mentors and helped many mentees. I learned something from everyone I spoke to. Mentors were instrumental in giving me career advice, teaching me the ropes in my career field, and reviewing paperwork that was necessary for career progression.

Discipline, Persistence, and Detail-Oriented Thinking

One day during a mental health team meeting, we were discussing a complicated case. The team discussed that the patient was not willing to put forth effort in work—or even brush his teeth. Our psychiatric technician remarked, "If you want to get better, you have to put the flippin' work in." Service members need to be willing to put the work in to achieve results.

There is a famous speech from Admiral McRaven who describes reasons to make your bed every day. He said making your bed is completing the first of many tasks of the day, a symbol that little things matter and preparation for conquering bigger things. He said if you have a miserable day, you come home to a bed that is made. Admiral McRaven's speech was about being disciplined, persistent, detail-oriented, and regimented. In the mental health clinic, my colleagues and I often counseled patients on sleep hygiene. His advice about going to bed and waking up the same time every day and night was also great health advice and helped maintain a good sleeping rhythm.

Keeping things clean and organized was also great advice. "Clutter in your home clutters your brain" was a pearl of wisdom passed on to patients during a mental health coping skills session.

Chinese Plate Spinning

Service members find themselves barraged with "taskings," often on short notice, with busted suspense dates. Service members are forced to context switch, which decreases productivity and increases stress levels. They are challenged with prioritizing and balancing military, work, and personal tasks.

An essential skill of serving in the military is learning to prioritize the things that need to be taken care of and filtering out the rest. The slang term for this is "cleaning off your plate." Recommendations for service members in this area include keeping a calendar with due dates, to-do lists, and good record keeping. These skills assist with long-term planning, anticipating when things are due, and beating deadlines. Tasks that are low-hanging fruit are easily accomplished. Service members figure out which tasks lead to bigger tasks and accomplishments, just as Admiral McRaven talked about in his speech about making your bed.

Chinese plate spinners twirl long sticks with numerous plates on top, simultaneously, in perfect balance. They rotate the plates to the front, back, in and out, and all over without dropping any of them. Often, I felt like a Chinese plate spinner, accomplishing the mission and getting my work done. To thrive in the military, service members must juggle tasks and balance plates.

Respecting the Chain of Command

A condition of service is that the service member follows orders and guidance from the command. The command, in turn, is charged with taking care of the service member. The command offers support with career growth, good performance reviews, and other positive personnel actions. There is an expectation that service members empower and assist leadership by making them look good and getting the mission accomplished in all situations. In my experience, it went farther than this.

At times, I experienced the military, especially the Navy, as mafia-like. There was an unwritten code of loyalty. My colleagues and I were part of the family and were punished if we were seen as disloyal. The punishment could be slight or severe. Sometimes the punishment was public and a warning for other members. The military has been criticized for having an unwritten code of silence. The culture of the military is such that everyone is afraid of retaliation from the person above them. Crossing the chain of command occurs when a service member is perceived as going against the command. I was told that crossing the chain of command is not taught in a textbook. Service members are wise to be sensitive and aware of these issues.

Surviving Poor Leadership

Most military leaders rotated every three years. If someone is really that bad, there is an unwritten rule to survive and wait until they receive a PCS to somewhere else. There are times when service members have a duty and find themselves in a situation where they have no choice but to file a formal grievance against their chain of command, but it comes with a risk of retaliation. In most situations, service members can find common ground and a way to survive poor leadership. Service members are urged not to let bullies win by granting them headspace or allowing them to get under their skin.

Engaging in Healthy Relationships

Breakups, infidelity, divorce, and relationship problems are a major source of stress for military service members. Service members are encouraged to practice healthy relationships, build support networks, and surround themselves with positive people, including family and friends. Positive relationships and support networks are a buffer to fall back on during times of stress. Service members are recommended to treat people with respect and communicate effectively and lovingly. A broken relationship opens doors for a better, more meaningful, and rewarding future relationship. Service members benefit from a healthy, strong partner. If a partner is dragging someone down—for example, encouraging their alcohol problem or irresponsible behavior—that is unhealthy. Often, a turning point for service members struggling with these issues was setting healthy boundaries or ending an unhealthy relationship. Service members are best to make wise relationship choices and engage in healthy relationships. I had great colleagues that suffered personally and professionally due to relationship choices.

Embrace Failure

A great piece of advice is that failure can be an extremely important teacher in life. Mistakes and mishaps are best viewed as opportunities. Getting passed over for promotion or having a mishap on the job are bad, undesirable things, but positive things come from the experiences. Those who fixated and got stuck on things that happened stagnated and fell into a deep hole. Service members are recommended not to be discouraged or afraid to fail. It is best to move forward, learn from experiences, and strive to achieve something greater.

Navigating the Helping System

The military helping system is a network of loosely organized and overlapping programs that vary depending on locality, service, available funding, and other factors. Finding good help is like a scavenger hunt. It also feels like Black Friday shopping, where one must pounce on available appointments before others scoop them up.

When obstacles are encountered, such as difficult people or broken systems for those seeking help, an essential skill is not to get discouraged. Helping personnel are human beings too. They have flaws, personal problems, biases, and bad days, and they have rubbed people the wrong way when they were only trying to help. Systems break, are underfunded, and need to be revamped and retooled. Service members experience missed opportunities because they get caught up and fixated fighting the system instead of taking advantage of available resources.

At a nonmilitary inpatient psychiatric hospital, homelessness was a familiar problem. A common approach for that issue was for a unit social worker to provide a list of homeless shelters and other resources. Ultimately, it was up to the patient to make phone calls and complete the legwork necessary to find housing. This approach had a therapeutic value because the patient practiced self-advocating and taking accountability. The military was a culture of self-help. In my experience, the military medical system was similar. Often, the burden was on the individual service member to do the legwork to get help.

Another core concept of getting help was to continuously evaluate the effectiveness of the help and not be afraid to cut losses and move on. If the mental health provider conveyed a bad feeling to the service member, was blaming, documented harsh judgmental statements, or set them up for discharge on the first visit, a provider change request might be in order.

Avoiding the Military Persona

I observed and heard from many service members about a military persona that worked in uniform but not outside of the military.

A forty-seven-year-old Army veteran explained to me that service members tend to be aggressive people who push their way through the mission and world. Senior personnel bosses around junior personnel, using rank with little or no consequence. They tend not to care how people around them receive them or react to them. He explained that the military persona hindered his ability to thrive in relationships in post-military life. Another sailor told me he learned to always look for problems, stay on top of them, and try to control them. He explained that he felt he needed to "do what is expected, or this will result in the death of everyone on board." He was trying to unlearn and change this mindset after leaving the Navy. A retired Navy captain told me going somewhere in the Navy meant being there five minutes early, and he had difficulty adapting to situations where people showed up late outside of the Navy.

Service members get away with a lot that they can't get away with in the civilian world due to rank and positional hierarchy. This includes being brash, confrontational, and micromanaging. After leaving the military, many discover that this persona doesn't work so well. Outside of the military, coworkers don't respond well if they are told what to do.

Art and Music

Art and music improve mental health and a feeling of wellness. Perhaps, like spirituality and religion, these activities stimulate a different part of one's brain. Research has shown that art and music can have a transformational power. During my medical training, I learned about and participated in art therapy. An art therapist asked everyone to draw and interpret how they were feeling. Another exercise was to draw your stresses; then draw a circle around them to close them off until the next day. Art and music help people express hidden emotions. In child mental health, children are asked to draw how they are feeling. They had difficulty talking about their feelings, but they were easily able to draw dark storm clouds.

Mindset of Service

Perhaps the most important key to thriving in the military is having realistic expectations and the right frame of mind. The purpose of the military isn't to serve the individual; it is to serve the country and the greater good. The military is a centuries-old organization whose purpose is national defense and public service. In the most extreme example, service is putting it all on the line and making the ultimate sacrifice for the country.

If one entered the military with an inflexible career path, the expectation that the military promised certain things, they were sorely frustrated and disappointed. For some, the promises and expectations turned out, but for most, they did not. It was important to have realistic expectations and temper them with patience.

CHAPTER 18

Clinical Pearls, Tips, and Techniques

I WORKED WITH many different people at many different places across many organizations. I witnessed what worked well and what didn't work so well. We strived to have a team approach to mental health, but many times it didn't work due to various obstacles and issues. Sometimes I hit grand-slam home runs, but other times I learned lessons the hard way. What follows are observations and lessons learned to provide great care and approach complex cases.

Listening

The military is a dynamic environment. People come and go and move around frequently. Sometimes an episode of mental health treatment was only a handful of appointments or even a single session. The most powerful tool for helping people was the simple act of listening and assisting people in telling their story. Just listening to people and helping them process situations, even for a few sessions, had a powerful impact. The simple act of telling a story could relieve burdens, provide validation and motivation, change perspective, and offer new insights into seemingly complex problems. One of the roles I had was to teach independent duty corpsmen, who were training to become the sole medical provider on a submarine, about mental health and substance abuse issues. My advice was to listen.

Assuming the Best in People

A lesson I learned was to assume the best in people, including their actions and intentions. Especially in the world of mental health. We think we know people and have insight into their thoughts and motivations. The truth is, as time goes on, it becomes apparent how little we know. It's best to assume people are telling the truth and wait for them to prove otherwise. Across my career, I've witnessed situation after situation where people didn't feel safe or ready to open up, and the truth came out at a later date, particularly for issues associated with shame and embarrassment. Service members are frequently reluctant to open up due to stigma and because they don't want to risk getting in trouble with the government.

In between my service with the Navy and PHS, I worked at a community inpatient psychiatric hospital. From time to time, active-duty service members would be hospitalized. Our facility had more solid privacy protections in place, and service members were in a much safer position to open up and discuss sensitive issues. It was eye-opening when active-duty service members at the community hospital told me, "I told the military provider this, but actually this was what was going on." Second-guessing the patient's motives and diagnosing malingering was almost always overly simplistic and didn't end well. From a broad perspective, feigning illness was a poor coping mechanism. Even if someone was truly malingering, they benefited from talking to a supportive mental health provider. The diagnosis of malingering should be avoided unless clear and convincing evidence was present.

Patience and Timing

One of the most important skills I learned during my career was patience. Timing was everything. When a patient was in an acute crisis, it was hard to talk with them or even formulate an accurate diagnosis. It was better to identify if they were in an acute crisis and work with them over time. When patients were in acute distress, it was more effective to listen, be validating, and offer encouragement. The real work and progress began after immediate needs were met and they were out of the crisis state.

Another related lesson was that forcing someone to open up when they weren't ready frequently backfired. I spoke to a service member who went to a retreat facilitated by a chaplain. She felt pressured to make disclosures about abuse she suffered from. The member wasn't ready for this, fell apart when she told her story, and experienced a mental health breakdown.

A case involving a Vietnam veteran I worked with illustrated the importance of timing and patience. He was a soldier who was awarded a Bronze Star from military combat in Vietnam. He was responsible for killing many people, lived under the constant threat of being killed, and struggled with psychological conflict about having done things he regretted. He was documented as not having dealt with and shutting out his experiences in Vietnam. His mental health providers wrote, he "needed to let the secrets out of the box." However, he wasn't ready to do this. In 2009 he participated in PTSD treatment, including flooding and exposure therapy. He told me he was forced to read a three- to four-page letter aloud about his worst experiences. Later that day, he experienced chest pain and was hospitalized for a heart attack. He felt that forcing the disclosure triggered his heart attack. Thankfully, he recovered.

Often, I observed that military mental health providers were rushed, pressured, and made premature judgment calls. A clinic visit was like a snapshot in time, like a single picture in an album of dozens of photos. Frequently, patients had bad days, and we saw them at their worst. We needed to give patients time to line up the snapshots to get a more accurate picture. The time spent also helped to gel and solidify the relationship between the service member and the mental health provider and improve communication. Sometimes it took weeks, months, or even years for patients to open up and address issues. There have been situations where a patient said their doctor told them to stop drinking, but they were not ready to stop until a year later.

When patients aren't invested in treatment, it's best to try to understand why. It was rarely worth fighting patients. Let the situation play out. There was a hard reality: Sometimes things needed to happen before someone was ready to advance to the next level. Sometimes patients had to suffer a second alcohol incident before they were ready to stop drinking. Patients were responsible for their own behaviors. When someone was noncompliant, it was best to contact them a couple times and document that in the record. After sufficient efforts to contact patients, chasing them was rarely helpful.

Recommending patients be separated from the military in an inpatient setting or the emergency room was a quick fix that didn't always turn out well. Patients benefited from at least a small amount of time—say, one month—to process experiences, reflect on some lessons, and give outpatient treatment a chance. Facilitating an administrative discharge to avert a mental health crisis was short-sighted. A lot of service members went to the emergency room on the worst day of their life. They needed time to calm down, get put back together, and have an adequate treatment trial. I worked with some service members who were initially desperate to get out of the military and then came to the realization that it was short-sighted.

Avoiding Viewing Situations through a Disciplinary Lens

Situation outcomes were best when viewed through a mental health lens instead of a disciplinary lens. In the community, there are situations where patients with severe mental illness, such as psychotic wandering behavior, are charged with petty crimes like trespassing. Arrests get them off the street but turn mental health disorders into crimes and overload jails. It is less expensive, and there are better outcomes when individuals with mental health issues receive mental health intervention. There have been bad outcomes when law enforcement responded to individuals with severe mental health issues (Kennedy 2023). The same was true of active-duty members, especially for the Navy. It was better to see service members as people who were suffering rather than trying to get out of work, out of trouble, gaming the system, and requiring a "corrective action." A related best practice I discovered was to err on the side of the service member when things were unclear. If something is unclear, it becomes apparent over time. If someone has a certain behavior pattern, such as severe alcoholism, the pattern repeats and becomes evident.

I witnessed situations where military mental health providers made harsh, invalidating statements to service members and pressured them to return to duty. There was a rare occasion when such an approach helped, but most of the time it backfired, especially when it involved a service member in distress. I observed situations where military mental health providers set patients up for administrative discharge, conspired with the command against them, and were involved in the prosecution of service members. Participating in those activities wasn't helpful, harmed the public image of military mental health providers, and contributed to mistrust.

Service members benefited from receiving positive support. Situations turned out best when facts and truth were a guide and drove decision-making. Service members had a right to tell their side of a story and participate in administrative hearings and proceedings. Processes worked out the best when they were allowed to play out and were not manipulated. The military had separate lanes, including legal, medical, and personnel actions. The best outcomes occurred when military mental health providers stayed in their lane.

A military mental health provider should always advocate for the service member and be a source of support. We should always try to make their lives better and advocate whenever possible. The system is stacked against individual service members. The government almost always wins. Mental health providers need to advocate for service members because, often, no one else will.

Whole Person Perspective

Resist the temptation to view people as numbers, lab values, constellations of symptoms, or through tunnel vision. Outcomes were most positive when people were viewed from a whole person perspective. A person was a collection of organ systems. The heart and brain were connected, part of the whole person. A person was impacted by their environment, command, relationships, and health. From the perspective of an operational command, a service member was either fit for duty or not. Medical board and military dispositions were ideally made from a whole person perspective. It didn't make sense to say someone with a catastrophic physical health condition was fit for duty from a mental health perspective. From a whole person and an operational health perspective, a service member is either fit or not fit for full duty.

Limited Duty and Medical Boards

For mental health conditions, a period of limited duty takes the service member out of an overwhelming stressor and gives them time to recuperate and improve coping skills. The frequency and duration of limited-duty periods varied from time to time throughout my career, depending on who was in charge and according to policy that underwent frequent revision. Sometimes the duration of limited-duty periods was decreased to try to decrease the number of service members on limited duty, but this resulted in more frequent appointments to evaluate limited-duty status and increased overhead. Sometimes the duration of limited-duty periods was increased to reduce system strain. The changes didn't make much difference in my experience. The trajectory and number of service members on limited duty remained about the same.

When limited duty was indicated, a good rule of thumb was a starting point of six months, especially for a more severe condition, such as PTSD, major depression, or anxiety disorder. The idea of shorter periods of limited duty for minor mental health issues, where an individual was overwhelmed by transient stress, was appealing, but there were issues with the implementation. It could take six weeks for a service member to receive an initial mental health appointment, and by that time, their three-month limited-duty period was halfway over. A second period of limited duty was usually only successful if the patient was moving in a positive direction and had significant improvement at the end of their first period of limited duty. Service members who were recommended for a second period of limited duty, with chronic, intractable symptoms, rarely improved. For those types of situations, it was best to proceed with a medical board rather than a second period of limited duty.

Reinforcing the Message that Getting Help Is a Good Thing

Making harsh, superficial judgments and writing stigmatizing comments in the medical record had damaging effects on people throughout my career. I witnessed situations where a patient experienced something like this and was discouraged from ever wanting to get help or talk to a helping professional again. Situations tend to go viral. Other service members and military leaders are always watching. If people witness a service member getting negatively impacted by the mental health system, this sends a viral message to others to avoid asking for help. While serving with Veterans Affairs, I spoke to many veterans who avoided seeking help on active duty because they witnessed the negative impact it had on their peers.

There was a situation reported where prosecutors called a marine's treating psychiatrist to testify against his patient at Camp Lejeune during a court-martial. The marine felt betrayed and wrote that he had difficulty with trusting as a result. The judge presiding over the case denied the prosecutor's request for the treating psychiatrist to testify (Brennan 2022). The full details of that situation are not known, but if a mental health provider testifies against their own patient during a legal proceeding, it spreads a viral message not to get help. Such situations reinforce fears that what is said in a mental health session could be used against them.

Recovery Can Be Scary

Sometimes service members are in a precontemplative state and are not ready for change. One way or another, the idea of recovery is anxiety-provoking. It is a radical change from the state they are in. Sometimes patients act out or rebel when faced with the proposition of making positive changes. It's helpful for the team to be patient and understanding with service members.

Command and Family Involvement

I learned to never underestimate the power of family and command in helping an active-duty service member. The command was the unidentified family for a service member. Sometimes a call home or to command made all the difference in the world for someone who was struggling. Strive to find a sweet spot or balance between the individual, the family, and the command. Include family and command when needed. Don't discharge a patient from inpatient care without command involvement. When someone is at high risk and has dropped out of treatment, call the command.

Ideal Military Mental Health Program

The ideal operational or military mental health program was constructed of critical elements. Often, military mental health initiatives failed because one or more of the components were missing.

A team lead is necessary to oversee operations, coordinate and communicate with leadership, advocate for issues, change, and act as a liaison officer. The team lead needs to have sufficient dedicated time to perform the role and associated administrative duties. When team leads got bogged down in clinical work, this negatively impacted their effectiveness. Issues were frequently identified that needed to be addressed by leadership. Without a dedicated or solid team lead to communicate and work out issues, they went unaddressed. For example, if there were facilities issues—service members were showing signs and symptoms of mental health issues because they didn't have hot food or there were issues with their work schedule—the mental health team lead met with the appropriate third parties and advocated for necessary changes. The team lead needs to attend meetings and be free to deal with administrative issues. Unless a military unit or mission was very small, one person can't do it all.

The team lead needs to have oversight of personnel, resources, and materials. I was part of a multidisciplinary team that included psychiatrists, psychologists, nurses, and psychiatric technicians. There was a different supervisor for each class of professionals who was outside of the team. This resulted in span of control issues because the team lead was unable to fully address situations. There were occasions when team members told the team lead to "talk to my supervisor" when there were issues.

The most effective mental health programs had regular communication, coordination, and referral pathways with local helping programs. These included the emergency room, primary care clinic, inpatient psychiatric unit, family services programs, and the sexual assault program. Communication and coordination with military chaplains were also beneficial. A lot of times, communication between departments fell on the team lead to facilitate. Without adequate crosstalk, programs became stovepiped, and this decreased their effectiveness. Sometimes interventions provided by different programs operating independently contradicted each other.

Mental health programs require a designated workspace that is clean and private. While serving with the Marine Corps, I was shocked when a patient complained that he could hear me talking from outside the room through a vent on the door. It turned out that the blueprint for the building identified the room as a storage area. I literally saw patients in a closet. I installed soundproofing over the vent as a work-around. The same applied for programs in the field. A mental health provider had to take someone outside and stand by a tree away from other service members to ensure adequate privacy.

A team approach is always touted as a great approach for mental health, but it didn't always pan out. Sometimes the notion was an elusive utopia, and achieving a cohesive multidisciplinary mental health team was an impossible task. Sometimes the team engaged in groupthink, and that made problems worse. A team approach assumed everyone was acting in good faith and had the best interests of patients, but it wasn't always the case. Mental health providers were people too and often acted in their own self-interest to fill their time and do the minimum, especially in a government-run health system. I observed mental health providers to have alternate agendas. When I worked for the Air Force, I was at a meeting where it was discussed that primary care providers filled their schedules with unnecessary follow-ups to minimize their workload. I witnessed similar things in mental health. Some psychologists I worked with filled their schedules with easy long-term patients to avoid taking new ones on. This contributed to a backlog of patients waiting for individual therapy appointments. I worked in a clinic once where it felt like a giant game of hot potato. I witnessed patients getting "merry-go-rounded." This happened when one psychologist referred the patient to a second psychologist. The second psychologist referred the patient to a third. Finally, the third referred the patient back to the first one.

A mental health team functions best with daily morning huddles and at least weekly team meetings to discuss challenging cases and situations and to achieve a battle rhythm. Meetings assisted mental health providers with staying connected, developing a sense of community and camaraderie, and facilitating collaboration to improve outcomes. When I worked on mental health teams that didn't have adequate meetings, it felt like the result was similar to a car engine's cylinders firing out of sync. Everyone stayed in their offices and closed their doors. Coordination was lacking, and care slipped. I worked on teams where there were unproductive meetings. The meetings sucked up a lot of time, were draining, and decreased productivity. It was best when meetings had an agenda that was followed instead of having open-ended around-the-room-type meetings.

Allocating time for walk-in visits and face-to-face meetings with military commands to support service members in distress was a best practice. Far too often, decision-making was centered around filling appointment slots instead of getting service members the right service at the right time from the right person. "Bean counters" advocated that mental health providers have back-to-back appointments, but mental health situations and the responses needed to optimally address them didn't operate that way. Time needs to be allocated to address patients in crisis and coordinate care. When such time was allocated, patients were seen as walk-ins for urgent situations, outcomes improved, and this took pressure off the emergency department. When I served with the Air Force, they had a best practice of assigning a provider of the day to have sufficient time to address urgent situations and walk-ins.

Outcomes of high-risk cases were best when compliance and participation was tracked in a database or spreadsheet. When individuals stopped participating or slipped through the cracks, outreach was conducted to recapture and provide intervention for noncompliant individuals. Sometimes dropping out of treatment and recapture was part of the process. Not tracking and intervening in high-risk situations worsened outcomes of situations.

Objective data and key metrics need to be captured and communicated to the team and management officials, including objective access-to-care standards. It helped when management officials knew about the good work the team was doing and about any issues or trends the team encountered.

Another key aspect of a successful military mental health program was being supported by responsive management officials in a timely manner. When access-to-care standards aren't being met, management officials need to assist and address staffing issues. Sufficient resources to manage and treat ailing service members are required.

Operational mental health providers require sufficiently staffed hospital or outpatient clinic-based mental health providers to refer complex treatment-resistant service members. The military medical treatment facility requires enough hospital providers to run a treatment program and maintain the educational pipeline to ensure the next generation of military mental health providers are trained. I observed situations where the operational mental health providers had better manning than the hospital-based ones. I experienced situations where an overseas location had better staffing or access to care than our facility in the continental United States. The overseas mental health clinic had a child psychiatrist, and ours did not. Once, I received a phone call from an overseas location, asking to transfer a patient to our military treatment facility. I agreed to do so but pointed out that they had better access to care than our facility.

A military mental health program required sufficient clinicians to do the work. Faran and colleagues wrote about their efforts in establishing an integrated behavioral health system of care at Schofield Barracks (Faran, et. al 2011). The authors wrote that, traditionally, the Army called for one adult psychiatrist for every

7,000 adults, but they found that one was required for every 3,000 adults. A rule of thumb was that one mental health provider per 2,000 service members was needed. Using these numbers, if 15 percent of service members suffered from mental health issues, that would equate to one mental health provider to manage 300 cases. Along those lines, I never saw an ideal patient panel size defined or enforced. Everyone agreed panel size reached a point that was too much, but no one would agree upon a number. I encountered situations where the panel size was too large. In these situations, the clinic would cut down the number of new intake appointments. I encountered situations where service members had difficulty accessing appointments, and this contributed to treatment failure. It was necessary for clinicians to have sufficient appointment time allocated for a face-to-face visit. In the private sector, a patient's needs could be met with a twenty- or thirty-minute appointment, but a military mental health provider required more time to address military-specific issues, such as fitness for duty, paperwork, and communication with commands to conduct interventions.

Approaching Complex Cases

The first step in addressing complex situations is recognition. A common pitfall was to oversimplify or generalize about a patient. When things didn't make sense, there was a good chance there was a deeper story that took time and patience to solve. Oversimplifying situations was an easy out and a temptation that had to be dealt with.

A sailor kept coming to the clinic complaining of severe treatment-resistant depression for many months. His psychologist and I couldn't figure out what was going on. One day he came to see me. He complained that he felt acutely depressed. I admitted him to the hospital, and he had a positive drug test for cocaine. It turned out that he had been struggling with cocaine addiction for over a year and had allowed a drug dealer to borrow his car, and it was stolen.

The clinical presentation of service members suffering from

mental health conditions is like geometric shapes missing sides. Sometimes only three sides of a rectangle are visible, and it is on the team or mental health provider to make the inference. The science wasn't exact. Once, I worked with a young patient who was diagnosed with a conversion disorder with adjustment disorder-like symptoms. He was suffering from weakness in his legs due to mental health issues. He was new to the Marine Corps, with less than six months military service, and was going through an unexpected and unwanted divorce. Thinking critically about the case, the overriding issue was anxiety, going through a divorce, and being new to the military. The conversion disorder issue was a red herring. Once the emphasis was on the issues that were bothering him instead of the weakness in his legs, his situation turned around and resolved.

On a different note, once, I saw a Navy psychiatrist cure a conversion disorder in a service member. The patient was hospitalized in a medical unit. He was a high-functioning senior enlisted service member. He had weakness and paralysis in his legs. A senior psychiatrist called me up, said he knew a cure for conversion disorder, and asked for my help. We went to talk to the patient. He offered encouragement and reassurance. We lifted the patient out of bed, into a standing position. The patient stood in between us and wrapped his arms around our shoulders. We walked up and down the hospital hallway a few times. To my astonishment, he regained strength and function in his legs. To this day, I've never seen or heard anything like that again.

When situations don't make sense, it is important to recognize this and think critically. Often, it is helpful to go back to square one, use objective data to drive decision-making, and reassess the diagnosis. Frequently, there is hidden substance use or some other factor the patient is having trouble opening up about. It was not uncommon for patients to be in denial, not able to open up about their secret drinking problem or other sensitive, potentially humiliating behaviors.

Service members are young. They are going through a dynamic time in their lives, and their clinical presentation is also dynamic. They seem healthy on the surface, but many suffered from a prodromal disease state, where they had early signs and symptoms of a mental health disorder, but the disease hadn't progressed enough to declare itself. Long-term, they might end up being diagnosed with a severe mental health issue, such as schizophrenia or bipolar disorder.

Mental health treatment is a team sport. Outcomes are best when there is teamwork, communication, and coordination with other professionals. Everyone brought something unique to the table. The Marine Corps was famous for its combined-arms approach to combat. The same dogma applied to the approach and management of complex mental health patients and situations.

When formulating a diagnosis, practical advice is to find the diagnosis that most logically accounted for all the systems. "Wild zebras" did exist, but they were ultra rare.

Often, patients were referred for psychological testing when the referring provider was anxious about making a judgment call. I've never met a patient I could not accurately diagnose with sufficient time and observation. Self-reported rating scales and psychological testing were useful, but the results had to be integrated into the clinical presentation.

In my experience, sedative medications and other controlled substances were best for short-term use, were rarely helpful, and had a tendency to make things worse. Controlled substances were used most effectively with care and caution. I witnessed situations where stimulants and sedatives were prescribed simultaneously. The practice of giving a patent an upper and downer at the same time didn't make sense, and clinical outcomes were almost always negative.

Depression, anxiety, and PTSD are very treatable conditions, but treatment responsiveness is less or slower for those conditions. Working with service members with ADHD was rewarding because their symptoms rapidly and markedly improved. I treated a sailor who had been struggling with undiagnosed ADHD his entire life. When he was a child, his teacher recommended his parents get him evaluated for ADHD, but they didn't believe in the condition. He had been in the Navy for over a decade. His career progression was stuck at E6. He hit every career milestone for advancement, including tough assignments and deployments, but was unable to do well enough on the advancement exam to achieve promotion to E7. He came to see me in desperation several months before his last attempt at the exam. I started him on ADHD medication, and it was like a light switch. Part of his brain came alive, he was able to study for hours, and he aced the exam. When he came to see me again, he looked like a different person. He was happy and confident, and everything went well.

CHAPTER 19

Burnout and Compassion Fatigue

SERVING AS A medical professional is a difficult job. The surgeon general of the United States published an advisory about addressing health worker burnout in 2022 (US Surgeon General 2022). He wrote that healthcare professionals are stretched too thin, fighting against ever increasing administrative requirements, and driven to the brink without the resources to provide patients and communities with the care they need.

Mental health professionals experience similar work stresses and contextual factors compared with the other medical disciplines, but the mental health field has its own subset of unique stresses. Mental health professionals experience stigma from the profession, patient suicide, personal threats of violence from patients, and demanding relationships with patients (Rossler 2012).

Military mental healthcare professionals are subjected to even more stress, over and above the normal pressures of being a mental health provider. We are on the front line, helping service members, and consulted when they are in distress, at their darkest hour and at their worst. We see the pain, trauma, and desperation in their eyes. Military mental health providers communicate with service members after they have a DUI or some other incident, not when there is a big organizational win. If there are 1,000 service members in a military unit, and a small percentage (10-15 percent) are struggling, we serve that patient population, approximately 100-150 service members. We don't see the other 900 service members who feel gung-ho, love their unit, and are thriving.

Organizational problems frequently impact military mental health issues. We suffer from those same bureaucratic and organizational problems just like everyone else. Military mental health providers are caught in Catch-22 situations alongside the service members and their families. We can identify upstream system problems impacting our patients but have limited ability to address them. This leaves the patients and military mental health professionals feeling frustrated, drained, and helpless.

The nature of the work of serving as a military mental health provider includes talking to patients all day and focusing on their problems. Hearing painful stories day in and day out and working as a mental health professional is taxing. We sacrifice a little piece of ourselves talking to them. Part of the job includes pushing personal problems to the back burner. It is difficult to get out of that mode and focus on personal issues and self-care. After talking to patients all day, there are times I shut down. At times I have grown so accustomed to talking to patients, it is difficult to talk about my own issues. It is critical to have a balanced lifestyle, feel grounded, have a solid foundation, and feel supported by the organization. It is helpful to experience all the parts of the military, especially the parts that are functioning well, and share in the wins.

Kennedy described challenges military psychologists faced compared with their civilian counterparts (Kennedy and Zillmer 2012). She wrote about mixed agency situations where the psychologist has responsibility to the patient and the government simultaneously. Military psychologists are placed into situations where they are recommended to balance the individual's needs, the military's needs, military regulations, and professional ethics codes.

I wrote about dual agency and trying to balance the rank and Medical Corps collar devices. Being pulled in so many different directions felt like being strung up in a medieval torture device at times.

Kennedy discussed issues with competence that result when military psychologists are required to hold disparately different jobs throughout their military careers. Another issue identified was having multiple, dual relationships and roles. These situations occur when a psychologist at a small, embedded, or deployed command enters into a clinical relationship with a coworker, friend, subordinate, or senior officer. A fellow psychiatrist told me about a situation where he was deployed with one of his patients and they shared the same tent. He had spoken with him about infidelity and observed him chasing women on deployment.

The same set of challenges that impact service members everywhere affect military healthcare professionals too. Life is unpredictable for us too. Service members frequently work, work, and work only to have all their work undone like a carpet being yanked out from under them. In an earlier chapter, I discussed the example of a military cardiologist who worked hard to achieve a prestigious chest pain certification for the hospital only to have the initiative set back due to a deployment. Just when it seems things have cooled off, something happens, healthcare professionals are deployed, and this wreaks havoc on the system and the people.

The Road to Burnout

Burnout starts before the oath of office is taken and the uniform is put on. Recruits receive their first taste of military bureaucracy when they are provided conflicting information from the recruiter, experience delays, and encounter organizational dysfunction.

When a military healthcare provider begins their career, they start off young, fresh, high energy, and idealistic, with a crisp set of uniforms. As their career progresses, they take hits, accumulate scars, and experience wear and tear.

Working as a mental health provider in and of itself is a challenging job. Mental health providers experience situations where they are short-staffed, the patients complain of difficulty accessing care, and it is demoralizing to see people suffer and not have the capability to see patients in a timely manner. The military environment adds to the challenge. Once, I spoke with a marine who had such a severe case of PTSD that he slept in his car, and it was tough to stomach not being able to do more. Frequently, service members did something dramatic to work around access-to-care problems, like threaten suicide and do harm to themselves. Experiencing those levels of desperation is upsetting and draining. There is also a moral injury aspect to experiencing these challenges. There is a feeling that service members and their families deserve better. Not being able to meet those expectations impacts military mental health providers psychologically. At its worst, it feels like working in a system of smoke and mirrors where getting help is more of an illusion. People had difficulty accessing care and got bounced around or merry-go-rounded between programs. For some, the illusion of help was therapeutic. From a mental health provider's perspective, working in a system like that contributes to burnout.

There are professional turf wars and tension between military officers of different mental health disciplines. Sometimes psychologists had an agenda to undermine psychiatrists, and vice versa. The hierarchy and rank structure made it worse. At Naval Medical Center Portsmouth, there was a feeling that physicians weren't valued. The command celebrated nurses' day and all sorts of days for every profession, but it was the only medical facility I ever served at where there was no doctors' day.

The military mental health professional advocates for patients by calling the chain of command to discuss workplace environment and other organizational issues. Often, intervention was successful, but at times efforts are met with hostility and dismissiveness, and that takes a toll.

A military medical leader spoke about working to one's capability, but the organization doesn't empower individuals to do this. It hurts not being able to work to full potential and being handcuffed by red tape and bureaucracy. Military mental health providers don't feel supported, and this is disheartening. The individual has the capability to work with a patient weekly, but this rarely happens due to organizational and system problems, such as poor planning, lack of resources, and an ineffective appointment scheduling system. For a mental health professional, seeing a patient once a month for individual therapy felt like being a grounded aircraft pilot. The reality is frustrating and wears on everyone. The same applies to other medical professionals too. Consider surgeons whose operating room times were canceled due to contaminated surgical instruments and unaddressed facilities issues, such as the hot water heater rupturing and taking weeks to be replaced. There is a learned helplessness among professionals as they grapple with a loss of control and a sense that they can't make happen what needs to be done. The military mental health provider lacks authority to make decisions or implement changes and has limited ability to control their program. It is difficult, if not impossible, to make hiring decisions, and there isn't a way to fix facility issues. Employees and other personnel are frustrated and blame leadership, although leadership does not have the authority to address the issues. The young professional tries to advocate for change but hits brick walls. The hits accumulate, and the burnout pathway progresses.

False guilt is another issue that impacts burnout. Good officers save the ship at all costs, but that mentality isn't effective for coping with chronic, complex system peacetime problems. A hard lesson I learned in my career was that the DoD, DHA, and individual services are responsible for chronic system problems that impact everyone. Programs fail and are retooled. It is not the fault of the individual healthcare professional if everything breaks when they deploy or take leave. Programs can't have a single point of failure. Success can't fall on the shoulders of an individual healthcare professional.

There were compromising situations where military health workers had to cross boundaries and standards to survive. It felt like one had to give up a piece of their soul to the government to survive. I described situations where military mental health providers were pressured and manipulated to make or not make certain diagnoses and to perform actions based on what was perceived as being in the best interests of the military. There was constant pressure to obey and support the chain of command, even if it didn't seem right. My grandfather was an Army physician in WWII and was asked to sign documents certifying that his unit was free of syphilis and other sexually transmitted diseases, although it wasn't the case. I think he coped with the situation by having a sense of humor. I recall a conference presentation where a Navy medicine flag officer introduced himself as a former psychiatrist. The implication was that he had to divorce himself from his professional identity to advance his career.

Military mental health professionals face scrutiny, second-guessing, and consequences that add to the stress. It feels like the system is set up for failure, and mental health providers are blamed when situations go bad. Witch-hunting is an unwritten military cultural tradition, especially in the Navy. If something happens or there is a near miss, perhaps the mental health professional could have handled the situation in a more optimal way. Often, the reality was that the patient had another incident due to their own decision-making and the situation was driven by work environment issues and system problems surrounding access to care. When a patient has an incident, it makes the department look bad. When the chain of command looks bad, they want to know who, what, when, and why it happened. What follows is intrusive questioning, micromanagement, punishment, and retaliation. It may be subtle, like a minor markdown, job reassignment, or vague comments on a performance review, but it was direct too. There was a medical officer who worked on a massive electronic records project that was mothballed. He felt blamed for the whole ordeal. He had a sign on his door counting down the number of days until he could get out.

The job of a military mental health provider has been described as plugging holes in a dam. Everyone sees where the dam needs to be overhauled, but the job is never done. The job becomes plugging holes for several years, barely scraping by, until a replacement arrives. The system is frequently crisis-driven, and there is never time for program development, retooling, and overhaul. Providers keep providing "downstream" interventions over and over. Providers experience an unfulfilled need to travel upstream to address underlying system problems and larger issues, but change and intervention are elusive. Not being able to get at the upstream issues takes a toll too.

Military mental health providers receive hit after hit. Unchecked, they find themselves on a downward spiral headed toward burnout.

Leadership Issues Contribute to Burnout

The master chief of the Navy was quoted during the *USS George Washington* suicide cluster news reports as saying the nation didn't have a whole lot of psychologists, psychiatrists, and other mental healthcare workers out there in abundance. He talked about young professionals being in debt and not wanting to come into the Navy as a lieutenant. The implication is that mental health manning issues are top problems the Navy faces. It implies recruiting, retention, and financial compensation. I participated in many similar discussions across my career. Frequently, the issues are simplified down to recruiting, retention, and not having enough mental health providers. The reality is that larger issues, including poor leadership and burnout, impact recruiting and retention of mental health providers. Poor leadership includes lack of direction, not being supported or understood by the organization, and just overall bad leadership. These issues spiked morale and were a retention killer.

My colleagues and I voted with our feet due to these issues.

Lack of leadership and direction is straightforward. Everyone agrees that mental health is important, but there wasn't a clear institutional vision or methodology of how military mental health should look or operate. There was an overall feeling that mental health and related issues were overlooked. Policies were lacking, and there were many gaps. I served a three-year tour with the Marines as an OSCAR division psychiatrist from 2005–2008. Once, at a meeting, the senior Navy psychiatrist apologized for not doing good staff work and not giving the program the time and attention it deserved. The Navy and Marine Corps failed to publish an instruction. We were left to our own devices to figure out what we were supposed to do at the local level and how to do it. Jesse Locke described the challenges, dysfunction, and pushback he faced serving as a Navy psychologist in the OSCAR program, on deployment with the Marines (Locke 2017). A decade after I served with the Marine Corps, he wrote about similar issues: stigma, working to get buy-in, being told "there were no OSCAR issues," and being turned away. Military mental health leadership was risk-averse, avoided putting things in writing, lacked expertise in program management, research, and statistics, and didn't provide specific methodology. Frequently, decisions were arbitrary and political, based on who was in charge, and that changed frequently. I spoke to a Navy psychologist about it. He told me he liked operating in a gray area and having freedom to do what he thought was helpful. Lack of leadership and direction had consequences. Programs and people clashed, there were bad outcomes, and the mental health providers and patients were caught in the crossfire.

A Navy psychiatrist I served with, a former submariner, worked with the Navy to implement changes to sleep and work schedules for submariners to improve sleep and reduce fatigue (Associated Press 2014). I was told around the same time frame that a similar proposal was submitted to senior admirals in the surface fleet, but they declined to sign off on it. A few years later, in 2017, the *USS John McCain* and *USS Fitzgerald* were involved in collisions where insomnia and fatigue were cited as contributing factors. The accidents resulted in a roughly $1 billion expense. It is possible the accidents could have been prevented if the sleep and fatigue issues were addressed. It was frustrating and disappointing when leadership did not buy in or support mental health.

Another leadership problem is identifying problems but not addressing them. There were many meetings where issues were identified, potential solutions were discussed, but the issues went unaddressed. Leadership didn't advocate for the team and was afraid of being seen in a negative light by the chain of command. It was demoralizing and felt like the leadership threw the team under the bus. I sat in many meetings where participants were asked to discuss "roles and responsibilities." Everyone suggested it was someone else's responsibility, and the discussions went nowhere. Leadership wouldn't provide clear direction, and everyone mentally checked out.

There is a feeling that the military hospitals and organizations are too top heavy (Kime 2023). There were plenty of administrators and leaders to push down taskings and work requirements but not enough providers to complete them. Most of the time, there was a backlog of patients. It felt like there was a disproportionate number of administrators compared with the medical providers in the trenches performing the clinical work. Many sought plum positions protected from workload. A lot of times, it felt like leadership wasn't invested or focused on success. I coined a term for a phenomenon I observed: "zookeeper leadership." Cages were left open, allowing the animals to escape, and the zookeepers had job security chasing them down. It was as if the higher-ups intentionally created problems to justify their employment.

The promotion system and ladder climbing drained everyone. It was easy to achieve promotion to O4, but above there were fewer and fewer promotions available, and competition became cutthroat. Perhaps it was like one of those zombie apocalypse movies where warring groups of individuals were fighting each other for scarce resources. The behavior of those trying to get promoted was appalling. There were those who were "title hungry" and would do anything or throw anyone under the bus to get promoted. They would place the value of the officer effectiveness report over the welfare of their own personnel and the patients under their care. These exact same behaviors I witnessed and experienced were well documented in a decades old study on military professionalism (US Army War College 1970).

There was an unwritten bad leadership playbook in existence that was passed down and perpetuated in a cycle of abuse. A common tactic of poor leadership was to turn problems back on the requestor. For example, if junior or field-grade officers complained about staffing and access-to-care issues, senior leaders would blame them for the problems and recommend they work harder. I was at a meeting where access-to-care issues were discussed. A senior Navy Capt./O6 recommended personal workload and working hours to be increased to evenings and weekends. Once, I worked at a small Marine Corps base that repeatedly sent infantry battalions to combat, and there was a need for mental health support due to acute PTSD. When local leadership and I attempted to advocate for the request, we were told productivity data didn't support that, knowing full well systems were grossly inaccurate. We were told there was no medical evidence to support the request. When we submitted a business case addressing those concerns, there were more excuses and pushback. We were told the request needed to come from a different person or it was not an official request. It was apparent to everyone involved that many of the more senior officials enjoyed protected positions working at the hospital and opposed requests for selfish reasons. Dr. Carl Castro described experiencing these behaviors from the surgeon general of the Navy when the release of an Army Mental Health Advisory Team study was blocked at multiple levels (Castro 2017). Dr. Castro wrote that the Navy surgeon general knew the marines would demand that the Navy provide more medical personnel to support the marines, and he did not want this to happen.

There was a perpetual war between Navy operational and hospital-based mental health providers. The hospital-based providers didn't want to deploy and opposed operational initiatives. On deployment, they would hunker down at the large base camps, refuse to conduct behavioral outreach, and claim they had no mission because no one came to see them. They would complain that they were not prescribing any medications and would request to be sent home. Not only did programs lack policy and direction, but there were those who tried to block implementation and undermine programs. The BHDP initiative was an example of that. The program was mandated by the DHA, but local leadership would drag their feet and make implementation as difficult as possible, with the hopes that it would go away. Marine Corps leadership was refreshing. Their mentality was to lead from the front, but military medicine leadership wasn't like that. Senior medical leaders had a reputation for not dealing with issues, frequently pawning off work and deployments onto someone else. Once, I witnessed a senior medical officer near retirement from active duty state that his career goal was to hire himself as a senior federal employee.

I encountered situations in my career where bad leadership would abuse authority and torture people. It was not uncommon to observe superiors abusing their authority to push work and deployments on others. Sometimes leadership was straight-up dishonest. Once, a senior medical commander told a military unit they were pushing forward and going into a combat zone. He was dishonest about it, knew it wasn't the case, stirred everyone up, and got a rise out of it. I witnessed situations where people were ostracized and banished for doing the right thing. I witnessed military leaders gaslight people. They would tell them they were helping them but then actively try to undermine them. There were situations where individuals were set up for failure and sent on wild goose chases. I worked with a senior military psychiatrist early in my career who was toxic and corrupt. Years later, I was at a conference and a colleague approached me. She confided in me how he repeatedly sexually harassed her to the point that she filed a formal grievance. We both shared our experiences with him, and it gave us both some peace.

Navy medicine had a cultural tradition of holding vendettas and being hard on people, which was different from the other services I worked with. I heard accounts from my patients and colleagues about getting poor performance evaluations out of spite. The Navy did not like medical providers who were perceived as "not following the Navy way." I was told a story about a psychologist who was targeted for over a decade, referred to as a problem maker, but the reality was, he was a team player and treated unfairly. I received an account of a PHS officer I served with at Naval Medical Center Portsmouth, who was loyal to the organization and punished with an average performance evaluation without justification.

A former marine and licensed clinical social worker wrote a book, entitled *Broken Promises*, about his experiences working in the VA's Vet Center Program (Blickwedel 2022). He described suffering from leadership issues, getting discouraged, and his efforts to advocate for change. He described feeling retaliated against. He described the personal toll, challenges, and burnout mental health providers face. He discussed his efforts to balance patients' needs, personal needs, and advocacy for improvement of organizational problems.

There were rarely ever repercussions or consequences for bad leadership. The annual performance review system lacked subordinate input into the evaluation process, and this allowed toxic leaders to thrive.

The Downward Spiral

Burnout is a progressive downward spiral of hits. It may be a death of a thousand cuts too. At first, the hits sting; then they start to hurt and begin to impact the individual. Individuals feel unsupported, undervalued, begin to check out mentally, and miss work. Burnout negatively impacts health. It causes stress, weight gain, poor decision-making, and unhealthy behaviors. It impacts relationships. Individuals would have affairs or develop issues with alcohol or substance abuse to cope. I observed senior leaders counsel service members who had "lost their way."

Individuals acted out. Sometimes there were dramatic displays, and individuals would ask to be reassigned. I received an email that was sent to all from a federal employee where he abruptly quit and blamed the department head. There was malicious compliance. I saw situations where mental health providers were directed to write a medical board they disagreed with. They would take out their frustration in the document, and on the patient, by writing negative and passive-aggressive remarks in the narrative summary.

I observed burnout impact the clinical judgment of military mental health providers and how they treated patients. It started with loss of compassion and empathy. Military mental health providers lost their ability to care and work ethic. They did the minimum to get by. They engaged in negative watercooler talk, including making harsh, superficial judgments that a service member was no good, trying to get out of work, and didn't deserve a medical board, and the clinical decision-making was focused on getting rid of them, not having to deal with them. I witnessed mental health providers trying to talk patients out of getting help. I saw psychologists who tried to discourage patients from seeking individual therapy because they felt overwhelmed by too many patients. I witnessed patients turfed to someone else like a *House of God*-style giant game of hot potato. On a rare occasion, I experienced situations where colleagues took delight in making patients suffer.

Burnout spreads. It starts with the individual but impacts relationships and spreads to the team. Work stress contributes to relationship problems, both at home and in the clinic. Burnout shuts down group communication. People go into their offices, close their doors, and stop communicating and collaborating. I witnessed colleagues attend meetings and participate in telephone conferences but not say anything. Burnout spreads through divisions and departments, resulting in a barrel full of crabs. There is tension in the workplace, and individuals send out condescending emails with inappropriate tones. Providers snap at each other and file complaints. Frequently, mental health providers quit, and retention rates declined.

The end state of burnout feels like the last few minutes of a soccer game, when the losing team flagrantly fouls the winning team and receives red cards. No one wants to play on a losing team. Many suffer from an instinctive feeling to quit and lash out against teammates. A turning point for me when I worked in a toxic situation was when a senior nurse pointed out that our clinic had devolved into an "every man for himself" situation. She left shortly thereafter. Teams turn on the administration too. At the Navy SARP program, employees banded together and filed grievances against management, who lacked authority and resources to implement the desired changes.

Burnout results in organizational rot. Perhaps the last step in burnout is attrition. Everyone fights as hard as they can to make things work, but individuals come to the realization that they can't do anything but quit. Sometimes quitting was vindictive. The only power an individual has in an unresponsive system is to create an unplanned personnel loss to get back at the system.

In July 2022, an Air Force surgeon, the commander of the 959th Medical Operations Squadron, submitted a fiery resignation letter that was publicized in the national media (Cohen 2022). The *Air Force Times* story documented that "Service cultures clashed and egos ruled, causing friction on matters large and small." In his letter, he wrote about his efforts to address issues with his chain of command and struggling with "Machiavellian maneuvering and counterproductive bureaucracy." His letter captured the struggle, pain, and frustration military doctors feel.

One day in early 2021, while working at Naval Medical Center Portsmouth, a medical student came to see me for a mentoring session. He was an ensign in the PHS. He was bright, pleasant, with a promising future. He felt that the military was positive and was soon to begin a military psychiatry residency. About two years later, I received a notification about his death and learned he died by suicide. No one saw it coming, and everyone was devastated. The death impacted many people. I can't say I really knew him, but it impacted me too. Suicide leaves everyone feeling a certain way, wondering what happened, why and how to process it. I, too, was left hanging with unanswered questions. The exact details of his situation were unknown. I can't help but wonder if burnout or issues in this chapter contributed to his death.

Military Burnout Is Preventable

The hits can't be stopped, but there is a way to reduce and mitigate burnout. Maintaining effective communication, conducting regular meetings, and fostering a team ethos are key elements in safeguarding against workplace stress. A best practice involves establishing a good battle rhythm, including regular meetings where leadership discusses current developments and is transparent about what can and cannot be addressed. When this occurred, everyone was on the same page, felt valued, their contributions mattered, and they were part of a unit. It was protective to know leadership was trying and is looking out for their people, even if they couldn't do anything about it.

The first line of defense is individual protection. This involved having an adequate support system, finding balance, and practicing good self-care. It involves making healthy choices.

Having good leadership is a critical protective factor. If leadership sits in an office all day, lacks transparency, and is perceived as disconnected, deceptive, dishonest, and malicious, that results in stress and tension in the workplace. There is nothing worse than having leadership value their annual performance review more than the welfare of their subordinates and patients.

Being looked after by leadership and having adequate career progression, advancement opportunity, and support is a critical protective factor. Nothing sends a worse message that personnel aren't valued when promotion rates are 10 percent or less, especially in junior ranks, where pay is abysmal. Competition to that degree creates a survival of the fittest, where nine out of ten are eliminated and only the strongest survive.

Being connected to the mission, actively participating in operational activities like deployments, and having funding for educational conferences can be both inspirational and protective. I participated in a meeting at the Veterans Affairs Medical Center where they took time to reflect on the life and military service of one of the patients and discussed how the organization was proud to offer him comfort and relief.

Another way to mitigate military burnout is to have a nice, clean, properly maintained facility. When a facility is badly in need of renovation, that sends a message to patients and healthcare professionals that they aren't valued. Not properly maintaining a facility is nonverbal communication that the organization doesn't care. Walking in the door and seeing the state of facilities, especially those in disrepair, sets the stage for failure.

Military mental health providers benefit from seeing the fruits of their labor and being provided positive feedback when they are making a difference. They need to taste and appreciate what they are accomplishing. A key moment in my career was hearing the chief of naval operations say he hated military medicine, it was too expensive, and he'd rather spend the money elsewhere. Hearing that was like getting stabbed in the chest. No one wants to always be scrutinized for the bad things that happen. The bad needs to be offset with the good.

Transforming Burnout into Empowerment

Working in the private sector was boring after a while. The money was good, but it was comparable to a well-oiled machine and an assembly line of patients with constant and increasing productivity. The sense of mission was lacking. Working in the military health system is unpredictable and exciting at times. There were times we did important work, saved lives, and helped accomplish the mission. The experience made us better people, improved our strength, and created new possibilities.

The way forward for burnout is for actions to be taken to empower individuals and to address the chronic problems that are under everyone's skin. The organization needs to provide well-thought-out and written policies that clearly define a vision of who is doing what and address the chaos that results from lack of direction and standardization. The organization needs to do its part to be solid, predictable, and better organized and take care of its people. Individuals need to do their part to improve balance and coping.

Personal Impact

I love being a psychiatrist, love the military, and believe in its mission. Serving as a military psychiatrist is a rewarding job, but it has also had a significant impact on me. I've found it to be isolating at times, particularly within the military system. Psychiatry is often referred to as a "low-density, high-demand" career field. I've frequently found myself in situations where I was the only psychiatrist or worked with few peers. I have felt under pressure to get the mission done. It is challenging to talk with others all day about their problems. It is desensitizing. Sometimes I have to block it out to push forward. I feel shut down and closed off, so I need to find a balance and enhance my social support system. Sometimes it is easier to talk with others about their issues than to talk about my own.

Serving in the Navy left an impact on me. Earlier in this chapter, it was discussed how Dr. Castro from the Army experienced the Navy surgeon general trying to block mental health research for the marines. Dr. Castro wrote how the Navy surgeon general unsuccessfully tried to block the research at multiple levels, including at the secretary of the Navy, assistant secretary of Defense for Health Affairs, and with the commandant of the Marine Corps. Dr. Castro had the advantage of approaching this as a senior Army colonel at the DoD level, while I experienced the other end of this from the perspective of a young LCDR in the field serving with the Marine Corps. The marines worked so hard, had such a fighting spirit, and it was a massive disappointment. The situation, especially the politics of Navy medicine, was a bitter pill to swallow.

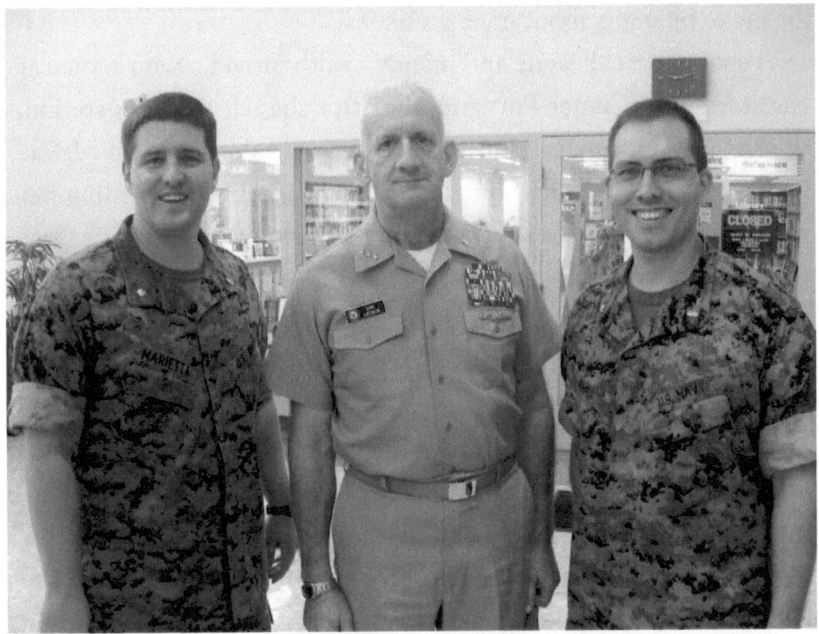

Pictured here are LCDR Bob Marietta (left) and LCDR Randolf Dipp (right) with their rolled Marine Corps sleeves and the surgeon general of the Navy in 2006.

Sometimes I have a light form of PTSD. I have trouble trusting people because of the bad leadership and maltreatment issues I experienced. During the height of the stuff I faced, I had anxiety and sleepless nights. I get triggered and become anxious when I start to sense I'm in one of those toxic military situations. I have bizarre military-themed nightmares. I feel anxiety when I walk into Naval Medical Center Portsmouth. I experienced carnage in a medical setting and patient suicide. I have never been shot at, but I encountered deployment trauma. What bothered me the most was toxic maltreatment and poor leadership, including experiencing things that threatened my career and hurt people. How the Navy treated its sailors and how the mental health system addressed their issues made me feel cynical and skeptical toward patients. I witnessed how my colleagues in the mental health system treated service members when they needed help, and that made it difficult for me to open up about my own issues.

I spoke to a colleague and mental health provider who served at Naval Medical Center Portsmouth. After she left the duty station, she had fear and anxiety due to the toxic issues she experienced. She felt a need to constantly update her new supervisor regarding her whereabouts and what she was doing. A turning point for her was when her new supervisor pulled her aside and told her she didn't need to provide updates, and the reason she was hired was because she was competent and trusted. We both went through a similar recovery process.

It was challenging to transition from the Navy's mental health system when I left active duty in 2008. I had to unlearn some of the military persona and associated behavior issues. I evolved to relax more, approach situations differently, and be less cynical. I had to learn a different diagnosing pattern and ways to document things in the medical record.

I went through a divorce in 2015. Words cannot describe the pain I experienced during the breakup of my nuclear family. It's not the military's fault I got divorced, but the military environment and my coping mechanisms contributed to the situation. I'm pretty sure I went through a major depressive episode at the time. A pivotal moment for me was confiding in my team lead about it while on deployment. He told me he was a big believer in divorce. At the time, I believed I would reconcile with my ex-wife, but his kind words set the stage for my recovery. I spoke to a Navy psychiatrist with an eating disorder who told me how hard it was for her to open up and ask for help. Neither of us were willing to receive care from a military provider due to our experiences working in the system and concerns about negative career impact. We both ended up receiving care. I participated in individual therapy with a nonmilitary provider, and there were times I just sat in the therapist's office and cried because it hurt so badly.

CHAPTER 20

Public Health Service

JOINING THE PHS was one of the best career decisions ever made. I was burned out after serving with the Navy the first time. I worked for a state and local mental health agency after leaving the Navy and then obtained a commission in the PHS.

The PHS falls under the Department of Health and Human Services (HHS). We have about 6,100 PHS officers in the United States. We are all healthcare-related officers that fall into eleven distinct professional categories: dietitian, health service officer, environmental health officer, pharmacist, scientist, engineer, therapist, veterinarian, physician, dentist, and nurse. The surgeon general is a phone call away from consultation with an expert in any healthcare-related field. The PHS falls under Title 42 and has a different mission set compared with the active-duty military (Title 10) and national guard (Title 32). Our role is to deploy under the secretary of HHS for urgent or emergent public healthcare needs.

I participated in a PHS officer promotion ceremony at the National Institutes of Health. The speaker said, "The job of a PHS officer is to stand by the side of those who have decided it was not yet time for nature to take its course." That was a powerful statement that resonated with me. PHS officers serve at numerous federal agencies. We serve at the National Institutes of Health, Centers for Disease Control, Indian Health Service, Bureau of

Prisons, Homeland Security, Coast Guard, Veterans Affairs, and DoD, to name a few. As a PHS officer, I was able to jump across agencies and services. I served with the Air Force, Coast Guard, and most recently Veterans Affairs, and this has helped me grow professionally and learn valuable lessons. I learned so much from serving with different agencies and service branches.

Every year, except during the COVID-19 pandemic, the US PHS Scientific and Training Symposium is held. Thousands of PHS officers around the world come to the conference and receive training. Early in my PHS career, I attended a leadership seminar hosted by RADM Boris Lushniak. He had a successful career and was deputy surgeon general. He served as acting surgeon general of the United States from 2013–2014. He started off his presentation by taking off his admiral shoulder boards, threw them on the floor, and proclaimed, "These don't make me a leader." He talked about checking your ego at the door and said PHS officers survive bad leadership. This was the first taste of PHS leadership I experienced, and it was refreshing. I have experienced Navy, Marine Corps, and Air Force flag officers before but never experienced anything like this. I became hooked on the PHS for life.

Another year, I was taking a Basic Life Support class at the conference and recognized the last name of one of the instructors, a PHS officer. Her name was "Elizabeth Lybarger." I swore I heard that last name before. After the class, I spoke with her. She had roots in Pittsburgh, Pennsylvania, where my grandparents were from. We both spoke to our families. It turned out, we were distant cousins! We had common ancestors in the Curry family. I'm convinced we have a healthcare warrior gene.

Around 2019 I was sent to Presidio, Texas, to provide medical support for a border patrol mission. The "guests" were each provided a medical evaluation and care as their needs dictated. We came across a group of Chinese nationals who paid exorbitant amounts of money to make it to the United States. They traveled through cacti and suffered splinters, which my team helped remove with precision and care. The team felt they tried so hard to come to our country and observed that they were motivated to become citizens. Privately, we felt their actions deserved a chance and hoped for their success. Shortly after that deployment, PHS officers at a detention facility were portrayed in the *Terminator Dark Fate* movie. The duties we performed were featured in a Hollywood movie!

One of the most memorable deployments I had in the PHS was to Liberia in 2014 to serve on an Ebola treatment unit for health professionals who were suffering from the virus.

The US Army was there too, but our service was the only one allowed to touch patients with Ebola. I had the best assignment. I spoke to every patient that was admitted to our unit. They had symptoms of possible Ebola and anxiously awaited their DNA PCR tests to see if they were positive or negative. There was a Liberian physician assistant and nurse who suffered from Ebola, both successfully treated at our facility and recovered. They joined our team after their recoveries and provided medical care to their countrymen who were suffering from the disease. This was the greatest example of force multiplication I had ever seen. We did not have any exercise equipment, but one thing we had plenty of was Meals Ready-to-Eat (MREs). Some clever officers created dumbbells out of MRE boxes. We used these to exercise, and they worked well. Our team remained deployed over the Christmas holiday. We all gathered in a tent, and the secretary of Health spoke to us by phone. She was tearful, told us she was thinking of us, and thanked us for our work. During 2014, *TIME*'s Person of the Year was named Ebola Fighters. My teammates and I all proudly carried that title.

The best thank-you letter I ever received came from a Liberian national, and I hung it on my wall:

> *Dear Dr. Sigh and Others,*
>   *I am so overwhelmed with excitement and I don't know*

how to begin; but one must always find a way...

It is with great delight and profound joy that I write to express gratitude to you all on behalf of my family. Words are inadequate to say how grateful we are.

Team 2 was such a great team which had wonderful people like Dr. Childs, Bob Marietta and others. They worked tirelessly to keep both Marphen and the late Elijah stable. Their selfless efforts in serving humanity will never go unnoticed. We appreciate everything you did to help Marphen and Elijah while you were here...

Many were those that went to various treatment centers, seeking cure from this deadly virus that has ravished the fabrics of our beloved nation, but very few are those that survived. We are very happy knowing that Marphen is among the survivors. We owe it all to God who is able to do all things through his infinite Grace. We owe it to you all as well, because of the enormous efforts you exerted to restore her fully...

Because of your passion, your sacrifices, your kind hearts and your love, my sister Marphen has fully recovered. Her survival tale would be incomplete without the mention of the Monrovia Medical Unit, without the mention of Team 2, Team 3, Dr. Childs, Dr. Sigh, and all the "Gallant Men and Women in BLUE" of the PHS of the United States of America. May the Lord bless you all.

Best regards and yours thankfully,
G. Joel Yardolo

In early 2020 I had a religious experience on a PHS deployment. I deployed to Maryland with Disaster Medical Assistance Teams from the National Disaster Medical System and the Army National Guard as a behavioral health provider. We conducted nursing home site visits at the height of the COVID-19 pandemic. Our teams provided assistance to facilities who were struggling. We assisted with COVID-19 testing, including swabbing and collecting samples. One day, I was on a team with the Army National Guard that drove up to a Catholic nursing home in a Humvee. We went into the facility, donned our personal protective equipment, and proceeded to assist nuns with testing the residents for COVID-19. When it was all said and done, there was a photograph of our team standing next to a group of soldiers and the nuns. I attended Saint Louis University, a Catholic school, for both my undergraduate and medical school. The mission and the associated photo were a religious experience. I felt that all the different parts of my life came together that day—religion, medicine, and military service. I also met my wife on that deployment, but that's another story.

CHAPTER 21

That Time I Became a Whistleblower

WHEN I WAS in training, we always joked that, to be truly successful in the Navy, one had to get in trouble and have an incident named after them. I never expected to experience anything like that.

My experience working with the Air Force and Coast Guard was that these services had a great track record of helping service members. When I served with the Air Force, I worked with service members, including VIPs, who got into trouble. The way these airmen were dealt with was overwhelmingly positive. The Air Force leadership held airmen accountable but always discussed positive steps and assisted service members in dealing with situations and getting back on their feet.

I went through a bit of a culture shock after returning to the Navy a second time, although, in retrospect, I wondered if my expectations were too high. A former Navy mentor once told me, "The Navy is 200 years of tradition unhampered by progress." It was disappointing but not surprising how sailors were treated compared to other services. I heard the stories and experienced, from an insider's perspective, the Navy mental health system problems that sailors from the *USS George Washington* and MARMC faced. My children participated in youth soccer, and I became acquainted with "sandbagging." This was a form of cheating where a team would stack themselves with ineligible players. I applied the same term to the Navy mental health system. Consider a boat that is sinking. Throwing sandbags onto the boat causes the boat to sink faster. It felt like my colleagues in the mental health clinic sandbagged sailors. They stacked the deck against them, through mental health documentation and personnel actions, to expedite their discharge from the Navy. In the *USS George Washington* investigation report, it was discussed that a sailor's diagnosis was changed from bipolar disorder to adjustment disorder and personality disorder. The report discussed how this impacted the medical boards process. I wrote about issues with underdiagnosing and misdiagnosing in the Navy's mental health system in an earlier chapter. I tried to cope by staying positive, focusing on what I could and couldn't control, and staying in my lane.

I provided mental health treatment for a command interest patient. Having experienced the Air Force and Coast Guard, I was a bit naive about the good intentions of others and was not prepared for the attention, interference, and negativity that came with the case. As the case progressed, I was peppered with emails from the convening authority and regional psychiatrist. I felt pressured and manipulated to change the diagnosis to personality disorder, which I refused to do. I was requested to testify in a Navy Board of Inquiry. When this became apparent, I felt pressured and guilted about testifying in the case. I testified in a number of military legal proceedings in the past and had never experienced anything like this. The hearing went by smoothly, from my perspective.

Up until this point, I had been working in Naval Medical Center Portsmouth's outpatient mental health clinic. Shortly after testifying in the hearing, my department head and his assistant came to see me. The department head told me a more senior and experienced provider was needed in the SARP and psychiatry continuity of psychiatric care programs and asked me to volunteer to take on the new roles. Historically, each of these roles was covered by a full-time provider, and I would be taking on the work of two people. It was presented to me as a choice and as something positive. A short time later, I was called into a meeting with the director of Mental Health. He asked me what my understanding of the meeting was. I told him it was to discuss the new roles. He said the purpose of the meeting was to discuss "performance issues." I was caught off guard and shocked by the meeting. I could see the look of a psychopath in his eyes and sensed the same toxic behaviors I'd witnessed at different points in my career. He proceeded to cite excerpts from my testimony in the hearing and tell me I made the directorate look bad. I thought to myself, *How does this guy know what I said in the hearing?* I knew what he was doing was wrong but had never experienced anything like it. He even threatened to fire me. During the meeting, I asked if the reassignment was a punishment for my participation in the case and the testimony.

A day later, I called the attorney, who called me as a witness. I asked for feedback about my performance in the hearing. She said I did a good job and was a victim of retaliation and that the command violated rules and regulations designed to protect witnesses in a legal hearing. She incorporated the retaliation in her legal rebuttal, which, of course, went nowhere. She asked me to file an inspector general complaint, but I was terrified. I experienced the Navy medicine mafia before. During the meeting, I tried to communicate to the director that I was part of the team and hoped the situation was resolved. Several weeks after this, my annual performance review was delivered electronically on a Friday afternoon without any discussion. I had been given an unsatisfactory performance evaluation without any formal or informal counseling. In the performance review, it was documented that I had difficulty with the "courts system" and complex cases, meaning the case I was involved in and the Board of Inquiry I participated in as a witness.

COER History (Recent Years Only!)

```
2023  Annual   6 7 7 7 7 7 7   S
2022  Annual   7 7 7 7 7 7 7   S
2021  Annual   7 7 7 7 7 7 7   S
2020  Annual   2 2 3 2 4 3 3   M  Rebuttal
2019  Annual   7 7 7 7 7 7 7   S
```

Pictured above are my annual performance reviews, illustrating a pattern of retaliation and reprisal

After this, I consulted with the Navy defense legal office and was told this was consistent with retaliation, and more specifically reprisal. Testifying in a legal hearing was protected speech, and my supervisors were wrong to confront me about it and take an adverse personnel action based on this. I asked the Navy defense counsel to talk to the Navy hospital attorney, but he refused. I was told they would only "ghostwrite" documents, and they weren't much help. I ended up hiring my own attorney. I was counseled that the behavior was consistent with black-letter unlawful command influence and reprisal, which I found to be 100 percent the case. The officers and civilians involved had personal relationships with the sailor. They did not want him to get his retirement, were trying to facilitate his discharge, and did not want me to testify on his behalf. They were trying to sandbag him out of the Navy, just like they did with other sailors. I wondered if the same individuals who pressured me to change the diagnosis in the case were also responsible for changing the diagnosis of the *USS George Washington* sailor who died by suicide. I was told unlawful command influence was "the mortal enemy of military justice." It was chilling, terrifying, and I would warn anyone who planned to testify in a Navy legal hearing about what I experienced.

I filed a Navy Article 1150 complaint. In my office, I had a full dress uniform ready to go. I was ready to meet with the hospital commanding officer or investigating officer, but the call never came. Weeks later, the Article 1150 complaint was returned without action, and I was told to file an IG complaint. I filed DoD and HHS IG complaints. The DoD IG told me the hospital commander had knowledge of reprisal and retaliation but failed to take appropriate action.

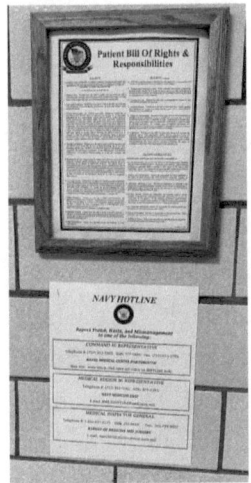
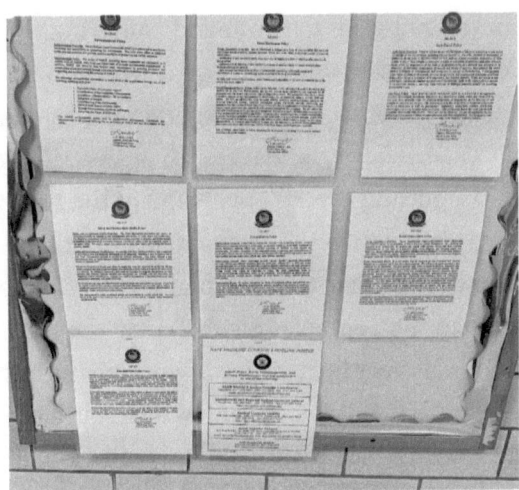

Shortly after the IG complaints were filed, the Navy hotline posters were updated all over the hospital. I did speak with both the Navy IG and HHS IG, but the complaints didn't go anywhere. Later, the Navy IG and DoD IG told me my complaint was transferred exclusively to HHS. The HHS told me they didn't have authority to investigate unlawful command influence. I was provided with a report from the HHS IG, but it was obvious the command tried to turn it around on me.

I got the feeling that the parties involved didn't want to deal with the situation, which was entirely consistent with numerous accounts from my patients who were active-duty sailors and Navy veterans regarding the issues they suffered from. A colleague offered an observation that the system was broken and service members who file complaints get tossed around until they give up. A retired Navy captain described a situation where a senior naval officer publicly threatened someone's career at a meeting, and an IG complaint was filed. The complaint was returned unsubstantiated, and it was felt that the IG did not speak with anyone in the room. The *USS George Washington* command climate and quality of life report (Caudle 2023) documented that there were IG complaints, and the DEOCS survey showed a command suffering from a chronically poor command climate, but those concerns never went anywhere either. I spoke to someone who experienced a similar situation. He told me his experience was that the IG serves the agency, and the situation is like putting the "fox in charge of the hen house."

I found myself experiencing firsthand a toxic military legal situation similar to what many of my patients had described and learned an appreciation for what they went through. The whole thing was very hurtful. I was working my butt off for the Navy, doing my best in a broken system with resource constraints. The situation was horrifying. I was told I would lose eligibility for my medical special pays and faced other negative career impacts. I was forced into a situation where I had to pay legal fees to defend myself. It was initially difficult for me to open up to and confide in my colleagues, but I did so. I received numerous letters of support. Many opened up to me about similar toxic behaviors they experienced. One individual told me how he wrote a letter of support for another command interest sailor who underwent courts-martial, how he was confronted about it, and how he was strongly discouraged from ever participating in a legal proceeding again. A colleague offered a letter of support: "In my entire Navy career, this was the worst leadership I have ever encountered. I served on a grueling carrier tour twice as the sole strike group psychologist and completed two back-to-back deployments. . . . I have no doubt the situation with Capt. Marietta is not because of anything he has done but is a direct result of the toxic leadership in the department."

I learned another PHS officer, LCDR Michell Sheedy, was retaliated against by the toxic leadership, fired from her job, and had to hire a lawyer to defend herself. She suffered an injury to her right leg, had to have surgery, and was recommended to participate in physical and occupational therapy. The command made it as difficult as possible for her to do so. After spending a considerable amount of money to defend herself, she never received justice either, but she was allowed to change duty stations. A couple years later, after leaving Naval Medical Center Portsmouth, she received a below-the-knee amputation of her right leg. She feels this was the result of toxic leadership interfering with her participation in her medical care. Her account is eerily similar to the issues Doc Jacobs faced, which was detailed earlier in this book.

The whole thing was eye-opening and discouraging. The evaluation was unlike any performance evaluation I had received in my lifetime. The department head and director who signed off on it really didn't know me. They sat in their office and had minimal interactions with me. The attorney who called me as a witness was suffering, and I could see it in her eyes. She complained that she was overworked and faced an uphill battle advocating for sailors. She felt the system was stacked against them. The behavior of the mental health providers I worked with was disappointing. They had a bias against the service member, lacked empathy and compassion, and were focused on pushing him out of the Navy.

During my internship at National Naval Medical Center in Bethesda, Maryland, every day I would get up early and arrive at the hospital by 5 or 6 a.m. for clinical rounds. I would walk by a bronze statue of a Navy corpsman carrying a wounded marine in the hospital's lobby. The statue was located in front of a backdrop of fifty flags, one for each state. The display was entitled "The Unspoken Bond" and was set during WWII in the Pacific. Walking by the statue of the marine and the corpsman every morning was inspirational. I'm sure, in combat, the bond between them was sacred and unbreakable, but it wasn't like that in the Navy's mental health system. One of the most disappointing things about the situation was how the Navy treated their own. One of the reasons I decided to pursue a legal complaint was the way they treated the sailor in the case, which captured the way the members in my directorate treated other sailors under their care.

I suffered injustice. I spent money on attorney's fees. I lost sleep and suffered from anxiety, especially around the annual performance review season. I have trouble trusting people. I heard far worse from my patients and am thankful I didn't have to go through what they did.

The closest thing I ever got to justice occurred when my lawyer threatened the hospital commander and attorney. It accurately addressed the situation and was one-hundred-percent justified. I never saw someone communicate with a commander like that in my entire career and just about fell out of my chair after experiencing it.

To the master chief of the Navy who spoke about issues with recruiting and retention of mental health providers, I would say how we are treated and valued by the organization is a huge issue. Two of the mental health providers who wrote me letters of support left the Navy because of how they were treated. A third retired when he hit twenty years instead of staying for another tour. As a result of this situation, I also changed assignments. How we were treated resulted in a net loss of four mental health providers.

I learned that testifying in a legal proceeding is protected speech. That was the time I became a whistleblower.

CHAPTER 22

Veterans Affairs

SERVING WITH THE NAVY a second time took its toll on me. The issues from the Navy's mental health system, fallout from the legal case I was involved in, and the suicide clusters contributed to a feeling of burnout. I was offered a position at a VA medical center and decided to take the plunge.

I was pleasantly surprised by the Veterans Affairs health system and felt immediate relief. The senior psychiatrist who ran the mental health and behavioral health service line had decades of experience in the VA health system and at the facility. She had worked in every program, was stable, and knew what she was doing. At the VA medical center, most of the leadership roles were held by seasoned, experienced federal employees. Most had been at the facility or working at the Veterans Affairs medical center for years. They were more stable and mature, having this type of leadership in place was a relief, and it improved patient care and business flow and protected against burnout.

At Veterans Affairs, I felt less pressure and no longer felt I had to defend myself constantly. Nobody was saying "How will this make us look?" Nobody was pressuring me on what to diagnose, not to diagnose, and the implications of certain diagnoses. On the contrary, patients would be discharged from the Navy and start receiving care at the Veterans Affairs medical center. Their diagnoses were updated, and the patients felt relief.

When I served at Naval Medical Center Portsmouth, I advocated for the use of Microsoft Teams and other information technology to improve operations, but I hit a brick wall. It contributed to burnout knowing we readily had access to technological solutions that could improve care we weren't permitted to access. Much to my surprise, Veterans Affairs had fully implemented Teams. Everyone used Teams instant messaging to communicate throughout the day, and it was more effective and efficient. There were far fewer back-and-forth emails. Meetings inside the Navy's mental health system were few and far between. At the Veterans Affairs medical center, every morning we had a fifteen-minute online Teams huddle that got our team on the same page and set us up for success. A big issue in the military system was long wait times at the pharmacy. The VA pharmacy had a mail option that solved this. At the end of each session, I could click an option to have prescriptions mailed or picked up at the pharmacy window.

Veterans Affairs had a fully functional telehealth platform called VA Video Connect that was used to communicate with patients via electronic video feed. Perhaps it worked too well, and there were issues. Once and a while, I would join a session and a veteran would be driving. If a veteran was driving, I would ask them to pull over for safety reasons. A variation on that would be if the veteran was a passenger in a moving vehicle. There were a few occasions where I spoke to veterans who were in bed and just waking up. As a mental health provider, I wanted to meet people where they were at, but talking to them in bed went too far. One day I joined a video session, and a veteran was at a car dealership; another time a veteran was being seated at a restaurant. Once, I was talking to a veteran on video. There was lag, and communications were garbled. It turned out, he was in Italy on vacation. This left me wondering if I could even legally provide medical care across international lines, including prescribing medication. On occasion it was challenging and frustrating to receive the veteran's undivided attention. It went the other way too. Once, a patient complained that their provider was at the beach during a session. Apparently, the virtual screen background stopped working during the appointment.

Veterans Affairs had another program the DoD did not, and that was peer support. The Veterans Affairs medical center had an active and well-managed peer support program. It was a group of veterans that met weekly and engaged in social activities together. I could write a medical consult for the peer support program, and a peer support specialist would reach out to the veteran, provide intervention, and encourage participation in the program. When I served with the Marine Corps, some of the best results occurred when the marines kicked the doctors, chaplains, and everyone else out of the room and worked on issues themselves. The VA peer support program was similar. When veterans had issues, often peer support specialists facilitated the process of veterans assisting and learning from each other.

Working at Veterans Affairs felt like working on a team of professionals helping veterans navigate out of deep, dark holes. I prescribed medications, a therapist helped them face their demons, the peer support program helped them reconnect and find camaraderie, the social worker helped find housing, and the vocational rehabilitation team assisted with employment issues. By addressing these issues simultaneously, our team was able to help veterans successfully climb out of "the hole."

I ran into a former Navy SARP counselor who also made the transition to the Veterans Affairs medical center. SARP had three full-time counselors who managed the treatment groups for the residential treatment program. At one point, I maintained a list of all the Naval Medical Center Portsmouth SARP counselors who left the facility during the time I served. I lost the list, but somewhere between three to six SARP counselors left the facility in a short period of time. That was over 100 percent turnover. We reflected on our time there and both felt relief. We discussed that the Navy had a mission-oriented mental health model, while Veterans Affairs had a recovery-oriented mental health model. We both felt the model employed by Veterans Affairs was more effective and resulted in an environment that was better for providers and patients.

At this point in my career, I was retirement-eligible, with twenty years of uniformed service. The focus of my career had been on providing care to younger, healthier active-duty service members. Now I found myself working with veterans, an older patient population I had little experience with. The assignment at VA was a godsend and a healing experience for me.

The patients at Veterans Affairs described how their experiences on active duty impacted them. They offered so much collective wisdom that I had to write it down to pass it on to younger active-duty service members and others involved in the care of veterans.

I spoke to a veteran who suffered the effects of a wrongful diagnosis. He was a seventy-year-old Army veteran who served in the 1970s to early '80s. He had been in the Veterans Affairs Health System for three decades. I read his first mental health note in the system. It documented that he was suffering from depression due to being treated unfairly and having been discharged due to no fault of his own. This soldier was talking to me about something that happened decades ago, and there were tears in his eyes like it happened yesterday. He said he wanted to make a career out of the Army, had been a good soldier for thirteen years, but had been diagnosed with a false personality disorder diagnosis. He felt the discharge resulted from racism. He was African American, had been promoted to E6, and felt his chain of command was dissatisfied that he was promoted and took it out on him. He recalled being told by a senior noncommissioned officer that the first time he stepped out of line, he was going to get him. He described a situation where a soldier didn't put oil in a vehicle, blew the engine, and was threatened with Army regulation 38-750 to pay for the vehicle. It was impressive that this soldier remembered specific Army regulations decades later. He received an Article 15 for missing formation. The patient felt that what happened to him was injustice, he suffered a psychological injury, he felt depressed, and he had a suicide attempt. He was accused of malingering, diagnosed with personality disorder, and processed out of the Army. I reviewed decades worth of mental health records in the Veterans Affairs electronic medical records system. I told him I couldn't find a single record that documented a personality disorder diagnosis and hoped it would give him some peace. By the way, the electronic medical records system I utilized to review the records, CPRS, is really that old. It is the exact same electronic medical records system I used when I was a third-year medical student during my rotations at the John Cochran VA Medical Center in St. Louis, Missouri, around 1998–1999.

There was a similar case of a Navy veteran in his late fifties who came to see me. He had a job, was high functioning, but struggled with anxiety. He served in the Navy from roughly 1980–2000. He complained shipboard life was toxic and he felt traumatized by bad leadership. He complained that he was harassed and threatened by leadership who said they would send his family back to the States while serving overseas. He witnessed other service members having suicide attempts due to the same behaviors. He felt stuck at E6 and psychologically injured by what happened, to this day. He takes medications for anxiety. He has just started to open up and discuss with a therapist what happened.

I talked with a thirty-nine-year-old Army vet who experienced stigma. He served on three deployments and struggled with a mass casualty situation that occurred on Christmas, 2004, in Baghdad, Iraq. He said he would never get help because "You are a bitch" for doing so." He complained that he became more and more socially isolated the higher the rank he went. He was working on his issues through the Veterans Affairs health system.

I spoke with service members who minimized and were

dishonest about their mental health and substance abuse history to join the military. I had never spoken with a service member who lied about their age. One day I joined a video call, and a Navy vet, age ninety-seven, was in the final hours of his life, in hospice with his family. His daughter discussed how he suffered from shell shock due to combat in WWII when his ship was pursued and attacked by Japanese ships. His daughter said their main concern was that his VA tombstone would be corrected. She explained that he had used an inaccurate birthday to join the Navy at age fifteen and wanted help to get his records corrected to reflect his actual birthday. I was able to connect them to the right place, and the issue was addressed.

A fifty-six-year-old Air Force veteran explained it to me. He said an idle mind was the devil's workshop. He talked about how not working and feeling underutilized negatively impacted his mental health. It was true. When I served at the Navy SARP program, many service members shared with me that a contributing factor for their unhealthy substance use was boredom, a lack of goals, and a sense of directionlessness. Additionally, many veterans discussed with me about how unemployment and a lack of purpose affect their mental well-being.

A seventy-seven-year-old Air Force veteran who served as an aircraft mechanic from 1966–1992 suffered from a "multitude of physical health problems." These included falls, a back injury, peripheral neuropathy, and diabetes. He received in-home care from the VA, including nursing, physical therapy, and occupational therapy. He was barely able to maintain independent functioning. Despite this, he was pleasant and still enjoying life. When asked what his secret was, he said it was to have the mindset not to worry about the things he couldn't control. The patients I worked with at Veterans Affairs who did the best had that exact mindset.

I spoke to a female Navy veteran, who had served in the Navy for ten years, in the late 1990s and early 2000s, on the twentieth anniversary of her trauma. She discussed how her ship was conducting drug operations with the Coast Guard in Ecuador, South America. She explained how $60 million worth of cocaine was seized in a drug bust. While in port, she got out of a taxi, and a car came flying down the road, hit her intentionally, and dragged her eighty feet. She was left for dead. She recalled locals chanting, "We got one." She felt it was attempted murder and retaliation for the drug bust. She recalled having a near leg amputation, discussed the medical care she received, and recounted the long recovery journey she made. She suffered from PTSD and traumatic brain injury. We discussed how the twentieth anniversary of her trauma was a monumental event. She said she was a role model to herself and her children. She reflected on the progress she made. She was a hero: strong, resilient, and a survivor. She thrived in her recovery. She achieved a good job, had a successful marriage with four children, and had grandkids.

A Vietnam veteran, age seventy-seven, came to see me for continued care of PTSD. He told me about his service in Vietnam during the late 1960s. He told me about a situation where a fuel and ammo dump were hit by the Vietcong. To this day, he lives near a military base, and when he hears jet and helicopter noise, he gets startled and feels he is back in Vietnam some forty years later. He said his advice for other veterans and what helped him best was to find a group at the Veterans Affairs medical center, open up, talk, and just listen in a nonjudgmental way. Hearing other vets vent and talk about their trauma and situations helped him best. He said, "Don't go it alone," and "Associate with people who are positive and good." He said to "stay away from alcoholics and drug fiends."

An Army veteran, age seventy-two, who served in the late 1960s, suffered from depression, PTSD, two bouts of colon cancer, chronic pain, and chronic obstructive pulmonary disease and was on oxygen. He suffered from the loss of his wife and son over a decade ago. He explained that he almost died multiple times from a car accident, his physical health problems, and by his own hand. When I spoke to him, he achieved remission of his symptoms. He said his secret was to go with the flow. He said having a sense of humor, having a positive perspective, and religion helped. He said there was no use crying over things you can't change. With a bright smile on his face, he said, "I'm so goddamn needy. God doesn't want me, and the devil is scared of me, so I'm stuck here." He explained that the prayer about God helping him understand the things he can change, the things he can't, and to help him let go assisted him.

I discussed the struggles of the Navy nukes throughout the book. A fifty-nine-year-old Navy veteran told me about his service aboard the *USS Orion*, a surface ship, called a submarine tender, that supplied and supported submarines. His opinion was that submariners eat themselves alive. I spoke to a Navy nuclear power veteran who struggled with mental health issues while on active duty, avoided seeking help, then went to Veterans Affairs for care. He was able to successfully deal with his issues. He continued in the nuclear power field. He completed his education, received a significant salary increase, and felt at peace.

I spoke to another WWII Army veteran at the Veterans Affairs medical center. He sat in a wheelchair with a bright smile. His daughter was with him for the appointment. He talked about being the last soldier to survive after his infantry company was wiped out. He told me he felt blessed. He said his secret to life was "to be happy, think happy." He talked about disability and physical health issues, including heart failure, diabetes, arthritis, and other problems. He said he learned to laugh to cope with his issues.

One day I was walking to lunch with my team's nurse. All of the sudden, a veteran walked up to us. He asked if I remembered who he was. Then he explained that I provided mental health care for him at the naval hospital. He told me I was a positive influence on his life and thanked me. He was disappointed about how his relationship with the Navy ended, but he found a good job and was doing well. It was rewarding to hear from veterans who were successful in moving forward and to receive a little positive affirmation in the process.

CHAPTER 23

Future Reforms

I'VE HAD THE unique opportunity and privilege to reflect on service across the Navy, Marine Corps, Air Force, Coast Guard, and Veterans Affairs. I listened to the voices of tens of thousands of service members and veterans. I considered the wisdom of military mental health colleagues I served with. I reflected on the issues I experienced across my career. In every review or discussion of military mental health, one of the top recommendations is to increase recruiting and retention of mental health providers. That is, of course, an important issue, but it's my belief that the issues with recruiting and retention are a secondary issue.

To evolve the mental health system to the next level, the issues raised in this book must be addressed. Utilizing a unified, whole-military approach to addressing mental health issues, delivery of mental health services, and fixing the underlying problems will make a stronger, more cohesive force. Here are recommendations for reform.

Create a Safe Channel for Mental Health

The situation exists where service members with significant mental health and substance abuse conditions are closeted. There are successful veterans who have come forward after they left military service, disclosed their issues, got help, and explained why they never asked for help while serving on active duty. The negative consequences for getting help include disqualification, career loss, and ostracism. These are a deterrent for getting help. Just like the general I mentioned in an earlier chapter who told the marines to be careful about getting help, many service members and their families don't trust the system and would never ask for help unless it was a last resort. The negative consequences experienced by those who seek help are real and have a ripple effect. Every time a service member experiences a negative impact, it is witnessed by other service members, and this discourages others from getting help.

There are several key issues that need to be addressed in policy to achieve the goal of creating a safe channel for mental health. First, involvement with command needs to be positive and supportive. Second, mental health providers should not be involved in actions that would be perceived as creating negative consequences for getting help. Finally, there needs to be stronger policy protection to reduce the consequences of suffering from mental health issues and participating in help-seeking behavior.

Positive Command Involvement

The best outcomes I observed for military mental health, especially high-risk situations, occurred when communication between commands, service members, and mental health providers was positive, supportive, nonjudgmental, and focused on reducing distress and risk levels. It was important for the right person at the command to be involved in the communication, including a senior O5 or O6 officer and senior enlisted who have the power to make changes if needed. There were times when mental health providers spoke to a junior officer or noncommissioned officer, and it wasn't productive. The command must be willing to listen to service members' concerns, be invested in their success, and make reasonable accommodations, including reassigning workspaces and changing shifts. When communication was negative, confrontational, dismissive, or with the wrong person, involvement from command went south and made situations worse.

DoDI 6490.08, Command Notification Requirements to Dispel Stigma in Providing Mental Health Care to Service Members, was referred to as the core instruction for the DoD's mental health system. It contained language about command notification, but in the field, communication was effective when it was positive and collaborative in nature. A good starting point would be to update DoDI 6490.08. The instruction should be renamed to "Command Collaboration and Positive Involvement in Providing Mental Health and Substance Abuse Care to Assist Service Members and Dispel Stigma." Updating this instruction to specify that interactions between command and mental health providers must be collaborative, supportive, and positive is recommended.

The Standards for Victim Assistance Services in the Military Community instruction, DoDI 6400.07, contains language prohibiting blaming, condemning past behavior, or making judgmental sentiments. It further directed that victims are to be respected, personal feelings would be distinguished from professional responses, and individuals were to be empowered rather than rescued. Similar language should be included in an updated DoDI 6490.08 to broaden the protection to mental health and substance use disorders. A service member complaining of suicidal thoughts should be offered the same protections. They should not be ostracized, judged, punished, or charged with malingering.

The best practice I observed concerning command involvement was the Air Force high interest list command meeting. After an airman was designated high risk by a mental health provider, a face-to-face meeting was conducted with the senior O5/O6 commander, senior enlisted, service member, mental health provider, and family members within a one-week time frame. This requirement should be in DoD policy.

Mental Health Providers Should not be Involved in Actions that Increase Stigma

A mental health provider-initiated discharge occurred when a service member presented to mental health and was recommended for discharge. The Navy's mental health system was notorious for identifying problems and facilitating discharges. Sometimes the mental health provider felt that they were doing what was in the best interests of the service member, but at other times the focus was on the needs of the military. Sometimes service members agreed with release from military service, but other times they did not.

Often, things went well in the military mental health system, and service members received appropriate care. At other times, things did not go so well. A colleague described some observations about a military inpatient psychiatry unit:

> *The inpatient psychiatry unit is currently the borderline personality disorder diagnosis team. Just about everyone on inpatient gets a borderline diagnosis. It seems to be the diagnosis of the day. Anyone needing inpatient behavioral health will look like a borderline owing to their distress. You can't diagnose it until you have had time to explore their history. Just reviewed a case of a service member sexually assaulted on deployment. No mention of the sexual assault program or offering to option. The notes say she is borderline personality with a recommendation to administratively separate.*

He also described one of the senior psychologists: She was "unethical, making rapid assumptions about patients, assuming diagnoses based on command's desire to administrative separate. She wants to please commands rather than protect patients."

A colleague shared an observation about Navy operational mental health providers: "Embedded psych seems to work for the command rather than the patient. I've found a lot of missed diagnoses and jumps to personality disorder are the standard diagnosis."

The struggle with bias regarding mental health diagnosing was real. There were many mental health professionals there to help, but I experienced and received accounts of others who focused on diagnosing personality disorder, malingering, and discharging patients. Many did not have the ability to put aside bias or harsh feelings toward patients.

There are occasions where mental health provider-initiated administrative discharges are helpful. An example of this is a service member with two years' time in service who should have never been allowed to join and clearly needs to be discharged. Unfortunately, by and large, mental health provider-initiated administrative discharges have been overused and abused. Regardless of the circumstances, service members witness mental health provider-initiated administrative discharges going wrong, and they are a negative public service announcement for why it's a bad idea to get help. It perpetuates the belief system that participating in mental health treatment will result in discharge. There's even a joke about military psychiatrists being wizards because they make service members disappear.

Clinical care should be focused on restoring service members to health. If a command feels that a mental health administrative separation is warranted, it should be done through the CDE process by an independent mental health provider. This process provides protection for the service member and delivers a wake-up call. I discussed how the Navy had effectively made wanting to quit a mental health disorder, as evidenced by a majority of separations resulting from mental health. If service members want to request early release from the military, a better way would be to submit a formal separation request to an authority outside of the command, as they have an inherent conflict of interest to prevent unplanned personnel losses. For the above reasons, I recommend that mental health provider-initiated administrative discharges be eliminated in DoD policy to reduce stigma and provide protection against misguided mental health providers.

Time after time, I witnessed service members suffer psychological injury after their military mental health provider colluded with the command regarding disciplinary, legal, and other negative personnel actions. They worked up their courage, opened up, discussed their painful issues, felt their mental health provider betrayed their trust, and were reluctant to ever participate in mental health treatment again. I was sitting in my office one day at Veterans Affairs and a forty-three-year-old Navy veteran came to talk to me. She was in tears as she described how she felt pushed out of the Navy via administrative discharge, how her mental health provider downplayed her PTSD and threw a wrench into the prosecution of her assailant. DoD policy should be revised to prohibit mental health providers from colluding with commands regarding negative personnel and legal actions, because these actions jeopardize trust with military mental health providers.

There are examples in this book about Navy mental health providers who participated in or were asked to participate in the prosecution of sailors under their care. There were limited protections regarding inclusion of mental health records in legal proceedings, but they didn't go far enough. The Manual for Courts-Martial, Rule 513, discusses the psychotherapist-patient privilege and limitations for use of mental health information in legal proceedings. The Air Force had the Limited Suicide Protection Program, where mental health records were given additional protection from utilization in disciplinary or legal actions. DoD policy needs to be updated to prohibit mental health providers from being involved in the prosecution of a patient under their care. DoD policy should go further in protecting service members' medical and mental health records from being utilized for prosecution.

I was at a Navy mental health conference in the early 2000s

during the time of "Don't Ask, Don't Tell." A Navy admiral, who was also a psychiatrist, said sailors who disclose homosexuality should be reported by their mental health providers. That would be unthinkable now, but it raises the point that there isn't clear guidance when a crime should be reported. Around the same time frame, I was reviewing an X-ray report, and a military radiologist documented in the findings section that a service member had a body piercing that violated military policy and reported this to the command for prosecution. Another situation occurred when a Navy senior chief with back pain, two years away from retirement, disclosed to a medical provider that he tried to self-treat with marijuana. He was reported and discharged. It was poor judgment on the part of the senior chief, but it didn't seem right. Policy needs to be clarified: Under what circumstances should a mental health provider conduct a notification to report a suspected crime or UCMJ violation?

Reduce the Consequences for Getting Help

There are real consequences for getting help, including disqualification and career loss. Some of it is common sense. If a service member cannot fly a plane, drive a vehicle, or arm up safely, they will be disqualified from their job. Disqualification protects the mission of the military and the service member. The balance was off in my experience. The organization tended to be risk-averse, and there were a lot of service members who were unnecessarily screened out and disqualified. When service members come through the door, the focus needs to be more on how they can be helped and strengthened. There needs to be less emphasis on whether they are fit, unfit, or need to quit.

While serving with the Air Force, I encountered an airman who was disqualified for overseas transfer because he had a diagnosis of insomnia and was taking sleeping medication. Disqualification wasn't as bad as participating in mental health treatment and being recommended for unwanted discharge, but unnecessary disqualification was another situation that resulted in the communication of a viral message: Why go to mental health and have documented mental health issues that could result in negative career implications? Duty status screenings taxed the mental health system. They ate up a lot of time and resources that could have been better utilized to directly assist service members.. Service members went through annual health screenings, and it would have been better to operate under a presumption that service members were fit for duty.

The Personnel Security Program instruction, DoDI 5200.02, contains great language: "No negative inference may be raised solely on the basis of mental health counseling." The sexual assault program instructions had service member protections that were off the scale compared to other instructions. If a victim was recommended for involuntary separation within one year of an unrestricted sexual assault case, they have an option to request a flag officer review. If a service member with mental health or substance abuse issues were to be under consideration for an involuntary negative personnel action, perhaps they could receive similar additional protections. In the Navy system, I witnessed flag officer reviews for mental health administrative separations. They were delegated to a mental health provider who conducted a chart review, and there were unanswered questions about their effectiveness.

Service members I worked with complained that unnecessary disqualifications amounted to discrimination. There were situations where removing a service member from work was the right decision, but often it wasn't and resulted in additional stress being added to service members, making their situations worse. There needs to be policy at the DoD level that broadens protections for service members struggling with these issues, to protect their duty status. What is needed is a comprehensive policy statement that service members who self-disclose significant mental health and substance abuse issues cannot face disqualification, job loss, denial of reenlistment, or other negative personnel actions solely due to these issues and that a CDE or independent fitness-for-duty evaluation is needed to provide protection. If a service member disagrees with a fitness-for-duty determination, they should have an option to request assessment by an independent evaluator.

Nerf Adjustment Disorder and Personality Disorder Discharges

The diagnoses of adjustment disorder and personality disorder have been overutilized and abused in the military, especially in the Navy's mental health system. This has negatively impacted readiness, increased stigma, and strained the relationship between service members and mental health providers.

There was a time in mental health when parents were blamed for their children's behaviors. It was said that the child had ADHD or some other problem due to bad parenting. Military personality disorder is a similar construct. The service member is blamed and considered to suffer from defects of character. It is a notion that the service member is flawed and incompatible with military service. Documenting that in a patient's chart was a career killer, and it negatively impacted the relationship between the helping professional and the service member. No gaining command would agree to accept a service member with that diagnosis. Far too soon and too often, in a patient's care, providers hit the easy switch with a diagnosis of personality disorder.

A doctorate-level psychologist confided in me that she would review the notes of her patients who were scheduled for the next day during her downtime. She would see a diagnosis of borderline personality, and this would cause her anxiety, dread, and apprehension prior to the visit, clouding her judgment and treatment recommendations.

Military personality disorder was a way for military mental

health providers to document someone who was incompatible with military service and facilitate their discharge. The diagnosis of personality disorder did more harm than good, on many different levels. Service members were fearful that they would receive a label and be recommended for discharge if they asked for help.

I'm told that the Army has a best practice in this area, and mental health providers diagnose personality disorder less frequently.

Adjustment disorder is temporary mental health symptoms that are associated with transient stresses. Any situation in military mental health can be described within the framework of an adjustment disorder because the only constant thing about military life is change.

The recommendation is to continue to reduce adjustment disorder and personality discharges. The Air Force had a best practice of utilizing a CDE to facilitate a personality disorder discharge. I would update adjustment disorder to limit administrative personnel actions to service members in boot camp, A School, C School, or within the first two years of military service.

Mental health provider-initiated administrative discharges cause more harm than good. There are better ways to deal with difficult people and facilitate their release from military service. If someone is failing at their job, they should be dealt with by personnel actions and be separated. A mental health provider is not needed to make that happen.

Separate Teams for Disability Evaluations and Clinical Care

Veterans Affairs has a dedicated team of mental health professionals who conduct specialized disability evaluations in the C&P branch. They receive training in conducting these evaluations. They have a dedicated schedule, with time carved out to solely focus on completing this mission. The C&P mental health professionals are in a better position to take a step back and conduct an independent, comprehensive, and longitudinal assessment of a veteran to achieve a deeper understanding. This practice frees up the remaining mental health providers to solely focus on clinical care to restore veterans to health. I experienced this as an effective best practice that reduced provider burnout and improved relationships with patients. I was told by a psychiatrist at Walter Reed National Military Medical Center, there was a similar best practice. Medical providers in the medical boards office author the narrative summaries instead of the treating providers.

Military mental health providers were constantly pulled between different tasks. At Naval Medical Center Portsmouth, we were doing it all—the clinical care, disability evaluations, and limited duty, and it was difficult to find time to get it all done. We were pressured from above and below by the command and service members regarding the outcomes of fitness-for-duty and disability determinations. When my patients disagreed with what I wrote in a medical board, it impacted our relationship and diminished my ability to assist them.

The quality and content of military fitness-for-duty and disability evaluations varied considerably. They varied depending on the service branch, from place to place, and from provider to provider. I reviewed a mental health fitness-for-duty evaluation on a service member with a severe medical condition like cancer. He was documented as being unable to perform the duties of his rate but "fit for duty from a mental health perspective."

Creating a separate lane for these evaluations and standardizing them would improve their quality and reliability.

Consolidate Policies into a Unified, Whole-Military Approach

There are too many policies pertaining to mental health and substance abuse, and they are fragmented. The number of policies in and of itself presents a challenge for any individual to fully understand and master. I reviewed an effort to inventory military mental health policies. There were 281 total policies documented on a spreadsheet. There were thirty-two DoD, eleven DHA, ninety-five Army, sixty-three Air Force, seventy Navy, and sixteen Marine Corps policies. The spreadsheet contained numerous columns documenting different policy aspects. The reviewers attempted to conduct a crosswalk of all the policies, but it was an impossible task.

I reviewed dozens of DoD policies and identified approximately 100 acronyms for this book. I utilized more on a day-to-day basis, and it was acronym soup. The number of policies and acronyms is overwhelming. The policies overlap in some areas and contradict each other in other areas. There are also a significant number of unaddressed policy gaps. Some of the feedback I received for this book concerned the nuances between the services, including how the Army does this better or how the Air Force does that better. Every service member should be treated in a similar way and afforded the same protections regardless of service. The result of not having the mental health system standardized is confusion, chaos, and a fragmented system that contributes to stigma and provider burnout. Policies regarding mental health, substance abuse, family advocacy, and sexual assault should be in alignment, offer similar protections, and form the backbone of a unified, whole-military approach that is standardized across services.

Set Clear Standards for Duty Status, Screenings, and Statute of Limitations for Prior Issues

When are service members placed on limited duty or on a profile? When are they referred for medical board? When are service or family members disqualified from different statuses, such as overseas duty? These issues are interpreted differently between services. Without this clearly being spelled out, the fate of service members is left in the hands of individual provider judgment calls. It isn't fair to the service member if they are told they are fit for duty but refused by the gaining command.

During any screening process, there needs to be a statute of limitations for prior behavioral health episodes. If a service member had a mental health encounter three years ago and was diagnosed with "borderline personality disorder" but hasn't had any behavioral health episodes or emergency room visits since, that is a good prognostic factor, and the diagnosis is likely inaccurate. The same would apply for substance use disorders. If a service member had a DUI five years ago and had a relapse, would the clock start over for treatment and relapse from a policy perspective, or would that be considered a treatment failure? If a service member stops drinking and successfully completes treatment, it doesn't make sense to disqualify them on the basis of a substance issue that has stabilized.

When service members are impacted by seemingly subjective decision-making that is inconsistent, the process feels unfair, and stigma results. When these situations happen, they reinforce the message that seeking help and having documented mental health issues negatively impacts one's career. I served in a Tri-Service area where there were Navy bases, an Air Force base, and an Army base. There were also Coast Guard bases. The DoD needs to update policy to standardize duty status across services to improve care, reduce confusion, and provide seamless care between medical facilities across different services.

Standardize and Franchise Mental Health Operations Across Sites

It was interesting serving with the different military branches. Mental health and substance abuse issues were universal conditions. Each agency and service had different approaches to managing them, including different sets of terminology and processes. The DoD and DHA would benefit from a clear vision, direction, and whole-military strategy for military mental health. Mental health clinics would optimally be run like a business franchise, with distinct geographic locations operating the same way, with similar staffing footprints, and delivering the same services using the same playbook. There would be regional and local practice managers who would track productivity and issues at each location and work issues as they arise. The quality and services rendered would be identical and subject to quality checks and inspections regardless of location. If a service member receives a mental health appointment on a Navy base and has follow-up a month later on an Army base, the care would be seamless.

How service members at increased risk are identified and managed needs to be done the same way across sites. Veterans Affairs had a best practice of using high-risk suicide prevention teams. This was a cell of mental health providers who would independently track and provide intervention for veterans who were designated at increased risk. They would assist veterans who might have otherwise slipped through the cracks and acted as a liaison between the treating mental health providers and other services. The DoD would benefit from suicide prevention teams at regional levels or national levels to track high-risk service members across sites.

Procedures for what happens when a service member no-shows an appointment, drops out of treatment, or transfers to a new base needs to be clearly defined. The Air Force had best practices in this area. If an airman was designated increased risk and no-showed an appointment, the mental health clinic would contact a senior O5/O6 at the command to do a welfare check and ensure the service members' needs were being met. The Air Force also scrubbed the records, identified service members who had not come into the clinic in a few months, and contacted them to make sure they hadn't slipped through the cracks.

How clinical information is documented would benefit from a standardized clinical documentation template that is used across all services. All clinics should use the same integrated electronic information systems to address the closed system and data fragmentation issues. It is important to note that there has been progress in this area. The military is implementing the MHS Genesis system to improve electronic medical records and provide integration with Veterans Affairs. The BHDP is used across services in the military's mental health system and has provided a way for clinicians to track mental health symptoms using measurement-based care.

Appointment standards, provider templates, and workload need to be standardized and spelled out with sufficient granularity. The roles and responsibilities of the personnel involved need to be spelled out. On many occasions, I witnessed situations where personnel pushed back when asked to perform certain tasks, saying it was not in their job description or within their scope of practice. When I served with the Navy's SARP program at Naval Medical Center Portsmouth, the Navy decreased the number of active-duty substance abuse counselors. Historically, the nonuniformed substance abuse counselors worked days but were directed to begin working nights. They were furious. Many quit, and those who remained fought the command tooth and nail on this. There needed to be a better game plan for who was doing what.

DoD policy should smooth and spell out the transition from inpatient to outpatient. The Army had great best practices in this area. A Friday or weekend discharge from the inpatient unit increased risk and was discouraged. The Army recommended Monday discharges, and soldiers received a face-to-face outpatient follow-up within a week. I would recommend it be written into DoD policy that service members are required to have a face-to-face follow-up one week after inpatient discharge and that group therapy appointments are not a substitute. Friday or weekend discharges should be discouraged in DoD policy. Policy should also direct meaningful collaboration and coordination with the command prior to discharge.

Similar standardization and uniformity should apply to substance abuse treatment programs. How they are staffed and operated needs to be clearly defined. Time targets, including the number of days after an incident to referral and the number of days after diagnosis to treatment start date, need to be specified. What constitutes a treatment failure needs to be more clearly defined.

The roles and responsibilities for embedded behavioral health providers need to be spelled out and standardized, including what they can and cannot do. I've been told that the Army does a great job of this. The rules of engagement between operational mental health providers and the clinic-based mental health providers need to be clarified and ironed out.

Overall, the DoD needs a better playbook and franchise system for how mental health operates.

Improve Integration and Crosstalk of Helping Services

In my job as a military psychiatrist, there were numerous programs that were stovepiped. We had ten or more information systems that didn't talk to each other. I had patients with complicated problems that crossed different realms. Consider a patient with severe marital problems, depression with suicidal thoughts, and alcoholism. It would have been optimal to see in real time what issues and services the substance abuse treatment program and FAP were identifying and have meaningful care integration, coordination, and crosstalk, but this was elusive.

If a service member was struggling with PTSD, alcoholism, and severe marital problems and had a child with special needs, they would benefit from a deep set of services with a team-based approach to address these issues simultaneously. Such a service member would benefit from therapy, medications for PTSD, treatment for alcoholism, marital counseling, and EFMP simultaneously, in a coordinated way, with meaningful communication between programs and professionals. A spouse or other family member would benefit from participating during family sessions in residential treatment for substance abuse. The

Marine Corps was famous for its combined-arms approach. The military mental health system could accomplish more if it was spelled out in policy about how mental health services were to work together, share information, and coordinate care with each service instead of acting independently of each other.

The idea of crosstalk between services fits into the notion of a scalable mental health system. The services directly provided to individuals have value, but so does the system of care. How services work, fit, and interact with each other has significant value. The rules of engagement need to be defined.

Reform of the Military Justice System

I participated in a captain's mast (Article 15 in the Air Force and Army) once in my career. That was in the early 2000s, and I will never forget it. The hospital deputy commander, Captain Matt Nathan, who went on to become the surgeon general of the Navy, presided over the proceedings. Strokes tend to happen in older adults around age seventy, but for some reason, a young sailor under my care in his early twenties had a hemorrhagic stroke. He described it as the worst headache of his life, just like what is written in medical textbooks. A hemorrhagic stroke has the potential to be lethal because internal bleeding inside the brain causes the brain to swell inside the skull, and there is nowhere for it to go. This sailor underwent a neurosurgical procedure where a coil was inserted into an artery in the brain to stop the bleeding. It worked; however, there was a complication, and he suffered an ischemic stroke where the blood supply was cut off to part of his brain. As I recall, he was staying in the hospital's behavioral care medical hold because he was having difficulty functioning and benefited from the extra support and structure the program offered. Some days, he didn't wear a uniform properly, or at all, and he was frequently stopped in the hospital hallways and confronted. He left the hospital to take leave but failed to fully complete the paperwork. He completed 90 percent of the process but didn't complete the final steps and, as a result, had taken an unauthorized absence. Anyone coming back from unauthorized absence was required to get a drug test, and his was positive for cannabis. As best we could tell, he only used it one time. The sailor was facing possible loss of his much needed Veterans Affairs benefits. I advocated for the sailor as best I could. It was a difficult case. The sailor understood right from wrong, was in control of his actions, but had difficulty with executive functioning, and it was hard to objectively quantify that. The hospital commander told the sailor he had to hold him accountable but was going to make some phone calls to make sure his Veterans Affairs benefits were not impacted.

At that time, I didn't feel that punishment and administrative discharge was the right answer. Years later, there has been recognition that mental health and substance abuse issues can be more effectively dealt with through justice diversion programs, where individuals receive treatment and support instead of punishment. A retired Navy captain told me the story of a peer who had a DUI while on active duty and was fired. He felt it mattered what was behind the DUI. He explained that, frequently, his peers turned to the bottle as a coping mechanism because they didn't feel comfortable asking for help and because help wasn't available. A thirty-nine-year-old Army veteran told me how she suffered two DUIs and was referred to a Veterans Treatment Court. She said the process saved her life. She learned how she was drinking to self-treat problems, how she was able to successfully address the root of her problems and achieved sustained remission of her drinking. The descriptions of sailors in the *USS George Washington* investigation reports suggested some committed disciplinary infractions and needed corrective action, but I was left feeling that there would have been better outcomes if a human being sat down with them and addressed underlying problems. Over the course of my career, I've witnessed numerous mental health and substance abuse situations where punishment and administrative discharge weren't the best answer, made problems worse, and increased suicide risk. A punishment approach where it isn't the right solution also increases stigma. The DoD should establish mental health and substance abuse diversion programs in policy and provide commanders better nonpunitive options for dealing with situations to improve outcomes.

A common theme I experienced working in the military's substance abuse and Family Advocacy Programs was that service members were terrified of getting in more trouble, and this hindered their participation in treatment. Frequently, there was an incident that resulted in the referral. The service members participated in treatment while their legal cases were unresolved. It was obvious that there was more that occurred, but service members were fearful to make disclosures. The DoD should provide protection so disclosures made during treatment cannot be used to expand or influence legal charges to assist service members in participating fully. Service members need protection so they can feel safe making disclosures and get the most out of treatment. Policy that prohibits mental health providers from participating in legal prosecution would assist with this as well.

In recent years, an independent prosecutor has been established for sexual assault cases. The command has inherent conflicts of interest and too much power. After an incident occurred, service members frequently told me they felt "railroaded," "piled on," or "dogged out" and found themselves in a cascade of negative personnel actions. They complained of no-win situations where they cannot move to a new duty station, reenlist, or do their job. The result was a feeling of injustice and increased risk of negative outcomes, including suicide. In my opinion, any action that could result in demotion, discharge, and career ruination should be vetted by an independent legal authority to add checks and balances. Such a legal authority could make independent judgments about maltreatment and other matters, such as issuance of MPOs.

An independent legal authority could function as a mental health and drug court and be better positioned to provide intervention for service members with such issues. A military mental health or drug treatment court could improve treatment completion rates and better define treatment failures. I observed discharge due to substance abuse treatment failure to be selectively enforced. There were service members who had numerous treatment failures, who remained on active duty, and others who were discharged at a much lower threshold. I wrote about the need for medications over objection for service members with severe mental illness, like what is done at nonmilitary psychiatric hospitals. A mental health and drug court could address this as well.

The DoD would benefit by establishing a justice diversion program, including a mental health and drug court in policy.

View All Substances the Same from a Policy Perspective

Substance abuse is a universal problem for everyone, everywhere, especially in the military. Across my career working in mental health, I talked to patients afflicted with alcoholism but also struggling with addiction from other drugs, such as pain pills, sedatives, and street drugs, including cocaine, heroin, and marijuana. From the perspective of a mental health provider, the problems are similar. The patient was taking a substance, often using it to self-treat mental health problems, it was having a negative impact on their life, and they had difficulty stopping.

People learn from their mistakes. A blanket zero-tolerance approach for substances other than alcohol is not the answer. The military has lost a lot of good service members due to zero tolerance. There are those who never got caught but self-referred, asking for assistance. There are service members who used illicit drugs, completed treatment successfully, and achieved remission. They would tell you they were stronger warriors and better human beings but were discharged. Consider a young service member in their late teens or early twenties who was immature and used cannabis a handful of times. If they were identified, they could receive brief education, advance their maturity level, and continue on in the military. On a rare occasion, I came across situations where service members didn't habitually use drugs but were desperate. They used illicit drugs one time, during a suicide attempt or to facilitate their discharge from the military.

A recommendation for the DoD would be to update substance abuse policies so all substances are treated the same and service members receive one strike, irrespective of the substance.

Changing the Culture of the Military

Every discussion ever written about military mental health recommends culture change to address issues. Updating organizational rules and standards will help, but ultimately, it needs to be organizationally and culturally okay to disclose problems and receive positive assistance addressing them. It must be culturally wrong to ostracize or make harsh judgments about service members who are struggling. If a service member can't function, instead of blame, there needs to be recognition, understanding, and a salvage pathway or a humane way to quit.

I learned a secret over my career: How people are treated and respected is a key factor and an intervention target for most cases. A lot of it boils down to the relationship a service member has with the chain of command and whether that person feels listened to, respected, and cared for. If service members feel valued, they will go above and beyond and bend over backward for people.

In 2022 a sailor was accused of igniting the *USS Bonhomme Richard* on fire. He was described as a young, arrogant sailor, angry about being assigned deck duty after failing to become a Navy SEAL (Watson 2022). He was accused of making the Navy pay in a big way but was later acquitted at trial. If the government's theory is correct, and he was disgruntled, it's possible the way he was treated contributed to a $3.2 billion expense.

If occupational demands are so high that it's breaking people, service members are fatigued because of their sleep schedule, there is maltreatment in the workplace, or the balance of self and service are off, those issues need to be addressed. The military could triple the number of mental health providers, and it won't fix workplace problems and personnel system issues. Negative work environment issues roll downhill, spread, and create a chain effect of negativity.

The military would benefit from a better sweet spot between not showing weakness, training hard, making the work environment more friendly, and making it culturally acceptable to get help. The "Mission First" mindset needs to include taking care of people, not just winning the battle. After all, part of the mission is recovering from the last fight and preparing for the next one.

Move Away from Zero Defect Mentality

Tradition is that a Navy captain who is in command of a ship when it runs aground is fired, along with the executive officer and command master chief. What happens to a military leader who fails and is relieved of command for "loss of confidence"? People learn, change, and evolve. Failure makes people better. There is a saying often in life: The test comes first, and the lessons come later. I met a Navy captain who was on a ship when it ran aground. His blood bled Navy blue. He was loyal and fully dedicated to the Navy. He learned a lot from the situation. There was an aspect to the situation of being treated unfairly, which made it an even more bitter pill to swallow. If he were permitted to sail again, there probably would be no better, more experienced individual than him. Instead, he found himself in a situation where his career was over two years prior to retirement, and he had no chance at career progression. I observed that the military had a cultural tradition of setting people up for failure and then punishing them when things didn't go well.

Diego Ugalde, a retired Navy SEAL, wrote in his book, *Leading from the Deep* (Ugalde 2023), "Most SEALs walk around with an invisible anvil hanging over their heads, feeling that leadership is willing and capable of ending a career over a perceived mistake."

I've observed that the military has high standards and an atmosphere where service members can't make a mistake. The pressure on service members to perform to a zero defect standard impacts their mental health. The promotion system is unforgiving. The stakes are high, and service members feel they are in do-or-die scenarios. Getting smashed with the career-ending anvil leaves a scar and impacts veterans even years after they leave the military.

Thomas E. Ricks wrote about a "swift relief" system in World War II where senior leaders failed, were removed, but were given second chances (Ricks 2012). They learned from their mistakes and redeemed themselves. Many went on to achieve promotion and had successful careers. He advocated that deviation from the relief system has contributed to leadership mediocrity in recent years. The military would benefit from looking at failure differently and developing salvage and recycling paths for service members.

Incentivizing Good Behavior, Health, and Readiness

The military was overly focused on negative reinforcement, including so-called good order, discipline, maintaining standards, taking corrective actions, crime, and punishment. There were familiar narratives heard over and over: "Punishment will ensue until morale improves."

Service members work hard to get the mission done. Either they accomplish it or hit a breaking point, "sad out," must be removed, or "med boarded." The system incentivizes the sick role.

The Army has a promotion point system that provides positive reinforcement. Soldiers who excel on the physical fitness test, achieve awards, or achieve educational goals and weapons qualifications can achieve promotion points. The military would benefit from restructuring the pay system to utilize positive reinforcement. Under such a system, service members could receive financial incentives for desired behaviors, including fitness for duty, physical fitness, and good behavior. If a service member was unable to perform their duties, didn't pass a physical fitness test, or got in trouble, their pay would be impacted. There is at least a small percentage of sailors at the limited duty commands who would have had increased motivation to recover and return to duty if there was fitness-for-duty pay and other financial incentives to do so.

At the medical center, having financial incentives for clinical productivity would have been a game changer. The mental health providers would have been motivated to produce more and see more patients.

There could be financial and other bonuses, such as promotion bonus points, for sustained positive behaviors. Leaders who received high marks on command climate surveys and subordinate evaluations could be rewarded with such bonuses. High performers need to be identified and rewarded.

Making It Easier to Quit

In discussing the issues in this book with mental health colleagues, it is apparent that a lot of issues come up because people start to spiral, feel trapped, and want to quit. People join the military for a variety of reasons. They want to better themselves, serve the country, escape problems at home, get a regular paycheck, get health benefits, and have a place to live. Some don't know what they want to do in life, and the military is a good starting point. It provides a structured environment with housing, insurance, and pay.

At a certain point, there is a percentage of service members who come to the realization that the military isn't for them regardless of the reason. Some of them realize they made a mistake joining. Maybe they don't like being away from home, their mind is somewhere else, their relationship is failing, they don't like the rules and regulations, they don't want to be on a ship or stationed overseas, or they don't like their rate.

As the Marine Corps general said, everyone reaches a point of quitting. Wanting to quit can be viewed as a personal preference, failure to adapt to military life, or poor coping. We can pull service members out of the environment, try to help them improve coping skills, and learn to think and behave better. Perhaps, from a broader perspective, it's simply just wanting to quit. The *USS George Washington* quality of life report documented that 99.7 percent of all recommended administrative separations of carrier sailors over the past five years were related to behavioral health issues. A sailor told me it's common knowledge that to quit, one needs to "say the magic words." She explained that if a sailor says, "I am suicidal," it could lead to their discharge from the Navy. Making wanting to quit a mental health issue is short-sighted. It taxes the mental health system and increases stigma. It contributes to a negative image of those who are struggling but want to remain on active duty. Quitting can be a good decision. If things aren't working out, it's best to cut losses and move on.

The military would benefit from an easier and more humane way out. It's a volunteer service. If someone doesn't want to serve, no one should stand in their way. Regarding the Ship, Shipmate, and Self code, wanting to quit isn't a betrayal, and it doesn't deserve retribution. It can be self-recognition, hitting a breaking point, or a needed change. Treating service members as quitters is short-sighted. It is not a good operational risk management strategy to hold someone hostage and trigger them to act out.

A lot of time and resources were invested in service members who wanted to quit or were not on a trajectory with continued military service. Forcing people to stay in against their will increased risk and was bad for the organization. I experienced situations where angry, bitter people impacted everyone else. I worked at an ICE detention center. The detainees would complete immigration paperwork, such as an I-589 form to request asylum, and they would be placed on the docket for a legal hearing for processing. I would recommend that the DoD eliminate mental health provider-initiated administrative discharges and establish a process where service members could request early release and have their case vetted by a panel or official outside the chain of command.

Maybe quitting isn't the answer. How about taking a career break or leave of absence? Service members could leave active duty, work in the private sector for a few years, and come back.

Rethinking Maltreatment and Intervention Strategies

The sexual assault program had some great best practices. They had a hotline to help service members, sexual assault representatives, peer victim advocates, and restricted and unrestricted reporting options. They had a database of perpetrators, called the CATCH program. The sexual assault program had special victim advocate attorneys to assist service members. The sexual assault program had an expedited transfer option, although it had its downsides. A female Marine Corps veteran, a victim of military sexual assault, told me she felt it was unfair that the perpetrator was allowed to remain in his position. She complained to me how she felt that an expedited transfer negatively impacted her career after the gaining command was less than supportive of her. She told me she successfully processed the assault, but what was really bothering her was how the command and Marine Corps treated her.

Across my career, I observed many different forms of maltreatment, including, but not limited to, domestic violence, verbal abuse, bullying, hazing, abuse of authority, harassment, discrimination, sexism, favoritism, retaliation, and reprisal. They all negatively impact service members and military readiness. I wondered if all the behaviors were interrelated and on a spectrum.

A recommendation would be to expand the sexual assault program services to other forms of maltreatment. A service member could report workplace violence, physical assault, harassment, or abuse of authority and have the claim investigated and prosecuted by an independent authority. Wouldn't it be interesting if five different service members at different commands all reported the same senior service member for bullying in the CATCH database? When I suffered retaliation and reprisal, I learned that other mental health providers had suffered similar issues and had even filed formal grievances against my chain of command. I would have benefited by having access to the victims' counsel. Instead, I had to hire my own attorney.

Implement Best Practices from Veterans Affairs and Others

The Department of Veterans Affairs had some great best practices, including a formal peer support program, high-risk suicide prevention team, virtual video appointments, the mailing of medication, and the utilization of Microsoft Teams. I encountered a couple other best practices across the services, including welfare checks and securing of firearms.

Implement a Formal Peer Support Program

When I served with the Navy and Marine Corps, I observed positive results when marines supported and assisted each other. The *USS George Washington* and MARMC reports documented issues with command involvement for sailors on limited duty. A formal peer support program would go a long way toward filling some of the hole, and Veterans Affairs has done exactly this. Veterans Affairs employed peer support specialists who facilitated group sessions and activities, where veterans were empowered to support and learn from each other. They were provided tools and a safe space to help each other out. The military, especially the Navy, would benefit from a formal peer support program like the one Veterans Affairs has implemented.

Veterans Affairs Video Connect

One of the big issues with the Coast Guard is it is a small service, with small bases dispersed across large geographic areas, where the cost of having a full-time on-site provider isn't justified. Using video technology, one mental health provider can provide regional coverage across sites and bases. Improved implementation of telehealth would improve access to services and efficiency. A centralized appointment call center could book unused virtual appointments for service members in need. A sailor in Virginia could receive a virtual appointment from Naval Medical Center San Diego if there was availability. I'm told the Army is already doing this in Europe, and the concept has broad applicability.

Mailed Prescriptions

When I write electronic prescriptions at Veterans Affairs, there is an option for window pickup or medication mailing. The practice of mailing medications was fast and convenient. Veterans were able to have appointments online and their prescriptions mailed to them. The practice of mailing medications helped the organization too. Veterans Affairs had a medication processing center where they were able to send out prescriptions across sites.

Suicide Prevention Teams

In my experience, the Air Force had a successful suicide prevention strategy. Airmen considered at increased risk were entered into an alpha roster that was distributed and tracked, resulting in an involuntary outpatient commitment-like situation. There were efforts in the Navy's mental health system to track and intervene on high-risk patients, but they didn't compare to what the Air Force or Veterans Affairs was doing. The Air Force system was effective but burdensome. The mental health providers in the Air Force clinic were tasked with seeing patients and running the suicide prevention program simultaneously, and it was challenging.

I mentioned previously how Veterans Affairs had a dedicated team of mental health providers that tracked and communicated with high-risk veterans to assist them. The Veterans Affairs approach of having a team of professionals with allocated time for this was more effective and protected the other mental health providers from burnout.

Securing Firearms

When service members were considered at increased risk, we would work with service members, commands, and others, including family and friends, to secure firearms. Sometimes firearms were secured by commands and placed into a base armory. I never saw a clear policy regarding securing firearms, and the DoD would benefit from this. The FAP instruction had language discussing securing firearms, and this could be a best practice for broader implementation. Previously, I suggested establishing a mental health and drug court in the military. In such a venue, service members could be legally mandated to secure firearms, and a mental health and drug court could collaborate with local law enforcement to make this happen.

Health and Wellness Checks

I wrote about the practice of in-home health and wellness checks. The practice was infrequent, but when it occurred—and commands were invested in a service member—it was very helpful. I described a situation where a command declined to go to a member's home to take him to the hospital. Local law enforcement was called, and their feedback was that the military should be conducting the wellness check. I never saw a clear DoD policy regarding this either. The DoD should establish and formalize health and wellness checks into policy.

Disability System Reform

We need a way to identify and prioritize high-risk cases to get them through the medical boards process faster. We had patients who were struggling with severe mental health disorders, including bipolar disorders and psychosis, who were noncompliant with meds. These cases had severe disability and no chance of return to duty. There were other cases where service members had recurrent suicide attempts and substance use relapses. The military environment was making their conditions worse. While the patients were waiting, their struggles worsened. They needed to be home, away from the military environment, to be near their support system, to recover optimally and begin their treatment in the Veterans Affairs medical system.

There are two separate systems for disability determination during the medical boards process, including a service determination and Veterans Affairs determination. I discussed several situations where the DoD and Veterans Affairs findings were not in alignment and the impact it had on service members. It isn't logical when the Navy finds someone fit for full duty and Veterans Affairs makes a finding of moderate to high levels of disability. I talked to a medical board reviewer for Veterans Affairs. He said the Navy is focused on whether to return a sailor to duty while the Veterans Affairs system assesses level of function by a professional who has received specialized training. He felt the system was ripe for reform.

I discussed how the system feels like it is engineered to increase disability and attrition. My experience was that the main driver for return to duty was high levels of internal motivation. Service members would benefit from financial and other incentives for recovery. Treatment compliance and the no-show rate would improve, with fees for missed appointments, like in the private sector. Another idea would be to designate a sizable portion of pay, approximately a third, as fitness-for-duty pay. Entering a limited-duty status would result in a loss of pay, and this would create financial incentives to return to a full-duty status.

360-Degree Performance Evaluations

There are a couple sayings about leadership that were passed on to me. The first is that leadership is a privilege. It felt like that was lost. Another saying is that there are two things that rise to the top—scum and cream. One never knows what will come up until it exposes itself. One way to rectify this is to make annual performance evaluations a two-way street. Subordinates would evaluate their leadership's performance. At promotion consideration time, each service member, including leaders, would have ratings from above and below. How military leaders are ranked by their subordinates would be racked and stacked against each other. Military leaders who are the cream—treating people fairly—would achieve faster career progression. The scum, with a bullying and abusive leadership style, would be forced to change their ways.

The chain of command has too much power. Just like the Stanford Prison experiment, unchecked power has led to maltreatment, abuse of authority, and negative impact on service members. A 360-degree performance evaluation would add balance to abusive power.

Strengthen Public and Private Sector Partnerships

The Military Health System has had successes with private sector partnerships. Medical professionals have had opportunities to train in the community to make up for lack of complicated cases, family members, and retirees. The Center for the Sustainment of Trauma and Readiness Skill (C-STARS) program embedded military surgeons in high-volume training centers, resulting in the improvement of expeditionary medical skills.

Personally and professionally, I have learned so much from jumping between agencies and services and serving with Veterans Affairs. There should be more opportunities for interservice career opportunities and collaboration in the military health system. The DoD health system would benefit greatly by establishing billets at

VA hospitals so medical professionals can learn more and broaden their clinical skill sets. The DoD would benefit from expanding the partnership with the Public Health Service to open to PHS officers outside of just mental health.

Elon Musk and NASA have done a great job with SpaceX. The Military Health System is up against difficult challenges, including the acquisition system and manpower issues. NASA alone was not able to achieve next generation space flight. Imagine if a successful large healthcare organization ran large military treatment facilities. NASA and SpaceX achieved this by working together in a private and public sector partnership. Such partnerships could take the Military Health System to the next level.

Education for Everyone at Every Level

When I served in the Navy, my colleagues and I developed a first aid- and CPR-like psychoeducational program called "Psychiatric First Aid" for marines and sailors. We developed a curriculum for service members, military leaders, and hospital corpsmen. We used flashcards that contained real-life vignettes to discuss mental health situations to assist service members in thinking about how such situations could be handled. Providing the training was a form of outreach and improved our relationships with service members and commands. We found, after we provided training, that our mental health referrals increased, and we were able to intervene in situations earlier, before they turned into crisis situations.

A retired Navy captain discussed his observations that military leadership often doesn't realize the impact their decisions have on service members. He explained that they don't realize the fires they create. He described a situation where a commanding officer of a ship decided not to give sailors a day off. When it was reviewed, it was determined that there was no requirement for a commanding officer to give service members a day off. There wasn't any consideration of how the decision would impact sailors' welfare. NBC published a story two years after the *USS George Washington* and MARMC suicide clusters, where the emails of those involved were reviewed (Chan 2024). One of the leaders was quoted as saying, "I myself, have an extremely limited understanding of mental health issues and have a very hard time understanding why." The military needs education and training about mental health issues for everyone, at every level, for prevention and training of what to do when situations occur.

Creating a Database Dashboard of Behavioral Indicators

For years, the idea of creating a meaningful behavioral health indicator dashboard has been discussed to provide senior leaders critical health intelligence data to assist in making informed decisions. Achieving this has been elusive. We need that Manhattan Project-like behavioral health database dashboard. We need a policy that defines what will be tracked, where the data will come from, who is responsible for pulling data, and how it will be put together.

Military Recruiting and Add a Feedback Loop

A professional colleague of mine worked at an Army Advanced Individual Training School in a mental health clinic. There was a small but significant percentage of soldiers who did not meet service entry standards that could have been screened out. Military recruiters are under pressure to make quotas, and it's an issue that needs to be looked at. From the perspective of a mental health provider, there is no feedback loop to the recruiter. There should be feedback, quality control, and accountability in some situations when service members are not screened optimally or are told "not to put it on paper." Service members deserve chances, but there were individuals that didn't meet standards of service and should have been screened out. Not dealing with these service members up front is setting them up for failure, kicking the problem down the road to operational units who are focused on the mission and burdening the system.

There are unanswered research questions regarding preservice screening. My colleagues and I observed that many service members who left the military suffered from preservice trauma, such as extensive childhood abuse or sexual assault. There were questions about whether these individuals would benefit from preservice screening and if prior service trauma would predict attrition from the military. Screening service members out and disqualifying them unnecessarily increases stigma and discourages members from seeking help. We need to use objective data to find a balance and drive decision-making.

Realigning Military Goals and Ambitions with Resources

A recurring theme I observed and was told about throughout my career, especially in the latter years, was that demands placed on service members were breaking them. I experienced this inside the military health system too. Increased operational requirements and the impact of the churn rate of personnel affected me, my family, professional colleagues, and service members under my care. I discussed that a senior operational mental health provider explained how increased operational demands led to a vicious cycle of increased mental health issues and unplanned personnel losses. If this is true, one possibility would be to reduce operational requirements. Another would be to increase the size of the military. Perhaps more of the burden of military service should be shared across more people, as seen in other countries, such as Israel, where military service is compulsory.

The WSJ editorial board published an opinion in Feb 2022, before the *USS George Washington* and MARMC suicide clusters, that the United States needed a bigger Navy (WSL Editorial Board 2022). The math is simple: With more sailors and ships, operational demands are shared across more people and resources.

Had the reforms suggested in this book been in place, I'm

confident there would have been better outcomes for the *USS George Washington* and MARMC situations. There would have been a mental health dashboard that would have shown an uptick in indicators to notify leaders about the problems before they went critical. Leadership would have been better educated about mental health, more invested, and more involved. There would have been better mentoring of junior service members. The issue of toxic leaders would have been addressed through the 360-degree evaluation process. Better protections would have been in place, and sailors would have felt more comfortable talking to Navy mental health providers. They would not have had to fear prosecution for malingering or being discharged. Revisions to limited duty and the medical boards processes would have helped sailors feel they were treated more fairly, get through the boards process faster, return home sooner, and reduce the pool of those on limited duty. Mental health provider burnout would have decreased, and retention would have been increased.

CHAPTER 24

Closing Thoughts

THE MILITARY'S MENTAL health system is ripe for reform. The same problems, especially stigma and negative consequences for getting help, have persisted for decades. Since 9/11, military suicides have been significantly higher than deaths in war operations. The military invests billions of dollars into service members and their families and achieves subpar results. Service members are disappointed because they experience difficult environments, have difficulty accessing care, and experience consequences for getting help. Military mental health providers are frustrated. We spend a lot of time caught in the crossfire, spinning our wheels, doing things that have questionable value, and trying to navigate broken systems. On the surface, the rhetoric is good. We are told that the DoD is "committed to fostering a culture that encourages help-seeking behavior and to dispel perceived stigma." The reality in the field and at the deck-plate level is otherwise. Efforts to address these problems have had limited success.

In page after page, I laid out how the military mental health system needs to be retooled. I provided examples, objective data, and references to back it up. I discussed how it impacted me, my patients, professional colleagues, and military readiness. A wise former mentor told me that output is the precise result of a finely tuned system. It feels like the system is engineered to make people sicker, worsen outcomes, and the military is shooting itself in the foot. Stigma exists and persists because there are consequences for getting help and having mental health issues in the military. Many have worked hard to advocate for and achieve policy revision, but continued efforts are needed to remove the consequences and establish greater protections for service members affected by these issues.

So much money is invested into military mental health and the issues discussed in this book, but there is a low return on investment. The military suicide rate is a great example of this. Service members have many positive protective factors against suicide. They go through a continuous, rigorous screening process. They are young, healthy, and physically fit. Service members have job security, housing, educational benefits, good access to care, health insurance, and extensive on-the-job training. They also have post-service benefits from Veterans Affairs. The military suicide rate is expected to be lower than the general population, but it is not.

The secret sauce of military mental health is how people are treated. The verbiage about reducing suicide is good, but then you read the horror stories in the news about how service members are treated. One of the reasons the trajectory never changes is because of this. If the issue of how service members are treated was addressed, the suicide rate would dip below the national average, but the system is never able to effectively address the underlying issues. A big tenet of emergency management and disaster recovery is taking care of the responders and preparing for the next disaster. The military needs to do a better job taking care of its people.

There are predictable, vulnerable pressure points frequently at the heart of mental health situations where stress is placed on service members. These situations include the performance evaluation system, promotion system, assignments process, medical screening process, and military justice system, especially when service members feel it is unfair. To really get at the problem, the military needs to find a way to make these pain points more bearable. We need a better balance between the individual service members' needs and the needs of the military.

Moving forward goes beyond taking morning personnel accountability, having a hotline people can call in a crisis, or giving them online training. It's revising policy to establish protections for confidentiality and prohibiting consequences for getting help. It is creating a safe channel where the military's strongest warriors can face their problems without judgment, without fear of losing their career, where they can get stronger. It's moving away from a zero defect mentality and establishing a positive environment where members can learn, recover from mistakes, and redeem themselves. It's finding a better balance between mission first and self. It's creating a framework, a system-based approach, including a modern information technology system where people can be tracked, including through periodic health screenings, and intervened on with meaningful crosstalk and care coordination.

The military would benefit from shifting its mindset from disability to health. I received feedback that people in the system are afraid to discuss disability reform because they don't want to be perceived as speaking out against veterans and heroes. The truth is, the current system is broken and incentivizes the sick role. Fitness for duty, good health, and good behavior need to be incentivized, reinforced, and rewarded. Approaching problems through a disciplinary lens, with a crime and punishment approach, has had limited success. We need to get away from the mindset that service members are broken or flawed and see failure and problems as stages of growth that make us stronger.

Suicide is a great example of a complex problem that is impacted by the confluence of numerous factors. Military suicide results when a service member feels they have no choice but to take themselves out. To successfully get at suicide, we need to improve the health of working environments, strengthen protections in policy to create safe channels where service members can feel comfortable getting help, and make sure help is available in a timely manner, both for intake and continued care. When service members hit a breaking point, there always needs to be a better option on the table than suicide.

We need to focus on the people we can help, but we also need to identify those who are not on a trajectory with continued military service, treat them humanely, and assist them in making a timely transition back to civilian life to set them up for future success.

We need to be realistic: We will never be able to eliminate mental health and substance abuse issues, but we must address the ones we can. By implementing the changes suggested, we can better address future problems, improve military readiness, and prepare for future combat and military operations.

As for me, I'm living in a golden age. Everything that happened to me took a toll and hurt, but I learned so much and have grown tremendously. I felt like a baseball player who kept stepping up to the plate. I kept striking out, getting hit by pitches, and flying out. Then, one day, I started making hits, home runs, then eventually hit a grand slam. The former acting surgeon general of the United States, Admiral Boris Lushniak, said PHS officers survive poor leadership, and I did exactly that. A big lesson I learned is that one has limited ability to fix broken systems. Another lesson, especially on a personal level, is you can't change others. Similarly, in both situations, time and energy is better spent moving in a positive direction.

I was told the Marine Corps OSCAR program I wrote about and served in, despite its struggles, expanded from the division to include the logistics group and wing. Instead of having a single team, there are now multiple teams for each MEF. My colleagues and I succeeded in advocating for mental health resources for the Marine Corps to be beefed up.

Regarding those who committed acts of retaliation and reprisal against me, I've chosen not to be bitter. I am happy I am not in their shoes. I'm confident the universe will deal with them. Like the guy told me at the soccer game, "Hate the game, not the player." A mentor in the PHS told me, when stuff rolls downhill, usually there are issues above impacting leadership. Rather than being bitter, I try to see things from a broader perspective and appreciate what others are facing. I'm sure those above me were feeling pressure and suffering too.

My relationship with my ex-wife has improved, and our kids are thriving. I remarried and have benefited from having a blended family. I have a new son, Robert Jr. I am a much better officer, doctor, father, spouse, and person because of my experiences. One of the things I enjoy best is that I learned how to help people recover from complex, seemingly impossible mental health issues. All this together empowered me and motivated me to write this book.

References

Associated Press. 2014. *US Navy approves changes for submariners' sleep schedules.* 21 Apr. https://www.foxnews.com/health/us-navy-approves-changes-for-submariners-sleep-schedules.

Bey, Douglas. 2006. *WIZARD 6 A Combat Psychiatrist in Vietnam.* College Station, TX: Texas A&M University Press.

Blickwedel, Ted. 2022. *Broken Promises.* San Diego, CA: ADZ Press.

Brennan, Thomas J. 2022. *Second Suicide Battalion: Where Military Justice Weaponizes Mental Health.* 15 April. https://thewarhorse.org/military-justice-system-weaponizes-service-members-mental-health/.

Castro, Carl A. 2017. "Research at the Tip of the Spear." In *Psychiatrists in Combat Mental Health Clinicians' Experiences in the War Zone,* by Cameron E Ritchie, Christopher H. Warner and Robert N. McClay, 99-107. Cham, Switzerland: Springer.

Caudle, D.L. 2023. *Investigation into Command Climate and Sailor Quality of Life Onboard the USS George Washington Inclusive of Systemic Challenges that Impact Carriers Undergoing Extensive Maintenance or Construction in Newport News.* Norfolk, VA: U.S. Navy Fleet Forces Command.

Caudle, D.L. 2022. *Investigation into Proximate Causes of, and Any Correlation Between, the Deaths of Three USS George Washington Sailors on or about April 2022.* Norfolk, Virginia: U.S. Navy Fleet Forces Command.

Chan, Melissa. 2024. *'Give them a verbal hug': Emails show how the Navy scrambled to manage a spate of suicides.* 16 April. https://www.nbcnews.com/news/us-news/give-verbal-hug-emails-show-navy-scrambled-manage-spate-suicides-rcna147206.

Cohen, Rachel S. 2022. *Military investigating possible 'dysfunction' at Texas medical center after colonel resigns.* 25 July. https://www.airforcetimes.com/news/your-air-force/2022/07/25/military-investigating-possible-dysfunction-at-texas-medical-center-after-colonel-resigns/.

Cordle, John P. 2023. *The Navy Must Double Down on Suicide Awareness and Prevention Programs.* September. https://www.usni.org/magazines/proceedings/2023/september/navy-must-double-down-suicide-awareness-and-prevention.

Davidson, Joe. 2018. *Public Health Service officers pay $25 for baggage fees and for no respect.* 2012 October. https://www.washingtonpost.com/politics/2018/10/12/public-health-service-officers-pay-no-respect/.

Department of Defense Task Force on Mental Health. 2007. *An Achievable Vision: Report of the Department of Defense Task Force on Mental Health.* Falls Church, VA: Defense Health Board.

DoD Inspector General. 2022. *Audit of Active Duty Service Member Alcohol Misuse Screening and Treatment.* Alexandria, VA: Office of Inspector General.

DoD Inspector General. 2023. *Concerns with Access to Care and Staffing Shortages in the Military Health System.* Alexandria, Virginia: Office of Inspector General.

DoD Inspector General. 2020. *Evaluation of Access to Mental Health Care in the Department of Defense.* Alexandria, VA: Office of Inspector General.

DoD Office of the Deputy Assistant Secretary of Defense for Military Community and Family Policy. 2019. *2019 Demographics Profile of the Military Community.* Washington, DoD: Office of the Deputy Assistant Secretary of Defense for Military Community and Family Policy.

DoD Under Secretary of Defense of Personnel and Readiness. 2022. *Annual Report on Suicide in the Military Calendar Year 2022.* Alexandria, VA: Defense Suicide Prevention Office.

Eyer, Kevin. 2016. *Charting a Course - How to Make Flag.* Jan. https://www.usni.org/magazines/proceedings/2016/january/charting-course-how-make-flag.

Faran, Michael, Albert Y Saito, Eileen U. Godinez, Wendi M Waits, Victoria W Olson, Christine, M Piper, Margaret A. McNulty, and Christopher G. Ivany. 2011. "Establishing an Integrated Behavioral Health System of Care at Schofield Barracks." In *Textbooks of Military Medicine Combat and Operational Behavioral Health*, by Martha K Lenhart, 563-576. Falls Church, VA: Office of the Surgeon General, Department of the Army.

Flory, Meredith. 2022. "How the Army Made Me Choose Between My Mental Health and Our Family's Dream Posting." *Military.com*. 17 May. https://www.military.com/daily-news/opinions/2022/05/17/how-army-made-me-choose-between-my-mental-health-and-our-familys-dream-posting.html.

Galinis, W. J. 2023. *Command Investigation into Causal or Contributing Factors in the Four Sailor Deaths Within 28 Days at Mid-Atlantic Regional Maintenance Center*. Washington Navy Yard, D.C.: U.S. Naval Sea Systems Command.

US Government Accountability Office. 2021. *Navy Readiness - Additional Efforts Are Needed to Manage Fatigue, Reduce Crewing Shortfalls, and Implement Training*. Washington, DC: Government Accountability Office.

Holt, Danielle B, Matthew T Hueman, Jonathan Jaffin, Michael Sanchez, Mark A Hamilton, Charles D Mabry, Jeffrey A Bailey, and Eric A Elster. 2021. "Clinical Readiness Program: Refocusing the Military Health System." *Military Medicine* 32-29.

J-9 Research and Development. 2019. *Management of Problematic Substance Use by DoD Personnel*. Falls Church, VA: Defense Health Agency.

Jacobs, Daniel. 2020. *There and Back Again Stories from a Combat Navy Corpsman*. Virginia Beach, VA: Koehlorbooks.

Jowers, Karen. 2018. "They sought help when their Army dad deployed. Now they're barred from joining the military." *MilitaryTimes*. 29 Mar. https://www.militarytimes.com/pay-benefits/military-benefits/health-care-benefits/2018/03/29/they-sought-help-when-their-army-dad-deployed-now-theyre-barred-from-joining-the-military/.

Kadet, Anne. 2022. *How Long Email Chains Can Make Us Frustrated - and Less Competent.* 12 Jun. https://www.wsj.com/articles/email-exchange-productivity-competence-11654784372.

Kellerman, Arthur L. 2023. *We Must Rebuild America's Military Health System-Before It's Too Late.* 14 March. https://www.healthaffairs.org/content/forefront/we-must-rebuild-america-s-military-health-system-before-s-too-late.

Kennedy, Carrie H, and Eric A Zillmer. 2012. "Ethical Dilemmas in Clinical, Operational, Expeditionary, and Combat Environments." In *Military Psychology Clinical and Operational Applications*, by Carrie H Kennedy and Eric A Zillmer, 361-390. New York, NY: Guilford Press.

Kennedy, Dan. 2023. *Mental Health Expert Calls for Change after Irvo Otieno's Death.* 23 March. https://www.13newsnow.com/article/news/local/13news-now-investigates/mental-health-expert-calls-change-irvo-otienos-death-virginia/291-b1661487-553a-4046-affe-4ddcf5a3ce3f.

Kime, Patricia. 2019. "His Suicide Note was a Message to the Navy. The Way he Died Was the Exclamation Point." *Military.Com*, 8 Jun.

—. 2011. "Navy Pay Delays Have Forced Some Sailors to Take Out Loans." *Military.com*. 19 Nov. https://www.military.com/daily-news/2021/11/19/navy-pay-delays-have-forced-some-sailors-take-out-loans.html.

—. 2024. *Navy Shutters Premier East Coast Substance Abuse Program Amid Staffing Shortages.* 19 November. https://www.military.com/daily-news/2024/11/19/navy-shutters-premier-east-coast-substance-abuse-program-amid-staffing-shortages.html.

—. 2023. *Soldiers Who Are Bullied or Hazed Are More Likely to Face Mental Health Issues, Study Finds.* 24 Jan. https://www.military.com/daily-news/2023/01/24/soldiers-who-are-bullied-or-hazed-are-more-likely-face-mental-health-issues-study-finds.html.

—. 2023. *Too Many Managers, Too Few Providers? Watchdog Tells Defense Health Agency to Reexamine Its Market Structure.* 2023 Aug. https://www.military.com/daily-news/2023/08/24/defense-health-agency-urged-reevaluate-administration-keep-treatment-facilities-fully-staffed.html.

Koffman, Robert L, Richard D Bergthold, Justin S Campbell, Richard J Westphal, Paul Hammer, Thomas A Gaskin, John Ralphi, Edward Simmer, and William P Nash. 2011. "Expeditionary Operational Stress Control in the Navy." In *Textbooks of Military Medicine Combat and Operational Behavioral Health*, by Martha K Lenhart, 121-136. Falls Church, Virginia: Office of the Surgeon General, Department of the Army.

Kors, Joshua. 2010. "Disposable Soldiers: How the Pentagon is Cheating Wounded Vets." *The Nation*.

—. 2007. "How Specialist Town Lost His Benefits." *The Nation*.

—. 2007. "Specialist Town Takes His Case to Washington." *The Nation*.

Lieberman, Oren, and Henry Klapper. 2022. "Sailors say aircraft carrier that had multiple suicides occur among crew was uninhabitable." *CNN*. 7 May. https://www.cnn.com/2022/05/06/politics/uss-george-washington-conditions/index.html.

Locke, Jesse. 2017. "Last of the OSCAR Psychologists in Afghanistan: An Expeditionary Model of Care." In *Psychiatrists in Combat Mental Health Clinicians' Experiences in the War Zone*, by Cameron E Ritchie, Christopher H. Warner and Robert N. McClay, 203-212. Cham, Switzerland: Springer.

Mansoor, Peter R, and Williamson Murray. 2019. *The Culture of Military Organizations*. New York, NY: Cambridge University Press.

Marshall-Chambers, Anne. 2023. *'People Feel Expendable' - Mlitary Could Lower Suicide Rate With Focus on Quality of Life*. 24 August. https://thewarhorse.org/military-suicide-prevention-could-improve-with-morale-focus/.

Martin, David, and Eleanor Watson. 2022. *Navy acknowledges suicides of 7 sailors assigned to the USS George Washington*. 28 April. https://www.cbsnews.com/news/uss-george-washington-suicides-navy/.

Martin, Gregg F. 2023. *Bipolar General My Forever War with Mental Illness*. Annapolis, MD: Naval Institute Press.

Mental Health Informed Consent Working Group. 2021. *Mental Health Informed Consent Best Practices and Guidelines*. Falls Church, VA: Navy Bureau of Medicine & Surgery Collaborative Care Board.

Moldavsky, Daniel. 2006. "A way out for the conscientious objector: "become" a mental patient." (BMJ) 332 (7548).

NBC Nightly News. 2022. "Former USS George Washington sailor speaks out about suicides among ship crew members." *NBC News*. 29 April. https://www.nbcnews.com/nightly-news/video/former-uss-george-washington-crew-member-speaks-out-about-suicides-138967621584.

Ricks, Thomas E. 2012. "General Failure." *The Atlantic*, November ed.

Rossler, Wulf. 2012. "Stress, burnout, and job dissatisfaction in mental health workers." *European Archives of Psychiatry and Clinical Neuroscience* 65-69.

Shane III, Leo. 2019. *MilitaryTimes*. 27 Aug. https://www.militarytimes.com/news/pentagon-congress/2019/08/27/whats-the-biggest-worry-for-military-medicine-in-the-next-few-years/.

Simmons, Laurie. 2012. *NewsChannel 3 Investigation: The Navy's $10 million mold problem*. 10 July. https://www.wtkr.com/2012/07/09/newschannel-3-investigation-the-navys-10-million-mold-problem.

Sullivan, Olivia. 2021. *US Navy punishes suicidal sailor who sought mental health treatment*. 4 Jan. https://www.federalwaymirror.com/news/us-navy-punishes-suicidal-sailor-who-sought-mental-health-treatment/.

Sullivan, Tom. 2017. *How the Coast Guard's ugly, Epic EHR break-up played out*. 26 April. https://www.healthcareitnews.com/news/how-coast-guards-ugly-epic-ehr-break-played-out.

Toropin, Konstantin. 2022. *10 Deaths in 10 Months: String of Suicides on a Single Aircraft Carrier*. 20 April. https://www.military.com/daily-news/2022/04/20/10-deaths-10-months-string-of-suicides-single-aircraft-carrier.html.

—. 2023. "'A 9/11-like Event': Navy Report on Carrier Suicides Cites Missed Warning Signs, Leadership Failures." *Military.com*, 18 May.

—. 2023. "Sailors Sent to a Maintenance Center Died of Suicide. The Navy Says it Wasn't Prepared to Help Them." *Military.com*, 22 May.

US Government Accountability Office. 2022. *Littoral Combat Ship: Actions Needed to Address Significant Operational Challenges and Implement Planned Sustainment Approach*. Washington, D.C.: U.S. Government Accountability Office.

U.S. Surgeon General. 2022. *The U.S. Surgeon General's Advisory on Building a Thriving Health Workforce.* Washington, D.C.: Office of the U.S. Surgeon General.

Ugalde, Diego. 2023. *Leading from the Deep.* Columbia, SC: Independently Published.

US Army War College. 1970. *Study on Military Professionalism.* Carlisle Barracks, PA: US Army War College. https://apps.dtic.mil/sti/citations/ADA063748.

Warner, Christopher H, George N Appenzeller, Todd Yosick, Matthew J Barry, Anthony J Morton, Jill E. Breitback, Gabrielle Bryen, et al. 2011. "The Division Psychiatrist and Brigade Behavioral Health Officers." In *Textbooks of Military Medicine Combat and Operational Behavioral Health*, by Martha K Lenhart, 89-105. Falls Church, Virginia: Office of the Surgeon General, Department of the Army.

Watson, Julie. 2022. *Sailor accused of igniting Bonhomme Richard puts fate in judge's hands.* 19 September. https://www.navytimes.com/news/your-navy/2022/09/19/sailor-accused-of-igniting-uss-bonhomme-richard-puts-fate-in-judge/.

Weinick, Robin M. 2011. *Programs Addressing Psychological Health and Traumatic Brain Injury Among U.S. Military Servicemembers and Their Families.* Santa Monica, CA: RAND Corporation.

Weiss, Kenneth J, and Landon Van Dell. 2017. "Liability for Diagnosing Malingering." *The Journal of the American Academy of Psychiatry and the Law* 339-347.

WSJ Editorial Board. 2022. *America Needs a Bigger Navy.* 22 February. https://www.wsj.com/articles/america-needs-a-bigger-navy-admiral-mike-gilday-pentagon-defense-spending-11645649492.

Ziezulewicz, Geoff. 2022. *'The worst command': Inside the submarine Scranton's dysfunction.* 20 September. https://www.navytimes.com/news/your-navy/2022/09/20/the-worst-command-inside-the-submarine-scrantons-dysfunction/.

—. 2020. "A troubled sailor was 'underdiagnosed' by mental health officials before mass shooting." *NavyTimes.* 29 Sep. https://www.navytimes.com/news/your-navy/2020/09/29/a-troubled-sailor-was-underdiagnosed-by-mental-health-officials-before-mass-shooting/.

—. 2023. *Inside the Navy's Pay and Personnel Crisis.* 4 May. https://www.navytimes.com/news/your-navy/2023/05/04/inside-the-navys-pay-and-personnel-crisis/.

—. 2023. *Investigation: Four sailor suicides from same command not connected.* 18 May. https://www.navytimes.com/news/your-navy/2023/05/19/investigation-four-sailor-suicides-from-same-command-not-connected/.

—. 2021. "Navy Denies Malpractice Claim Filed by Family of Sailor who Killed Himself in a Military Jail." *Navy Times,* 18 Oct.

—. 2022. *Three deployments. Two mental health visits. One attempted separation.* 13 December. https://www.militarytimes.com/news/your-navy/2022/12/13/three-deployments-two-mental-health-visits-one-attempted-separation/.

www.ingramcontent.com/pod-product-compliance
Lightning Source LLC
LaVergne TN
LVHW091540070526
838199LV00002B/147